AṢṬADAḶA YOGAMĀLĀ

AṢṬADAḶA YOGAMĀLĀ

(COLLECTED WORKS)

B.K.S. IYENGAR

Volume 7

Questions and Answers

ALLIED PUBLISHERS PVT. LTD.
NEW DELHI • MUMBAI • KOLKATA
CHENNAI • BANGALORE • HYDERABAD

ALLIED PUBLISHERS PRIVATE LIMITED

Regd. Off.: 1/13-14 Asaf Ali Road, **New Delhi**–110002
Ph.: 011-23239001 • E-mail: delhi.books@alliedpublishers.com

17 Chittaranjan Avenue, **Kolkata**–700072
Ph.: 033-22129618 • E-mail: cal.books@alliedpublishers.com

15 J.N. Heredia Marg, Ballard Estate, **Mumbai**–400001
Ph.: 022-42126969 • E-mail: mumbai.books@alliedpublishers.com

No. 25/10, Commander-in-Chief Road, Ethiraj Lane (Next to Post Office)
Egmore, **Chennai**–600008,
Ph.: 044-28223938 • E-mail: chennai.books@alliedpublishers.com

P.B. 9932, 1st Floor, Sunkada Chickkana Complex,
Loop Lane Off Race Course Road, Next to Hotel Maurya,
Gandhi Nagar, **Bangalore** - 560009
Ph.: 080-22262081 • E-Mail: bngl.books@alliedpublishers.com

Sri Jayalakshmi Nilayam, No. 3-4-510, 3rd Floor (Above More Super Market)
Barkatpura, Telangana, **Hyderabad**–500027
Ph.: 040-27551811, 040-27551812 • E-mail: hyd.books@alliedpublishers.com

Website: www.alliedpublishers.com

First published, 2008

Edition, 2025

ISBN: 81-8424-283-2

Cover design : The Author

Artwork : S.M. Waugh

Published by Sunil Sachdev and printed by Ravi Sachdev at Allied Publishers Private Limited, Printing Division, 1/13-14 Asaf Ali Road, New Delhi - 110 002

Invocatory Prayers

ॐ

Yogena cittasya padena vācāṁ

Malaṁ śarīrasyaca vaidyakena

Yopākarottaṁ pravaraṁ munīnāṁ

Patañjaliṁ prāñjalirānato'smi

Ābāhu puruṣākāraṁ

Śaṅkha cakrāsi dhāriṇaṁ

Sahasra śirasaṁ śvetaṁ

Praṇamāmi Patañjaliṁ

I bow before the noblest of sages Patañjali, who gave yoga for serenity and sanctity of mind, grammar for clarity and purity of speech and medicine for pure, perfect health.

I prostrate before Patañjali who is crowned with a thousand headed cobra, an incarnation of Ādiśeṣa (Anañta) whose upper body has a human form, holding the conch in one arm, disk in the second, a sword of wisdom to vanquish nescience in the third and blessing humanity from the fourth arm, while his lower body is like a coiled snake.

Yastyaktvā rūpamādyaṁ prabhavati jagato'nekadhānugrahāya

Prakṣīṇakleśarāśirviṣamaviṣadharo'nekavaktrāḥ subhogī

Sarvajñānaprasūtirbhujagaparikaraḥ prītaye yasya nityaṁ

Devohīṣaḥ savovyātsitavimalatanuryogado yogayuktaḥ

I prostrate before Lord Ādiśeṣa, who manifested himself on Earth as Patañjali to grace the human race in health and harmony,

I salute Lord Ādiśeṣa of the myriad serpent heads and mouths carrying noxious poisons, discarding which he came to Earth as a single headed Patañjali in order to eradicate ignorance and vanquish sorrow.

I pay my obeisance to him, repository of all knowledge, amidst his attendant retinue.

I pray to the Lord whose primordial form shines with peace and white effulgence, pristine in body, a master of yoga, who bestows on all his yogic light to enable mankind to rest in the house of the immortal Soul.

BY THE AUTHOR

This volume of *Aṣṭadaḷa Yogamālā* published by Allied Publishers, Delhi, is the sixth volume of the second part of the "Collected Works" of Yogācārya B.K.S. Iyengar. Each part comprises several volumes which are arranged according to the following scheme:

Articles
Interviews
Question and Answer Sessions
Techniques of *Āsanas, Prāṇāyāma, Dhyāna* and *Śavāsana*
Therapeutic Applications of Yoga
Garland of Aphorisms and Thoughts
General Index and Analytical Dictionary
Addendum

Also by the Same Author

Light on Yoga
Light on Prāṇāyāma
Concise Light on Yoga
Art of Yoga
Tree of Yoga
Light on the Yoga Sūtras of Patañjali
The Illustrated Light on Yoga
Yoga Dipika (Marathi)
Yoga Ek Kalpataru (Marathi)
Ārogyayoga (Marathi)
Light on Aṣṭāṅga Yoga
Aṣṭadaḷa Yogamālā (Vols 1 to 6)
Yoga: The Path To Holistic Health
Yoga Sarvānasāṭhi (Marathi)
Basic Guidelines for Teachers of Yoga (co-authored with G.S. Iyengar)
Yogacandan (Marathi)
Light on Life

Also on Iyengar Yoga

Body the Shrine, Yoga Thy Light
70 Glorious Years
Iyengar His Life and Work
Yogapushpanjali
Yogadhārā

TABLE OF CONTENTS

SECTION I – YOGA IN GENERAL

SECTION II – ON PATAÑJALI AND YOGA

SECTION III – ON *AṢṬĀṄGA YOGA*

III.1. – *Yama*

III.2. – *Niyama*

III.3. – *Āsana*

III.4. – *Prāṇāyāma*

III.5. – *Pratyāhāra*

III.6. – *Dhāraṇā*

III.7. – *Dhyāna*

SECTION VI – ON MY PRACTICE

SECTION VII – THE PRACTICAL PSYCHOLOGY OF YOGA

SECTION VIII – ADJUSTMENTS IN PRACTICE

SECTION IX – ON PRACTICE – THEORY

PLATES

TABLES

ACKNOWLEDGEMENTS

The Author wishes to extend his gratitude and thanks to my students for their assistance, enthusiasm, interest and time which they willingly gave for the presentation of this volume. Without their help the volume would not have seen the light.

Geeta S. Iyengar – For her valuable suggestions and assistance in seeing this subject that is difficult to present, was conveyed without distortion and also for going over, researching, checking, re-checking, correcting and overseeing the entire editing process of this volume.

Faeq Biria – Travelling to India every year for reading, editing as well as overseeing the project.

Patxi Lizardi – Also who out of dedication travels to India every year, for editorial work and giving suggestions.

John J. Evans – Who graciously looked into the volume bringing a cohesive English throughout.

Stephanie Quirk – Editing assistance, book design, layout and preparation of the plates.

Uma Dhavale – For editing assistance.

Raya Uma-Datta – Assisting with tables and plates.

Mr Kokate – For artwork of the front and back covers.

Surojit Banerjee – Overseeing editorial work for Allied Publishers (Delhi).

The various subjects depicted in the plates who willingly allowed themselves to be photographed for this volume in order to express with clarity so that the readers adopt with ease to follow in their practices.

FOREWORD

Inquisitiveness is an inborn trait in man. Without the knowledge of knowing and understanding his life becomes odourless and tasteless. The urge to know *(jijñāsā)* is inherent in each individual. Even a child wants to know, explore and understand everything that it sees. We all like to know things around us as our mind, intelligence and consciousness are caught in the whirl-wind of what life is and why it has been bestowed. These inquiring thoughts, ideas and queries also convey an absence or a want of knowledge. Yet it is this same inquisitiveness that triggers and leads us towards constructive thinking for intellectual and spiritual development.

Fear, confusion and doubt activate the mind to know the value of life and the truth of its living. Innovation and invention help and guide man to discover and re-discover life's meaning.

In the *veda* and *upaniṣad* we see the same curiosity to know the truth through dialogues, discussions, debates and arguments.

The word *veda* comes from *vid* which means to know. It means the thirst for *jñāna*. The seers *(ṛṣī)*, astonished at the wonders of the world, wanted to know of themselves as well as the universe. They wanted to know how and why the universe was created and their connection to it.

In the *Ṛgveda* there are certain *sūkta*, in the form of a direct discussion with the deities. They indicate a praise and glorification with pure emotional feel sprouting from their hearts, for those deities.

The word *upaniṣad* means to sit closer. The *śiṣya* comes nearer to the *guru* physically, mentally, intellectually, he sits closer to the *guru* to study and learn. The *upaniṣad* contain dialogues in the form of questions and answers. The *Praśnōpaniṣad* is an apt example wherein the *śiṣya* goes to the *Guru* to get the right answer. In *Kaṭhōpaniṣad,* Nachiketa talks to Yama, the God of death, to clear his doubts. In the *Bṛhadāraṇyakaōpaniṣad,* Yājñavalkya and his wife Maitreyī discuss together. Yājñavalkya, being the *Guru,* answers his wife convincingly. Similarly, between Yājñavalkya and King Janaka, who is well versed in spiritual knowledge. Yājñavalkya proposes questions to the King. As a King should never be questioned, he answers the questions himself, instilling the finest of the finest knowledge in the King. In *Taittirīyōpaniṣad* the *ācārya* advise the *śiṣya* through discussion to know the truth. In *Muṇḍakōpaniṣad,* Angirasa advises Śaunaka. There are instances in almost all the *upaniṣad* where questions and answers lead to the development of knowledge and wisdom (*viveka-jñāna).*

The *Bhagavad Gītā* is also in a dialetic form where Shri Krishna instructs Arjuna. The reputed Socrates, explains the philosophical approach towards life to his disciples through argument, question and answer.

In *Caraka Samhitā* (an *āyurvedic* text), *ṛṣī* like Atreya, Angirasa, Bhṛgu, Vaśiṣṭa, Jamadagni and others came together to discuss and deliberate on the subject.

When it comes to yoga most of us, though not well versed have a plethora of questions in our minds. Wherever I went, people used to bombard me with questions. Their queries and doubts made me realise that there is a big gap in understanding the subject concerning its theory and its practical aspects.

Their questions were interesting, provocative as well as evocative, and I tried to convince them. Answering them helped me to bring to the surface my hidden experiences.

In this volume I have structured the questions systematically, codifying them through titles and sub-titles into main themes on the subject. With this classification and elaboration on yoga the *sādhaka* can see the philosophical vision behind his *sādhanā.* It will help aspirants to accede to the subject with ease and guide them to practise and know precisely how to reach the further finer aspects of yoga, from where doubts and confusions that taint their search evaporate. I hope this format will convince all readers to know the subject as a pre-requisite in practice, experimentation, deliberation and analysis.

In the *Vishnu Sahasranāmam*, after listening to the thousand and eight names of Lord Vishnu, Pārvatī asks Lord Shiva:

Kena upāyen laghunām viśṇurnāma sahasrakaṁ I
Paṭhyate paṇḍitai nityam śrotrum icchāmi ahaṁ prabhoḥ II

Oh Lord! I would like to know how the Vishnu *Sahasranamam* is recited by the *puṇdits* in short everyday.

Lord Shiva tells her; *Srīrāma, Srīrāma, Srīrāma. Srīrāma* is the only name that is equivalent to the thousand names of Vishnu.

Similarly, if at all I have to answer in short everything that is in this book, I will say;
Do practise with calmness! – *Sādhanā, Śāntiḥ, Sādhanā, Śāntiḥ!!!*

B. K. S. IYENGAR

SECTION I

YOGA IN GENERAL

SECTION I – YOGA IN GENERAL

I.1. – Yoga its origin and aim

The *Yoga Sūtra* begins with *atha yogānuśāsanam* (I.1). It covers the entire scope of yoga. *Atha* means 'now' and *śāsanam* means 'codified disciplines to be practised'. Yoga is as old as civilisation. It was passed on from generation to generation and that is why it is still with us. Yoga is the creation of God as all *Veda* are. God is its *guru,* the *guru* of all *gurus.* According to the *Veda,* Brahmā – the Creator, created yoga along with all other creations. As creation evolved, yoga too came into existence. Hence, it is known as *hiraṇyagarbha yoga.* Patañjali codified yoga from various existing sources. He condensed and compiled it in to the form of *Yoga Sūtra* for us to understand its essence. He gave us a clear picture in the form of a concise treatise. It is meant for the whole of humanity.

Yoga is meant not only for gaining health but for encountering the vision of the Self *(darśana).*

Our energy is often sapped by desire, anger, greed, infatuation, pride and hatred *(kāma, krodha, lobha, moha, mada* and *mātsarya).* Our thoughts move in these six spokes of the emotional wheel creating inner disturbances and yoga minimises these turmoils. Like the waves of the sea, our thought waves, knowingly or unknowingly, move from one end of the body to the other, hitting the physical and spiritual bodies, creating psychic problems and physical diseases. They are either from the somatic to the psychic or from the psychic to the somatic. These are known as *pañcavṛtti* and *pañcakleśa* in yoga.

Practice of yoga minimises or controls not only the physical disturbances but also mental modifications. One even gets freedom from onslaughts of mental disturbances and bodily afflictions, which originate from our actions *(karma)* and their reactions *(parikarma). Tataḥ kleśa karma nivṛttiḥ* (*Y.S.,* IV.30) – yoga is meant to end all afflictions of *karma.* If *karma* brings psychosomatic diseases, *parikarma* in the form of yoga makes us regain balance and harmony in body and mind. Now, let us see where yoga leads one.

Yoga is a journey from the body towards the mind and from the mind towards the soul.

First some background knowledge is needed. From *cit* (soul) comes *citta* (consciousness). The sprout of the *citta* is *asmitā*, or pure "I-consciousness". It projects as a duplicate in an unripened intelligent man. Besides the duplication, intelligence *(buddhi)* springs forth. From *buddhi*, the mind, from mind, the senses of perception and organs of action spring out. Like this, man is like a healthy tree. As the fragrant fruit comes out at the top from a healthy tree, the essence of life flows from the top of the head to savour through yoga.

Mind is the link or bridge between the body and soul. Mind belongs to the element of fire *(tejas)*, which has form *(rūpa)*. Mind connects the gross body *(bāhyakaraṇa)*; organs of action and perception, mind, five elements and their five infrastructures, to the subtle body *(antaḥkaraṇa)* composed of intelligence *(buddhi)*, 'I' and consciousness. The first five aspects of yoga *(yama, niyama, āsana, prāṇāyāma* and *pratyāhāra)* regulate the gross body and connect it to the subtle body to receive the right knowledge and auspicious imprints leading one towards the core of one's being.

The other three subtle aspects of yoga *(dhāraṇā, dhyāna* and *samādhi)* discipline the inner body. By using skilfull intelligence with proper practice *(sādhanā)*, it is possible to reach the goal, i.e., to come in close contact with the soul. This is the aim of yoga.

Though we use the terms body and mind, the yoga philosophy dissects the body and mind into twenty-four segments as the principles of *prakṛti*. The aim of yoga is to connect these twenty-four components of nature by filtering and purifying them, and then to merge them in *Puruṣa* (Self).

There is one more important component – conscience *(antaḥkaraṇa)*, which acts as a bridge between the consciousness and the soul. The journey from the body to the soul is possible only when all these twenty-four aspects become as pure as the soul.

As the *citta* is tainted and tinged by the *saṁskāra* of body, mind and intellect, the soul itself appears as veiled and clouded. For this *citta* has to become as pure as the soul,. Once these taints of our actions are subdued, *citta* becomes pure and hence the soul becomes pure. The track of the yogic journey is to lead one towards clarity, purity and sanctity, at all levels of life.

a) – Is yoga a religion

Yoga though originating in India, cannot be defined as part of the Hindu religious culture, but it is definitely a self-culture. Yoga in a nutshell has the disciplines of all religions.

Yoga, is a universal religion. It is religious because its aim is to culture the body, mind and self of man to realise the true SELF.

You and I, irrespective of our country or religion, are made up of the five elements (earth, water, fire, air and ether) as well as body, mind, intelligence, consciousness and the individual self all covering or veiling the SELF. Hence all these veils need to be cultured for one to become a true and real human being. As we are all made of the same principle components, there is no difference between us whether one is an oriental or an occidental. Probably the customs, culture, traditions and different interpretations on religion have caused changes in our way of thinking, which shows differences in our outlook and way of living. Otherwise, our bodies, mind, intelligence and natures are undoubtedly universal. Even our physical problems, emotional turbulences, conceit, ego and vanity are almost identical. Each one of us needs healing and wants solace and happiness in life. Yoga does that and this is what yoga did for me.

In order to learn and understand the subject from scratch one has to use the visible part of the self, the body. One has to start from the body as base to reach the Self. Is it not the essential source of all of us?

Just as it is impossible to hold water without a container, the Self too needs a container. The container of the Self is in the form of the body. As the Self is carried by the body, one certainly cannot neglect the body. The moment the holder of the Self – the body is neglected, know that immorality has set in. God has given us this body not only for worldly enjoyments but to understand and move towards that infinite which is hidden within all.

As we like to know, study and understand the external world, we have to give a thought to knowing and understanding the internal world.

Today technology has touched the optimum level of studying and knowing the external world, but spiritually we are empty. When the water gets filled completely in the vessel, not a single air bubble remains. In the same way yogic practices help the self to touch in totality our senses, mind, intelligence, consciousness and self to engulf vertically and horizontally so that the real Self is one with the container without gaps or bubbles. Without using the cognisable and conative body (the container of the Self), it is not easy to know or feel the Self. The Self cannot exist without a body and body without the Self.

The self expresses itself through the instruments of body, mind and intelligence, which act as well as reflect and react. By this the self gets tainted and one may lose sight of the right path and end up in confusion. The real Self is never tainted, but the taints in the individual self throws a shadow over the real Self.

A raw beginner who comes to the class to learn *āsana* is innocent. While learning he does not know the difference between body, mind or self. As he is not aware of such divisions, the teacher divides the parts of the body to make him understand, so he may know each and every part of his body and function of his mind, and be guided towards right action. As the body is the base for all actions, it becomes the abode of righteous and virtuous actions *(dharma-sādhanā).* Therefore, care has to be taken of the body, so that our actions turn towards purity.

How fortunate are we to know of *āsana* and their significance for the well-being of the body! I am sure that from this state we will soon taste the immortal Self that is within.

The body is made of five elements; we have to understand how they work. If there is a slightest imbalance in these, then it shows signs of diseases in both the body and the mind. These diseases distract one from the path of spiritual culture. Whether one is a common man or a saint *(sādhaka* or a *siddha),* when elemental distortion takes place diseases set in. To eradicate these, one needs the power of endurance, tolerance and patience, which develops only through *āsana* practice.

Here, I would like to bring to the attention of all that the ultimate goal of yoga *sādhanā* can be read in *sūtra* 19 and 20 of chapter II.[1] Through them Patañjali mentions how important it is for a *sādhaka* to work to bring the five *bhūta,* five *karmendriya,* five *jñānendriya, manas, tanmātra* (odour, taste, shape, touch and sound), *ahaṁkāra, buddhi, mahat* (cosmic intelligence) with the *guṇa (sattva, rajas and tamas)* to dissolve in the unevolved matter *(mūla prakṛti)* so that the Self shines without depending upon these.

When disease sets in, one has to forget the great billboard of "freedom". Religiosity in one's practice truly begins when the body's mechanism is disturbed. The disease brings religiosity in one who begins to discipline himself due to the imbalance in health. When discipline sets in, mind becomes religious and that journey from indiscipline towards discipline begins through yoga.

Yoga is a three-tier discipline – the ethical discipline, the neuro-physiological discipline and psycho-spiritual discipline. Thought process is dependent upon the above three-tiered discipline. The flow of life force in the cellular organism brings healthy physical, physiological, neurological and psychological reactions as well as the interactions to experience harmony in these three tiers.

---

[1] *Viśeṣa aviśeṣa liṅgmātra aliṅgāni guṇaparvāṇi* (*Y.S.,* II.19) – The *guṇas* generate their characteristic divisions and energies in the seer. Their stages are distinguishable and non-distinguishable, differentiable and non-differentiable.

Draṣṭā dṛśimātraḥ śuddhaḥ api pratyayānupaśyaḥ (*Y.S.,* II.20) – The seer is pure consciousness. He witnesses nature without being reliant on it.

The first tier is ethical discipline. The great principles of morality are followed from sacred books like *Bhagavad Gītā, Bible, Koraṇ, the Upaniṣad* and sayings of the Saints. They are the foundation for a righteous balanced life. Indiscipline defies religiousness in life. Ethical disciplines of yoga are explained in *sūtra* thirty of chapter two.[1]

As far as my experience of practice and teaching goes, *āsana* bring significant transformation ethically, mentally and spiritually in the practitioners. When one does *Uttānāsana* he experiences a state of silence. When one does *Sālamba Śīrṣāsana* one experiences alertness. In *Uttānāsana* one feels the state of passivity in the brain while in *Sālamba Śīrṣāsana* one becomes active and dynamic. No matter what man is aiming for he can find value in the practice of different *āsana* by adjusting the body with measured intelligence to experience their effects. I tried and learnt and it opened avenues for new knowledge and experience. The experiences that come through *āsana* are sanity, sanctity, silence, serenity and wholeness. In this way one sensitises with *jñāna, vijñāna* and *prajñāna* in *sādhanā*. If *jñāna* is to know oneself, *vijñāna* is to know the methodology. Combination of *jñāna* and *vijñāna* leads one for direct experience as *prajñāna*. One can liken this to the acquisition of academic knowledge as *jñāna;* the methodology used in laboratory tests as *vijñāna;* and subjective experience as *prajñāna*.

When I practise, I use the body as a laboratory to experiment and observe which part gets the feedback in different *āsana*. From this feedback I study and react to feel at all places in the *āsana*. Hence I practise and study each *āsana* with respect as it is the door for insight. No one *āsana* is great or insignificant, or unimportant. Know that each *āsana* carries different rays of knowledge.

In *Uttānāsana* the mind becomes pensive, but that pensivity is quite different from that of *Halāsana*. Compare and measure the quality of pensivity as well as silence in these two. Then, study the quality of silence in *Setu Bandha Sarvāṅgāsana* which is quite different again. Study these chemical reactions that happen in the brain and mind in each *āsana* and note the changes.

In *Ūrdhva Dhanurāsana* one expresses the stretch by extending the body and expanding the chest. The most interesting thing that happens in this *āsana* is that though the body extends and expands, the mind moves inside the body. Watch this inward movement, which is the same as it happens in *dhāraṇā*. Such experiences do not come from books but through direct observation and reflection. When attentive stability is built up, naturally it makes one move towards *dhyāna*.

---

1 *ahiṁsā satya asteya brahmacarya aparigrahāḥ yamāḥ.*(*Y.S.,* II.30) – Non-violence, truth, abstention from stealing, continence, and of greed for possessions beyond one's need are the five pillars of *yama*.

Nowadays *dhyāna* (meditation) has become like instant coffee. Meditation has been mistaken for tranquillity and quietness of the mind *(citta prasādanam)*, which one can get in *Uttānāsana, Setu Bandha Sarvāṅgāsana* and *Halāsana. Sālamba Śīrṣāsana* keeps one fully active. In backbends one becomes an introvert. These experiences and feelings are the starting points to imbibe *dhyāna.*

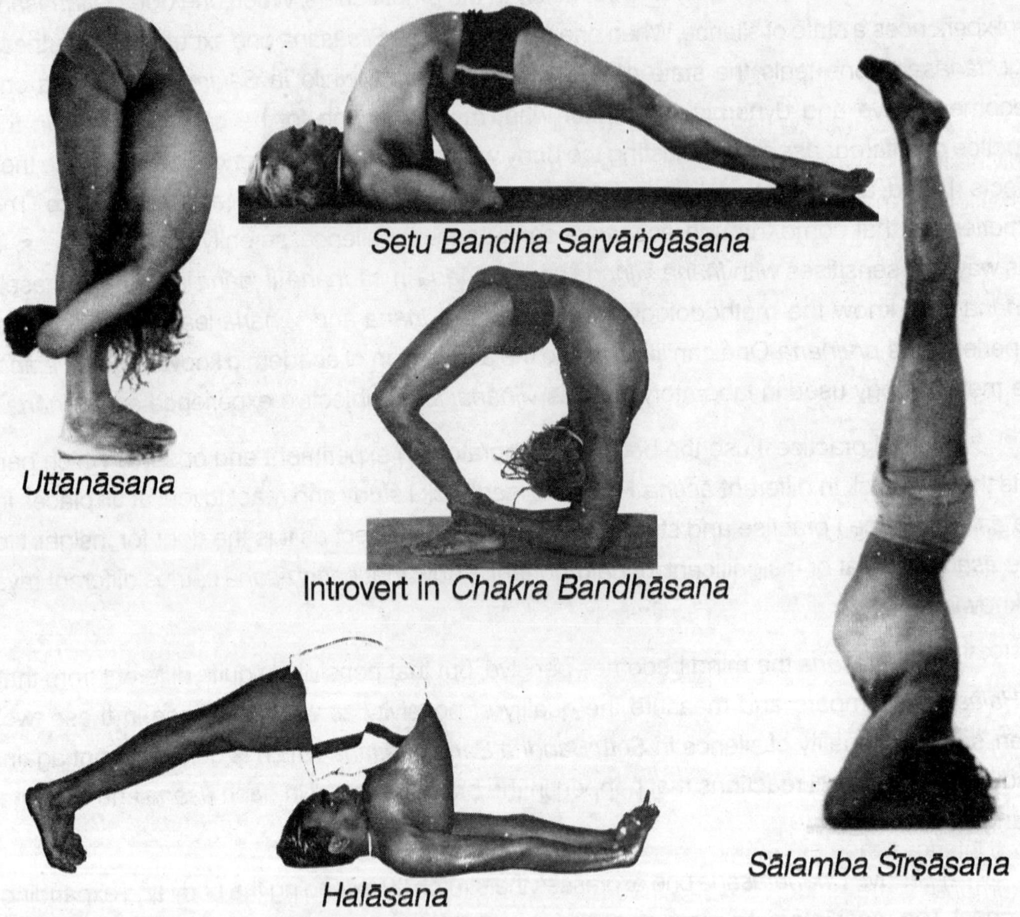

Uttānāsana

Setu Bandha Sarvāṅgāsana

Introvert in *Chakra Bandhāsana*

Halāsana

Sālamba Śīrṣāsana

Plate n. 1 – *Āsana* as starting points to imbibe *dhyāna*.

Today the term meditation is misunderstood and misinterpreted. All begin yoga with *dhyāna*, though *dhyāna* is the seventh state in *aṣṭadaḷa yoga*. Give a thought to Patañjali's approach, why he begins with *yama* and proceeds towards *dhyāna* and *samādhi*. According to him *dhyāna* is close to *samādhi*. The state of consciousness in *dhyāna* gets transformed into *samādhi*. *Dhyāna* is meant to eradicate intellectual pride and intoxication, but today *dhyāna* is taught for "peace of mind".

If a beginner comes to a class and immediately starts with backbends without even knowing the basics of *āsana,* he will end up in a hospital. Similarly, an unprepared and unripe mind will not be able to bear the state of *dhyāna* or *samādhi.* On the contrary they may damage the nervous system, which may not be repairable in spite of hospitalisation. When one plants a seed he nurtures that seed for it to germinate. If he pours water more than what the seed needs, it dies. The same thing happens to one who jumps to complicated and complex *āsana.* The primary course in yoga is *yama* and *niyama,* secondary course is *āsana, prāṇāyāma, pratyāhāra,* the college course is *dhāraṇā,* and the university course is *dhyāna* and *samādhi.* This way one gets stabilised from the gross level towards the subtlest and finest level in yoga.

The foundation for meditation has to begin from the practice of *āsana,* so that when the divine light dawns through *dhyāna,* one does not get frightened, but glad to accept and face the light of that luminous Self.

Please understand that meditation is not for tranquillity, but for sublimating the pride and ego. A lot of attention is needed while practising *āsana* as they lead us towards *dhāraṇā.*

The sky *(ākaśa)* is immeasurable, known as *mahat-ākāśa.* Similarly, the space inside us is immeasurable, known as *cidākāśa.* As one cannot measure the sky, one cannot measure the space that is within as *cidākāśa.*

To understand *mahadākāśa* and *cidākāśa,* the fourth petal of yoga, *prāṇāyāma,* teaches us to connect the *cidākāśa* (Self), with *mahadākāśa* (the frontier of the Self, the skin). In *prāṇāyāma* before inhalation, something moves giving room for the in-breath to cover the torso. This moving-out force is the Self. In letting out the breath, one raises the torso, holds it firmly and releases the breath gradually. As the breath releases, the Self recedes to rest in its abode. This is the meditative state in *prāṇāyāma.* In inhalation, watch how the empty space within expands and comes into contact with the outer layer of the body. This contact of the Self with the external body is nothing but the union of *cittākāśa* with the exterior *mahadākāśa.* In retention of breath *(kuṁbhaka),* union takes place with these two spaces, while in exhalation the outer space moves towards the interior space of the body, connecting the outer space with the inner space. In both types of *kuṁbhaka,* the union between the individual self with the real Self takes place. This union is known as the meeting place between nature and soul *(prakṛti* and *puruṣa).*

The internal space is *ākāśa tattva. Prāṇa* that is drawn-in, held or let out is *vāyu tattva* (the feel of touch). The feel of warmth is *tejas tattva.* The feel of coolness and soothness is *āp tattva* and the feel of firmness or fullness is *pṛthvī tattva.* Exhalation begins from the earth element (the solid physical body), then moves to the water element or the fluid body (physiological body), creating gas from the flame of fire as fire element reaches the point where the last particle of air *(vāyu)* rests in the abode of the soul *(cit),* the space inside the body *(ākāśa).* Study the mind at the beginning of exhalation; observe where the mind is in the middle of exhalation as well as between the median plane of right and left lungs and at the end where it reaches.

Watch inhalation. It also touches the *cit (ākāśa),* then *vāyu,* then *tejas,* the flavour of the breath as *āp,* and firmness at the end – *pṛthvī tattva.* If inhalation is the grace of God, exhalation is the surrender of oneself to God. In *kuṁbhaka* all the five elements harmoniously meet, uniting *prakṛti* and *puruṣa* as if they are married. This is how *prāṇāyāma* develops one's state of consciousness and makes *puruṣa* to embrace *prakṛti* in inhalation while exhalation makes the *prakṛti* to embrace the *puruṣa.*

Bhajan is singing the name of God in various tunes (sound). *Nāmasmaraṇa* means recalling the name of God. In *prāṇāyāma,* there is a kind of unintentional *bhajan* or *nāmasmaraṇa.*

Sapta svara (the seven notes) namely *sa, re, ga, ma, pa, dha, ni,* are the basis for the keys and scales to form the musical *rāga* in which the songs of devotion *(bhakti)* are chanted. Patañjali uses the same concepts with different words: *japa, artha* and *bhāvanā.* In *prāṇāyāma* each *pūraka, kuṁbhaka* and *rechaka* produces the *praṇava mantra.* Whether one says *āuṁ* or not, it just happens in *prāṇāyāmic* breathing. This *praṇava japa* comes with meaning *(artha)* and feeling *(bhāvanā).* If *japa* is listening *(śravaṇa),* reflection is *manana* and feel is *nididhyāsana.* The *āuṁ* has three letters; *ā* stands for inhalation, *u* for retention and *ṁ* for exhalation.

Having said that yoga works as a tool for the (w)holistic growth of man irrespective of geographical divisions, it is meant for all living beings on this planet.

Imbibing oriental wisdom, and having taught for years in the occidental world, I find that the urge for self-realisation appears as the goal in all cultures. For this goal one need not demarcate oriental ways of life with the occidental way of life. The ways of the East and the West are like two branches of a trunk growing in different directions. Let us not divide, but go to the trunk. The aim being identical for one and all, I do not think that yoga divides man from the religious point of view. As thousands and thousands practise in the West, it is enough assurance that yoga as a Universal religion fits irrespective of geographical divisions.

b) – Why so many yoga's

Any science, art or philosophy has its own depth. But in order to understand them one has to study and build from the base. Take chemistry, it is a single subject, yet it is demarcated into physical chemistry, inorganic chemistry and organic chemistry. Each science at a certain point branches out for further specialised detail and depth. This is perspectival concentration. In the same way if one has to know the body's depth, its structure, anatomy; he has to have the knowledge of how the various systems function. One needs to know how ageing and disease take place, as well as the ways to alleviate and remedy them. There is chemistry as well as physics in the body. In the body the physics lie at its core, and its chemistry is the change that takes place in the content. As it is natural to branch out compartmentally to know and understand each aspect in detail, so it is in yoga. The science of yoga begins from the body; it leads one to study and penetrate further the inner layers and sheaths with the journey ending in the realisation of the soul *(jīvātmā)* and surrender to the Universal Soul *(Paramātmā)*. This requires study, culture, purity and sanctity in the body, organs of action, senses of perception, mind, intelligence, I-ness, consciousness, conscience and the individual self. It is a journey from the microcosm to the macrocosm – the individual to the Universal. In order to reach this goal different techniques and different names such as physical yoga, spiritual yoga, *jñāna* yoga, *karma* yoga, *kuṇḍalinī* yoga, *rāja* yoga were given as a way of describing the path. But the beauty is that the word 'yoga' remains common in all the paths.

One is required to study the fundamentals of science to become a master of a branch. In yoga one cannot drop any branch or aspect, the approach has to be thorough and total if it is to attain the goal.

People brand the practice of one aspect of yoga, *āsana,* as physical yoga. The same people fail to acknowledge that *āuṁ* or any *mantra* too needs physical organs for their very pronunciation. Self has physical, moral, intellectual and spiritual bodies. Yoga is meant for mankind to use in a right way for a right purpose.

In the *Bhagavad Gītā* each chapter concludes naming yoga in different ways; *arjuna viṣāda* (yoga of dejection), *sāṁkhya yoga* (yoga of knowledge), *karma yoga* (yoga of action), *jñāna karma sannyāsa yoga* (yoga of knowledge with the disciplines of action) and so forth. But the message of all the eighteen chapters is to unite the individual self *(jīvātmā)* with the Universal Self *(paramātmā)*. This covers the whole scope, range and aim of yoga.

Actually, yoga has no varieties. But authors of different intellectual levels presented yoga according to their calibre and gave different names. This is how the branches of yoga sprouted. Some choose certain subjects to study in depth. In medical practice, there are specialists in cardiology, urology, dermatology, neurology and so forth. Similarly there are branches as part of yoga. If one predominantly takes one part of yoga and concentrates on it, he may name it according to how he associates with that branch.

Specialists in the medical field desire to help patients to derive maximum benefit of their knowledge. It is the same in yoga. One wants to gain the depth of yoga for themselves, also wish to help those who come to them.

Man is made of three important components, namely, organs of action and perception, the brain and the heart. With these components, he acts, thinks and develops knowledge to become divine. If hands and legs are meant for work and service, brain is to avoid faulty acts, and heart for emotional human touch. Action *(karma)*, knowledge *(jñāna)* and devotion *(bhakti)* evolved on this basis. Yoga is derived to keep the body to act clean, brain to think pure and heart to feel and respect all as children of God. Due to these three characteristic components in man, yoga is described as different paths; but I consider them all as branches of a single tree – the Tree of Yoga.

I.2. – All can embrace yoga, but does yoga embrace all

Many from various parts of the globe ask me whether yoga is international or secular or universal. As yoga can be embraced by all it is universal, as it guides and shows the right way of living.

The ocean is one but for the sake of convenience man divides and names it with various names. Like one ocean and one earth, yoga is a single unit. As human beings we are one, but we get divided by our petty minds and thoughts. But beyond the labels we are all simply human beings.

Yoga texts claim it as universal *(sārvabhauma)*. It builds up in all of us right knowledge so that we live a spiritually happy contented life.

Our physical and mental problems are the same, but the differences are in the beliefs, outlooks and conditions that shape the mind and intelligence.

As yoga uplifts man from the physical, ethical, mental and intellectual drawbacks, it belongs to all irrespective of one's religion, class, caste, creed, colour, age or gender. The distance between God and man is on account of man's weaknesses. Yoga helps to close this gap and gets man to unite with the divine. At the very least it guides one to become a better human being.

Patañjali classifies consciousness *(citta)* into five categories, which are; dullness *(muḍha)*, negligence *(kṣipta)*, agitation *(vikṣipta)*, one-pointedness *(ekāgra)* and restraint *(niruddha)*; along with the three qualities that govern nature *(sattva, rajas* and *tamas)*. Patañjali does not deny anyone but shows ways of approach. He wants not only to uplift those who are blessed but also those who lack stability and tranquillity to live in a wholesome state of consciousness *(samāhita citta)*. A wandering consciousness *(vyutthāna citta)* needs culturing, cleansing and polishing. This is achieved by the eight petalled yoga, which transforms one from an unsteady mind to a steady state of mind or *citta*.

First of all, yoga starts in helping an unhealthy person to become a healthy person, arresting the decay in him. I have taught yoga to those who were tender in age up to ripe old age, as well as invalids. So I feel that all are fit for yoga, but to reach the end aim of yoga may be hard and difficult.

It uplifts the afflicted to a state of health, it guides the neophyte seeker to practice with ardour and develop skill to refine the gross and unstable body and mind so that it becomes fit for further penetration of the intelligence into the inner sheaths of man. For the intense practitioner it guides him to seek the ultimate, the sight of the Self.

The adage, "where there is a will, there is a way" applies well for yoga. For one who has courage and willingness to face hardships, there is no bar in practising yoga. Only one should know what to do, how much to do and which way to do according to one's capacity and capability.

I.3. – Is yoga a path of *karma, jñāna* or *bhakti*

At the outset Patañjali declares that the goal of yoga is to be directly attained through the unconditional surrender of all our forces to God. Such surrender is nothing but love; it is love free of lust *(bhakti)*. Knowing that this is almost impossible for many, he incorporates the paths of *jñāna* and *karma* under the name of *kriyā yoga*.

To quote *citta vṛtti nirodha* is quite different to the actual state of experiencing *citta vṛtti nirodha*. In order to understand *citta vṛtti nirodha* one has to comprehensively adopt the principles of *karma, jñāna* and *bhakti* – through the fountain of *Pātañjala yoga*.

Citta is the composite of *manas, buddhi* and *ahaṁkāra,* and *vṛtti* is movement, so *citta vṛtti* means movement in the consciousness. In order to restrain the movements in the consciousness the path of *karma* is advised, as right action stabilises the mind *(manas)* and intelligence *(buddhi).* The intellect gets cleansed through understanding and right knowledge to such a state that one is able to surrender *(bhakti)* to God. With its three components the *citta* is tamed and remains without movement *(vṛtti).* This is how yoga transforms *citta vṛtti* into *citta* without *vṛtti* through its practices.

The tangible body is the vessel *(ghaṭa)* of the soul. We must keep our vessel in a perfect, healthy and compact shape without disturbances or ruffles so that its contents – consciousness, intelligence, mind and senses – are brought to a well balanced state to think on the higher levels of consciousness. If any vessel is placed at a crooked angle, there are going to be ripples, but if the vessel is stable on its base, it doesn't shake. Similarly the vessel of the body is to be trained to be stable and steady for its contents to remain steady and stable.

We have been endowed with three instruments, body *(kāya),* speech *(vāca)* and mind *(manas),* a thinking faculty for evolution. Our actions, behavioural patterns and thinking processes depend upon the senses of perception *(jñānendriya)* and the organs of action *(karmendriya).* As they are close to the mind, the mind gets fed by them and it inevitably gets more involved. The triune of *karma, jñāna* and *bhakti* gets coloured and influenced by instincts, intuitions, emotions and afflictions. Therefore if the energy of this triune has to be channelled in a right direction, one needs to utilise and activate all the three aspects through yoga to reach purity of the body *(kāyaśuddhi)* by *karma,* purity of speech *(vācāśuddhi)* by *jñāna* and purity of the consciousness *(manas-śuddhi)* by *bhakti.*

As we enjoy wearing new clothes by discarding the old ones, Self too says, "I want to proceed, but this cloth, the body, is wearing out. Let me discard this and have a fresh body to think and act afresh." This is what yoga does in fulfilling and accomplishing the desired path in this very life: it renews, revitalises and enlivens the vessel of the Self.

All religions emphasise action, knowledge and devotion *(karma, jñāna* and *bhakti)* as pathways towards a noble and worthy life, yoga is a means for uniting *karma, jñāna* and *bhakti* through its methodology of ethical discipline *(nīti),* action *(kṛti),* power *(śakti),* inventive skill *(yukti)* and devotion *(bhakti),* which lead one to live in a noble way.

As Patañjali begins yoga with surrender, it is nothing but a travesty of truth to say that *karma, jñāna* and *bhakti* are different from *Pātañjala yoga.* Whatever has been said, found and practised, Patañjali brought them together under one roof. Paths of *karma, jñāna* and *bhakti* are definitely implicit in yoga. *Tapas* involves *karma, svādhyāya* leads to *jñāna,* and *Īśvara praṇidhāna* to *bhakti*. Hence, yoga is the uniting factor of *bhakti, jñāna* and *karma*. In *Samādhi Pāda, sūtra* 23, the word *Īśvara praṇidhāna* explicitly indicates that it is the path of *bhakti*. In *Sādhana Pāda* the explanation of *aṣṭāṅga yoga* as *kriyā* yoga or yoga of action covers action, knowledge or study of the self, and surrender to God: *Tapasvādhyāyeśvarapraṇidhānāni kriyāyogaḥ* (*Y.S.*, II.1).

He interweaves *karma, jñāna* and *bhakti* from *yama* through to *samādhi*. *Yama, niyama* and *āsana* make the aspirant skilfully tread the path of *karma; prāṇāyāma, pratyāhāra* and *dhāraṇā* the path of *jñāna;* and *dhāraṇā, dhyāna* and *samādhi* the path of *bhakti*. It is a journey from body to brain and from brain to the self.

According to Patañjali, *yama* are mighty universal vows *(mahāvrata)* to be followed as *tapas*. *Niyama* encases everything from cleanliness, contentment and resignation to God. Similarly, *karma, jñāna* and *bhakti* are all inherent in *āsana*. Culmination of effort *(prayatna śaithilya)*, in *āsana* and *karma* without seeking the fruits of action implies purity of action as described in the *Bhagavad Gītā*.

Lord Krishna says,

Yogasthaḥ kuru karmāṇi saṅgaṁ tyaktvā dhanaṁjaya I
siddhyasiddhyoḥ samo bhūtvā samatvaṁ yoga ucyate II (*B.G.*, II.48)

Fixed in yoga, do thy work, O winner of wealth (Arjuna), abandoning attachment, with an even mind in success and failure, for evenness of mind is yoga.

Yadṛcchālābhasaṁtuṣṭo dvandvātīto vimatsaraḥ I
samaḥ siddhāv asiddhau ca kṛtvā'pi na nibhadhyate II (*B.G.*, IV.22)

He who is satisfied with whatever comes by chance, who has passed beyond the dualities (of pleasure and pain), who is free from jealousy and remains the same in success and failure, he is not bound in action.

This is the hidden meaning of *prayatna śaithilya* in *āsana*. *Āsana* leads one towards *ananta samāpatti,* towards the threshold of *bhakti*. All these indicate that yoga is devotion-oriented action *(bhaktipūrvaka karma)*. That is why I often say that *āsana* takes one from the skin to the soul. When this state is reached, the dualities drop out like weathered leaves. This way Patañjali brings *karma, jñāna* and *bhakti* in the three *sūtra* on *āsana* (*Y.S.*, I.46, 47 & 48).

Concerning *prāṇāyāma,* he says that the veil covering the *sattva guṇa* diminishes and the knowledge dawns. Does this not indicate that *āsana* and *prāṇāyāma* are the paths of *jñāna? Pratyāhāra* inverts the vision of senses and mind to flow towards the seer. *Dhāraṇā* keeps on eliminating the destructive and interruptive thoughts from the senses and mind. *Dhyāna* maintains a continuous uninterrupted flow of attentive awareness *(ekatānatā)*. In *samādhi* one gets to feel the presence of Divinity *(bhakti)*. *Jñāna* and *dhyāna* go hand in hand as *samādhi* and *bhakti* go hand in hand *(samādhisiddhiḥ Īśvarapraṇidhānāt).* No doubt, it is *samādhi* that leads one towards surrender of oneself to God or it is through God's grace, one experiences *samādhi (Īśvara praṇidhāna) (Y. S.,* II.45). Hence, this yoga embraces *karma, jñāna* and *bhakti* and therefore yoga has this triune of *karma, jñāna* and *bhakti.* If these three elements are not brought to function, practice of yoga is incomplete, one falls short of the goal and efforts are wasted.

I.4. – What does *āuṁ* stand for

Āuṁ is the first primordial sound pronounced by the Creator. *Āuṁ* is the origin of everything and it is "the sound of the soundless Absolute".[1]

The world was created by Hiraṇyagarbha, a universal golden womb or golden embryo, also called a golden egg.

When opening the mouth the first sound to form is *ā*, then when we prolong and extend the tongue, it moves towards *u*, and then as we end, closing the lips the sound ends with *ṁ*. Hence, *āuṁ*[2] becomes the root of speech *(śabdabrahma* or *nādabrahma).* When the golden egg broke and the universe came into existence, its breaking sound was *āuṁ*. It is on account of this that the *Upaniṣad* say; *āuṁ* is the seed *(bīja)* of speech and *āuṁ* represents God.

According to tradition, the science of yoga was abiding in Universal Thought, and when Hiraṇyagarbha was born from the navel of Lord Viṣṇu, Universe and yoga came at the same time. The *Mahābhārata* says that *Hiraṇyagarbha Yogasya proktā na anya purātanaḥ* – Yoga was pronounced by none other than Hiraṇyagarbha. The word *āuṁ* connoting God, and the universe were created by Hiraṇyagarbha.

Patañjali says that God is represented by the sacred syllable *āuṁ* as praṇava (the mystic syllable), and it has to be repeated constantly with feeling, realising its full significance; *tasya vācakaḥ praṇavaḥ* (I.27), *tajjapastadarthabhāvanam* (I.28).

---

1 *Maitrāyaṇīya Upaniṣad,* VI.22.

2 See the author's *Light on Yoga,* pp. 28, for an explanation of *āuṁ* in detail.

I.5. – Is the yogic path hard and painful

The yogic path is not actually hard or painful. It is the mind that induces such feelings.

Man has learnt to tame cats, dogs, serpents, lions, tigers and elephants; but he has not learnt to tame himself. On account of this he feels that the yogic path is hard, difficult and painful. It only demands discipline and if he accepts to practise with discipline and determination, then these ideas do not surface at all.

It is the nagging mind that expresses that yoga is hard. It is the mind that has the problem and not yoga. Do not children feel hardship and pain to go to school? Does one allow them to follow their wishes or coax and cajole them to go to school? In the same way, one has to discipline and tame the negative thoughts and approach yoga practice with a positive mind. Then I am sure that the ideas on yoga will be different.

a) – Have we to strive or not in yoga

To strive or not to strive in yoga is nothing but twisted information. No yoga texts say that without dynamic action and attention things happen. Yoga is not a passive non-demanding subject.

Let me take my favourite theme, *āsana.* The three aphorisms (46 to 48) in the second chapter of Patañjali's *Yoga Sūtra* convey that whatever *āsana* is performed it should be done with the will of intelligence of the head along with delightful intelligence of the heart. When this is the fact can anyone achieve this by allowing it to happen? The effort has to be there. As practice stabilises, effort transforms into an effortless state, which draws the self to experience its state. This experiencing state is realised only when the intelligence and consciousness are made to spread and feel the interior carpet of the skin touching longitudinally and lattitudinally in the *āsana* without leaving any part untouched from the self on the interior layer of the skin.

When the subject matter is as clear as daylight, I cannot comprehend how such ideas spring out for things to just happen without effort. As bees come to the flowers to suck their fragrance, it is we who have to approach yoga to savour its flavour.

See what Patañjali says; *tatra sthitau yatnōbhyāsaḥ,* and; *sa tu dīrghakāla nairantarya satkārāseveto dṛḍhabhūmiḥ (Y.S.,* I.13 & 14) – yoga practice is a steadfast effort to still the mind and stability comes only with long uninterrupted and alert practice. *Viṣayavati vā pravṛttiḥ utpannā manasaḥ sthiti nibandhani (Y.S.,* I.35) – one may equally attain an exalted state of consciousness by becoming totally engrossed with dedication and devotion in an object of interest. As I practise with dedication and devotion, I am totally in it.

I.6. – Do not demarcate yoga as physical and spiritual

Yoga has a wholeness of its own without division. It covers the physical, mental and spiritual phases of life of man. The physical facet of life is recognisable through the functioning of the organs of action, senses of perception and mind. The other components of the human being, namely, intelligence, I-ness and consciousness are mercurial and to be traced to feel the eternal Self.

Whether one is an oriental or an occidental, he or she will believe in what he/she sees and grasps of the tangible known sheaths of the body. This is the physical aspect. To involve further on the subtle sheaths of man, he/she has to trace and reach the source of all movements to experience the finest facet of life, the Self.

Hence, one will be limited in thinking that the essence of yoga is stretching, strengthening or relaxing at a physical level. Inference is one thing and fact is another. For me the body is the visible self, mind the subtler self and 'Self' the subtlest of the subtle and the finest of the fine. Yoga *sādhanā* is to uncover all of man to live in the eternal flow of life that has no divisions or branches.

This is the hierarchy in yoga. A practitioner cannot jump at once to the highest level of the hierarchy. He has to gradually progress step by step, from the physical to reach the spiritual height. If yoga is treated as exercise it is not the fault of yoga.

Secondly, it is a dilemma for many to demarcate yoga as physical or spiritual. It covers both. When I began on this path of yoga, I was under the same impression as many. I was a sick boy and I thought I should develop physical prowess to be free from sickness. Probably, it is the same with majority of people who like to solve their physical problems through yoga. There is nothing wrong if such people take to yoga to recover health. The moment we think of yoga is it possible for us to think on spiritual aspects? Naturally we begin with health, earn it and then move towards higher and nobler thoughts. First we have to have physical health, and then think of inclining towards spiritual nourishment.

Is not the body the main instrument for spiritual practices? If one wants to meditate, as if it is the only one for spiritual aspects, one needs the body to be able to sit straight and mind to be steady. Is it not necessary to culture the body, the mind and intelligence before one thinks of spiritual aspects?

Nowhere in any text is it ever mentioned that *āsana* are physical. Why do you bathe each day? Because we want to be clean. It is the same in yoga. We have to bathe not only the body but also the senses of perception, mind, intelligence and consciousness, so that we remain clean inside and outside so that divinity is felt from the body to the core of our being.

One cannot concentrate or meditate on an empty space. By *āsana* practices one understands the space of his inner body and practises the *āsana* to increase that inner space. This approach in *āsana* cannot be physical. We are made up of five elements and we penetrate these elements and reorganise them while doing the *āsana*. We engage our mind and intelligence to reach and experience the indivisible that exists within.

Let us not divide yoga but live in yoga to discover ourselves. Let us involve ourselves totally and wholly in the *āsana* practice and see where our doubts take us.

Āsana and *prāṇāyāma* helped me to develop defensive energy to fight the offensive forces that were affecting my body, mind and self.

If one understands of what is being said so far, I am certain that one's intelligence will lead him further towards the internal awareness to live in the core of his being so that he is free from the dilemma or doubt that *āsana* are beyond physical boundaries.

Yoga is a journey from the phenomenal to the noumenal. *Prakāśa kriyā sthiti śilaṁ bhūtendriyātmakaṁ bhogāpavargārthaṁ dṛśyaṁ* (*Y.S.*, II.18) – nature, its three qualities *(sattva, rajas, tamas)* and its evolutes, the elements, mind, senses of perception and organs of action, exist eternally to serve the seer, for enjoyment or emancipation. All the phenomenal *(liṅga)* aspects evolve from and are supported by the unevolved noumenal matter *(aliṅga)*. If one gets a background of the physics of the body and its chemistry, then one cannot demarcate yoga, as it is a journey from body to the soul.

Know that the body is the primary instrument with which we proceed on the journey. It trains the mind and intelligence to touch the ultimate, the establishment of the Self. Yoga practice cultures the container – the body – as well as its content – the Self.

Fortunately yoga is a practical subject whether one believes it or not; but the moment one experiences the beneficial changes, faith sets in. To expect and experience these changes, uninterrupted practice for a long time is needed as nature takes its own time, which appears excruciatingly long. Yet with patience, if one perseveres, he is bound to reduce and minimise the sufferings and afflictions and move towards enlightenment.

I.7. – Is yoga an addiction

"Addiction" is not a relevant word for yoga. An addiction is when one gives oneself up powerlessly to something that makes him dependent. Even if one gets accustomed to good things, good habits and good words, it is not addiction but a cultivation of what is good for life. Addiction to bad habits is one thing. "Addiction" to yoga for health and happiness is another. If someone suffers from pain or disease, do we call it addiction if they take to yoga? By chance if one develops a passion and aspiration to yoga, as it is a self-educative subject, then do we consider this an addiction or education?

The difference between addiction to drugs and getting "addicted" to yoga is that yoga removes doubts and confusions and exhilarates one towards positive life.

One who is addicted to drugs feels: "No drug, no peace"; and one who is addicted to yoga says: "Know yoga, know peace". The more one goes towards poise and peace, the more he gets involved. Drugs are psycho-toxic and yoga is a psycho-elixir. If drug addicts miss the required dose, they develop abstinence syndrome and become sick whereas by stopping or missing yoga, nothing is lost except the guilt of non-practice. Addiction to drugs clogs the brain, yoga clears the brain. A smoker puffs the lungs with nicotine breath. One puffs oxygenated air in yoga. A smoker takes the toxins of tobacco and a practitioner of yoga takes the aroma of cosmic nectar.

a) – Does yoga affect an unborn baby

As drug addiction affects a new born baby, so too does yoga.

The baby in the womb rests as in *Garbha Piṇḍāsana*. It breathes in the *āsana*. If the mother practises yoga before and at the time of pregnancy, the unborn child may have an imprint that is yet to be born. If yoga is practised by both (husband and wife), not only does the alchemy of the blood improves but also the brain's sensitivity of the expected baby develops. When the parents are healthy, the child is bound to be healthy.

The unborn baby is imprisoned in the womb. It has to rest in that small narrow place. When the mother does *āsana*, she creates room for the baby to unconsciously kick, stretch and expand and the child experiences space in that limited area.

The farmer before sowing the seed loosens the soil. By loosening the soil, the seed receives water, air and minerals to sprout. Similarly, the baby within needs oxygen, movement and supply of blood to grow healthily. Yoga helps the child to feel the affectionate contact of the mother as her moods get balanced for the baby to breath with these imprints.

By *āsana* practice we can know how to face the ultimate relinquishing of all our attachments and addictions. In Śavāsana we begin to train and educate ourselves for surrender.

Fear of death is worse than death. Death is certain; then why fear? I have spoken about fear of death and clinging to life, which does not leave even a learned and wise person (*Y.S.*, II.9). Learn how to do *Śavāsana* well, that simulates death and brings silence and non-movement. After all what is death? It is a non-existing and a non-feeling state that one experiences often in *Śavāsana*. Therefore, better taste life with education and not addiction.

I.8. – How the gates of the West opened to yoga and made it popular

No doubt, in the beginning, I encountered many problems, which I do not like to go into. But one thing I would like to say is this. India, which was ruled by the West, was considered as a slave country. Even though we had won Independence a few years before my first visit abroad, the idea that Indians were slaves had not faded from their minds. On account of this I had in me an inferiority complex. With this complex, to be a driver of the slave drivers was not easy, I had to surmount enormous difficulties. But as time went by, I began cultivating strength to face them and began conveying the message of yoga to their physical and mental levels.

The content of man is divinity, but the container of this divinity is the body. The majority of people perceive with ease the pleasures of the body and mind. I began guiding the western students in a way that sooner or later they could move from the pleasures of the external joys towards the bliss of the internal world. It was, no doubt a herculean task to take them from the known towards the unknown, that is Self or Soul *(puruṣa, draṣṭā, ātmā)*. I am happy to say I did it and transformed many towards the higher goals of life.

In those days people of the West were proud of their intellectual prowess as well as their arrogance of being masters of the World. Though it was a hard job, fortunately, they quickly grasped the subject in its perceivable and conceivable aspects and it took them beyond their mental frame. I took the path of explaining of what real health is and what peace means. Yoga as a science is very straightforward; it could easily achieve their wants. Reading their mental pulse I attracted them to yoga by satisfying their mental wants. As they soon realised the value of my teaching they left off all their arrogant attacks and they embraced it.

As they went on practising they realised it is not a religion, a creed or a cult. It is not a cult of the body alone, but shows ways of culturing the mind, intelligence and consciousness to merge in the self and then with the Supreme.

The human body is the finest machine created by God. Millions of cells are produced each second and die out swiftly. They give strength, fitness and calmness. Each cell has its own intelligence. The orchestra of bones, muscles, tissues, nerves, blood vessels, limbs, organs and physiological systems are tuned to a veritable dance and surge qualitatively as a fountain of energy. In one sense, yoga begins with the cult of the body towards the culture of the mind, civilising the intelligence and consciousness to finally feel and live in the Self.

The West had all material richness but was literally unhappy. Yoga with its spiritual background filled that gap. Therefore it became popular.

I do not hesitate to say that yoga thrived in the lap of the West. The West had a big hand for yoga to rebound back in India.

I.9. – The five sheaths of the Self

The seed is the cause for the tree to grow, but the surprising thing is that in the seed there is nothing visible for one to know how the tree grows and with what content. From this apparent 'nothingness' of the seed the tree shoots up. In the same way, the seed of our life force, at its core is the Self.

Man is made of causal body (*kāraṇa śarīra*), subtle body (*sūkṣma śarīra*) and gross body (*sthūla śarīra*). These three bodies are like the envelopes to the soul. They encase the five sheaths or *kośa* of the body. *Taittirīya Upaniṣad* is the first scripture which reveals the five sheaths or envelopes that cover the light of the Self.

Man's structural body is *annamaya kośa*. *Anna* means food. The body with its muscles, bones and tendons is built on food and hence is known as *annamaya kośa*.

The first purpose of yoga is to tune and tone the body *(annamaya kośa)*. This *kośa* is like the foundation of a building, a foundation that is equated to *pṛthvi tattva*.

We do not survive on food and water alone but also on air, without air we cannot survive. This part is connected to the *prāṇamaya kośa* or physiological body as energy *(prāṇa)* vibrates in this *kośa*. The respiratory, circulatory and the other systems come under this *kośa*. This *kośa* is equated with *āp tattva*, because of spongy and fluid nature of it.

a) – The breath acts as a link between body, mind and Self

Here, let me bring to your attention the value of this vital body *(āp-tattva)*. "Breath is life and life is breath. As long as there is breath in the body, there is life; when the breath departs, life departs", says the third stanza of the second chapter of the *Haṭhayoga Pradīpikā*.

There is an intimate relationship between breath, mind and Self. They are like twin brothers. The other term for breath is *prāṇa*, commonly known as energy. Wherever energy is focused, there mind, intelligence and consciousness get focused and wherever the mind or intelligence or consciousness is attentive, there the energy gets saturated and helps concentration.

Prāṇāyāma is the churning of the gross breath, which is a raw material that acts for the production of *prāṇa*.

The five sheaths of the body are interwoven and work in unison. The Self has five sheaths, representing the five elements with their atomic qualities and seven constituents.

As one constructs a bridge to cross over the river, in our system the *prāṇamaya kośa* or the physiological body is the bridge between the physical and mental bodies. The physiological body is nothing but the vital organic body. This vital body is the one that filters energy from the gross atmospheric air that we draw in. This filtered energy *(prāṇa)*, stimulates the thinking faculty of the brain for higher thinking and simple living.

This *prāṇa* is the key to open the gates of the mind connecting body and Self. Hence, breath is the bridge between body and Self.[1]

Then comes *manõmaya kośa*, which is connected to the fire element *(tejas tattva)*. Mind belongs to *tejas tattva*, which creates emotional disturbances causing anxiety, blood pressure, cholesterol variation, diabetes, as well as for peacefulness and quietness. As yogic practice mainly affects the mind, one experiences the inner poise, serenity, lightness and freshness. Here the mind moves towards gaining a benevolent state *(saumanas)*.

Vijñānamaya kośa is the intellectual sheath. It belongs to the element of air *(vāyu tattva)*. This *tattva* interweaves one's intelligence from the body to the Self. Through yogic practice the intelligence remains crystal clear in the heart and head. This sheath being close to the *jīvātman*

[1] See *Light on Prāṇāyāma*, published by INDUS, Rupa and Co.

helps one to identify the individual self *(jīvātman)* and the eternal Self (Puruṣa), as this *kośa* has the power to develop exalted knowledge *(viśeṣa jñāna).*

Ānandamaya kośa is the conscience (*antaḥkaraṇa*). It is of the element of ether or space *(ākāśa tattva).* Due to the purity in intelligence and purity in consciousness purity in the conscience takes place. From this purity in intelligence, consciousness and conscience the sight of soul takes place bringing untainted inexplicable and inexpressible bliss. Then one lives in space; hence it is termed as *ānandamaya*, which has no frontier. This way the practice of yoga penetrates all the five *kośa,* leading one to live in the experiential self.

While practising *āsana* one starts from the *annamaya kośa,* positioning the *āsana* properly and accurately according to the anatomical structure of the joints and muscles. Then he proceeds to penetrate into the organic body *(prāṇamaya kośa)* adjusting each part to rest in its place. Then with steadiness on the physical and organic body, he makes the mind to 'feel' the body along with the extension to be at ease *(sukhatā).* From this state of equilibrium *(samaṁkāya)* and benevolent mind *(saumanas),* he moves his intelligence *(vijñānamaya kośa)* to feel and touch the inner frontier of the body evenly. This intellectual touch with *tej, āp* and *pṛthvi* (psychological, physiological and physical bodies) alerts the self to attention by making it to engulf the five sheaths and five elements as if everything is *ānandamaya* and *ākaśamaya.* This is *ātma prasādana.*

I.10. – The seven states of consciousness and health

Yoga is not only meant for gaining health but to understand the seven interior states of consciousness. Health and consciousness are closely linked. Health is equated with an undiseased body and well being. In the yogic sense, health has many connotations; health is wellness in moral, physical, physiological, mental, intellectual, conscientious and spiritual levels. When one is not at ease in any of these seven stages of health, it is disease.

Body is one but it functions at different levels. Similarly, the mind is one but it gets affected with lust, anger, greed, infatuation and so forth. Intelligence and consciousness also have their own defects.

As there are seven stages of health, there are seven states of consciousness. The seven states of consciousness are; raising consciousness *(vyutthāna citta),* restraining consciousness *(nirodha citta),* tranquil consciousness *(praśānta citta),* fabricating consciousness *(nirmāṇa citta),* attentive consciousness *(ekāgra citta),* split consciousness *(chidra citta)* and flawless consciousness *(divya citta).* All these states of consciousness are closely connected to the seven stages of health. These seven states of consciousness and seven stages of health uplift and transform man from the mundane life to a divine state of life. During these transformations there could be moments of unease that in turn create health problems and disturbed states of consciousness.

Let me speak on health first, which is easier to understand than the states of consciousness. Health has to be maintained at all levels. Whatever one's goal may be. Whether for worldly pleasures or spiritual bliss, one needs health. Married life or a spiritual life, both need sound health. Man is endowed with seven evolutory instruments, namely: body, senses, mind, intelligence, I-ness, consciousness and conscience. All these evolutory instruments need to be cultured and cultivated in a right way to maintain health.

Medical science has two forms of treatment. One is through conventional treatment and the other through drastic invasive treatment, which is surgical. Treatment through yoga depends on *pañca bhūta* and *tanmātra, pañca vāyu, ṣaḍsampat, bhāvanā śakti, jñāna śakti, icchā śakti* and *kriyā śakti.* These aspects need to be understood and administered in a practical way known as *abhyāsa, sādhanā, anuṣṭhāna, tapas, tejas, viveka-prajñā* and *vairāgya.*

First duty is to know the symptoms and cause of a disease. Ego, pride, carelessness, heedlessness, I-ness *(ahaṁkāra),* attachment and aversion are the causes for different ailments. The signs of disease, or uneasiness are: sorrow, despair, unsteadiness of the body and irregular breathing. In order to eradicate the causes of ailments, one has to know the meaning of yoga *dharma* or religiosity of it in life.

Today, for me discipline is religiousness and indiscipline is irreligiousness. Health leads us from bondage to liberation and it has to be earned through strict discipline.

Now let me explain the levels of health, one by one.

Physical health: Body is made up of five elements (earth, water, fire, air and ether), with their atomic potentials (odour, taste, form, touch and sound). Energy forces *(prāṇa)* function in five categories as *prāṇa, apāna, samāna, udāna* and *vyāna.* These act as fuel on the five elements with their atomic potentials and the elementary systems. *Prāṇa* controls the nervous and respiratory system, *apāna* – excretory and reproductive system, *samāna* – digestive system, *udāna* – nose, chest, throat, organ of speech and *vyāna* – circulatory and nervous system.

—

The three qualities of nature are *sattva, rajas* and *tamas.* Body and mind get engulfed by these *guṇa* and imbalance in them disturbs the health of the body as well as the mind and the consciousness.

The metabolism of the body depends upon the three humours; wind *(vāta),* fire *(pitta)* and water *(kapha).* The body has seven ingredients *(sapta dhātu).* These are: chyle *(rasa),* blood *(rakta),* flesh *(māṁsa),* fat *(meda),* bone *(asthi),* bone marrow *(majjā)* and semen *(śukra),* and three excretes: sweat *(sveda),* stools *(mala),* urine *(mūtra).* All of these get disturbed when imbalance takes place in the body. Practice of yoga brings back balance.

Psychological health: Psychological problems and disturbances take place on moods, moulds, habits, emotions, cults, character and conduct. Yoga being a psychosomatic science helps to recover and regain a well functioning metabolic system.

Ethical health: Ethical health depends upon the value based conduct, culture and tradition. Its implementation is dependent upon the society and words of trustworthy people *(āpta vacanam* or *āpta vākyam),* which are within the frame of the principles of *yama* and *niyama.* If we plan life within the frame of these principles, we gain ethical health.

Mental health: Mental health is the total awareness of the mind itself. This is done with attentive awareness. Fluctuations affect the mind. Movements in the mind are like strong tides creating imbalance in body and ripples of disturbance in the mind. Waves in the lake do not occur if there is no wind. When actions lead towards valid experiences, it is to be considered as a healthy action and thought. Otherwise, the erroneous, mistaken, illusory knowledge and twists distort the mind and lead towards unhealthy actions and thoughts. A watchful attention that synchronises actions with thought and thought with action is mental health.

Intellectual health: Rationality, reasoning judicial discrimination and wisdom are the essential qualities of intelligence. Man is highly intelligent among all creations. When intelligence fails, sensitivity gets lost. Misunderstanding and misconception cloud the intelligence, perverting and creating intellectual confusions. Even if you see something clearly through your eyes, still the confused intelligence will infer that the seen is something else.

Dhāraṇā and *dhyāna* bring clarity in intelligence and correct the wrong notions into right notions. This is intellectual health.

Conscientious health: Conscience is called *antaḥkaraṇa* or *dharmendriya* in *Sanskṛt.* Its function is to be aware of good and bad deeds and save one from falling from the threshold of ethics. Its job is to uphold, sustain and support man. It is a special sense where it witnesses all actions and weighs them, and guides judiciously to live with religiousness and virtuosity. This conscientious health comes through wisdom *(viveka)* with dutiful action and conduct. We often say, have clear conscience because it has the quality of admission and confession of guilt feelings. It takes the practitioner towards equipoise *(samādhāna citta)* or the state of *samādhi* where all afflictions, taints and fissures in the consciousness terminate leading to the last stage of health – divine health.

Divine Health: It is the highest, subtlest and the finest state of health. It leads one to salvation. Here all the parts of the self remain serene like the mid-ocean.

As I said before, these seven stages of health are inter-related with the seven states of consciousness. The consciousness undergoes this ascending transformation in health or it may act as a stumbling block if one is careless and heedless and slack in efforts *(pramāda* and *avirati).*

Having explained the seven stages of health let me take you to know the seven states of consciousness *(citta).*

Vyutthāna citta: Its tendency is outgoing. When the consciousness is dull, in disarray, agitated, distracted, attached, envious, infatuated, it disturbs the outgoing tendencies and movements creating imbalances in the consciousness. These movements are to be noticed and disciplined.

Nirodha citta: Means restraining thoughts in the consciousness. It also means to obstruct, oppose or suppress the wandering thoughts.

Praśānta citta: Is a state in between wandering and restraining states of *citta.* This pause is like the bogies of a train, which have space in between them so that they do not crash with each other while in motion or at the time of braking. If the pauses between wandering and restraining thoughts are increased for a longer period of time, it is known as *praśānta citta.* Here *citta* gets impregnated with quiet and silent moments. Then this state becomes the base for culturing the *citta* to reach *samādhāna citta.*

Ekāgra citta: Is one pointed attention. We are often only able to concentrate for a short while on a thing, or a point. Hence it has to be cultivated gradually. It has to undergo transformation to reach *ekāgratā citta (eka* means one and *agra* means the first principle – the *puruṣa.* This *puruṣa* is without a second). *Ekāgra citta* is no doubt a blessing, but there are chances of slipping due to arrogance in this state of achievement. This arrogance or pride intoxicates the superior state of the consciousness and taints it with an egoistic consciousness *(ahaṁkāra citta).* This state may create splits or fissures in the consciousness as *chidra citta.* If those who are blessed intellectuals remain humble, they are angels on earth. Otherwise it brings a downfall in their evolution, creating room for fissures to appear and making them lose the purity of intelligence in their consciousness. Hence health in this sheath is a must.

Nirmāṇa citta: Ekāgrata citta causes *chidra citta* (split consciousness), or *nirmāṇa citta* (auspicious, ripe consciousness). Cultivation of sprouted *citta* to reach its highest state is *nirmāna citta.* Due to the power of concentration one often gets intoxicated, which becomes a stumbling block to reach towards *nirmāṇa citta. Nirmāṇa citta* is *samāhita citta* or the auspicious state of the 'I' *(asmitā citta).* This too may act as a stumbling block due to the feel of purity and auspiciousness in the 'I'-ness.

In the normal walk of life, *citta* is full of moods, emotions, pride, prejudice and malice. Sometimes it likes to be quiet, silent, non-interfering, tender, soft, affectionate and sincere. On account of the sense of pride of purity and auspiciousness, this state of *citta* acts as the impostor of the Self. It fabricates and acts as if it is the Self. Then the *sādhaka* must know that by this behaviour ill health may set in, in this sheath. So one has to go back and re-start to the yogic *sādhanā* to sublimate this impostor that cheats the *sādhaka* as pure Self.

Chidra citta: Means splits or fissures in the consciousness. Even a small fissure or a hole is enough to disturb the consciousness towards deformation or regression. The pride of success in one pointed attention can split the *citta.* Like the hair at its ends has splits, it is the same in the case of the *citta.* Like a glass when dropped breaks into pieces, *citta* too splits and cracks at this ultimate stage of refinement. Hence, Patañjali cautions the *sādhaka* to be humble and not to be proud of success.

In the fissure or hole of *chidra citta* old impressions rise up their hoods again and may lead the yogi to become a *yoga bhraṣtan.* If he crosses over this bridge, he reaches that health, which leads him towards the divine consciousness *(divya citta).*

Divya citta: Means divine. When the *citta* is purified it becomes the receptacle of the *ātman* as *divya citta.* At this stage, no hurdles occur. The consciousness becomes equal to the *ātman* remaining always in a pure state *(kūṭastha citta). Kūṭastha* means immoveable, perpetual and universal. Hence, it is termed as *divya citta.*

When this divine health in *citta* is earned and achieved, the *sādhaka* becomes a *muktan;* he experiences freedom, beatitude and emancipation.

Many are long time students of yoga; it is beyond my understanding why most *sādhaka* live only on the physical and mental levels. As practitioners, one has to move on to the wholistic level to live in holiness. As there are seven states of consciousness and seven aspects of health learn to understand the importance of health in each stage or in each state of consciousness. Fissures may form at any level. Yoga has means to remedy at each level and make one to cross the hurdles with patience at each level. For this divine state of health and consciousness, the energy and awareness *(prāṇa* and *prajñā)* have to play a great role in the *sādhaka* on his *sādhanā*. *Prāṇa* and *prajñā* work in unison through yoga on all the seven states of consciousness.

Now let me take you to understand *prāṇa-śakti* and *prajñā-śakti* and how they are generated through the interaction of the seven properties of life:

a) *pañca bhūta (bhūta śakti):* earth, water, fire, air and ether; its counterparts *pañca tanmātra;* odour, taste, form, touch and sound;
b) *pañca vāyū (vāyū śakti): prāṇa, apāna, samāna, vyāna* and *udāna;*
c) *ṣaḍsampat śakti:* six spiritual wealth: tranquillity *(śama);* power of restraint *(dama);* power of endurance and patience *(titikṣā);* power of keeping away from sensual pleasures *(uparati);* power of reverential faith *(śraddhā)* and lastly to set the mental energies to flow in a right way *(samādhāna);*
d) *bhāvanā śakti*: these are friendliness *(maitri),* compassion *(karuṇā),* gladness *(mudita)* and indifference *(upekṣā).* These conducive emotional aspects generate healthy emotions;
e) *jñāna śakti*: deliberation of intelligence *(vitarka),* reflection *(vicāra),* thoughtfully encountering the wrong and evil tendencies *(pratipakṣa bhāvanam).*
f) *icchā śakti* : will-power to stop thoughts, which otherwise create an ocean of desires *(vāsanā);*
g) *kriyā śakti:* will behind actions, which are to be done whole-heartedly with a clear, powerful and effective mind.

These seven *śakti* generate *prāṇa* and *prajñā.* They are upheld and sustained by the practice of *aṣṭāṅga yoga* as its role is to destroy the impurities and bring light of knowledge *(aśuddhikṣaya* and *jñānadīpti).*

Similarly, practice of yoga has seven layers: *a) abhyāsa, b) sādhanā, c) anuṣṭhāna, d) tapas, e) tejas, f) viveka* and *g) vairāgya.*

a) *Abhyāsa* means to establish with repeated attempts and zealousness. Practice *(abhyāsa)* has to be maintained uninterruptedly with cheerfulness and enthusiasm.
b) *Sādhanā* is to utilise the body, mind and intelligence as an endeavour to animate the *prāṇic* energy in the body, senses and mind. *Sādhanā* is three-tiered. They are external (*bahiraṅga),* internal (*antaraṅga)* and innermost *(antarātma).* All the three-tiered *sādhanā* are to be utilised and moulded instantaneously and simultaneously to serve the purpose of reaching freedom and beatitude.
c) *Anuṣṭhāna* means practice with religiousness in mind, followed not as duty but with auspiciousness.

d) *Tapas* is a burning zeal or desire to eradicate the impurities of the body, mind and speech. It acts as a blazing fire that lifts one from darkness to light.

e) *Tejas* is the fire element as *asmitā*. It is needed to fuel our endeavours as it is close to *jīvātman*. It helps in taking one from 'I-am-ness' to 'am-ness' generating *prāṇa* and *prajñā* towards the spiritual health.

f) *Viveka* is qualitative study *(guṇātmaka svādhyāya)*, which guides one in judging what is right and what is wrong, what is correct and what is incorrect, what is real and what is unreal; charging the *sādhaka* with the luminosity in his *sādhanā*.

g) *Vairāgya* is the study to distinguish the difference between bondage *(bhoga)* and emancipation *(apavarga)*. This study makes *prakṛti* to gravitate towards the Self *(puruṣa)* and God *(puruṣa viṣeśa)*.

Yoga *sādhanā* is a *dharma* (religious spiritual study), which minimises or eradicates disturbances that occur from four types that are dealt with below.

These are:

a) *Pañca vṛtti:* valid and correct knowledge *(pramāṇa)*; perverse knowledge *(viparyaya)*, imaginative or fanciful knowledge *(vikalpa)*, state of void *(nidrā)*, memory *(smṛti)*.

b) *Pañca kleśa:* spiritual ignorance *(avidyā)*, ego *(asmitā)*, attachment *(rāga)*, abhorrence *(dveṣa)*, adherence to life *(abhiniveśa)*.

c) *Citta vikṣepa:* physical and psycho-physiological diseases *(vyādhi)*, mental sluggishness and laziness *(styāna)*, doubt *(saṁśaya)*, callousness *(pramāda)*, idleness *(ālasya)*, incontinence *(avirati)*, mistaken notion *(bhrāntidarśana)*, missing the point *(alabdhabhūmikatva)*, unsettled state *(anavasthitatva)*, sorrow *(duḥkha)*, dejection *(daurmanasya)*, shakiness of body *(aṅgamejayatva)*, disturbance in breathing *(śvāṣa praśvāṣa)*.

d) *Ṣaḍripu* or six emotional upheavals: desire *(kāma)*, anger *(krodha)*, greed *(lobha)*, infatuation *(moha)*, pride *(mada)*, jealousy *(mātsarya)*.

The action of yoga is meant to arrest all these disturbances that take place along with *guṇa (sattva, rajas* and *tamas)*.

In addition to these, one has to understand the following duty of man. It has class *(varṇa)*, stages in life *(āśrama)*, and aims *(puruṣārtha)*.

As our nature is dependent on *guṇa dharma*, it has a bearing on *varṇa dharma*. If *varṇa dharma* is intellectual wisdom *(brāhma dharma)*, prowess and power *(kṣātra dharma)*, managing with supply and demand *(vaiśya dharma)*, capacity to labour *(śūdra dharma)*. Similarly, *āśrama dharma has;* a) *brahmacaryāśrama* – education for gaining knowledge, b) *gṛhasthāśrama* – a house-holder's life for the good of the society, c) *vānaprasthāśrama* –keeping aloof and with non-attachment help the family and society in the art of right-living, and lastly, d) *sannyāsāśrama* where one withdraws from the worldly activities and devotes on God. Though the *varṇa dharma* has lost its significance *āśrama dharma* is still persistent as it is designed to maintain the individual health as well as social health and healthy state of consciousness.

The *puruṣārtha dharma*, has four-fold aims. These are righteous and virtuous science of duty *(yoga-dharma)*, utilisation of means *(artha sādhana)*, fulfilments of desires *(kāma)*, and lastly emancipation *(mokṣa)*.

Thus *guṇa dharma, varṇa dharma, āśrama dharma* and *puruṣārtha dharma* are meant for us all to proceed from mundane health towards divine health. Divine health is freedom from all afflictions. Hence, the importance of the seven states of health and seven states of consciousness are essential to come out from the realm of bondage in order to enter the kingdom of untainted bliss or *mukti* – the end of the *sādhanā* and the fulfilment of real health and real consciousness.

I.11. – Commentary on Patañjali was a challenging task

Sanskṛt words have rich lexical semantics. Different meanings on a single word are conveyed according to the context of the subject matter.

It is my good fortune that my attentive practice, reflective thinking and felt experience guided me in reading the aphorisms and studying them when they coincided with my practice. This helped me grasp the real evolutary essence of yoga on my life's progression.

The thought I have in mind is to bring these terse *sūtra* for an average *sādhaka* to understand the basic views as a background and as a means to practise to feel their views.

When I had to encounter the challenges of explaining the third chapter – the *Vibhūti Pāda* I depended upon the guidance given by Patañjali himself: *tasya saptadhā prāntabhūmiḥ prajñā* (*Y.S.*, II.27) – through this unbroken flow of discriminative awareness, one gains perfect knowledge which has seven spheres. *Yogāṅgānuṣṭhānāt aśuddhikṣaye jñānadīptiḥ āvivekakhyāteḥ* (*Y.S.*, II.28) – by the dedicated practice of the various aspects of yoga impurities are destroyed: the crown of wisdom radiates in glory.

I took my *āsana* practice and the inflow and outflow of the breath in *prāṇāyāma* as my *japa* and practised them repeatedly with full significance of their meaning and feeling *(artha bhāvanā).* This helped me get a clear picture for writing on the *Vibhūti Pāda.* A further guidance came from: *etena bhūtendriyeṣu dharmalakṣaṇa avasthā pariṇāmāḥ vyākhyātāḥ* (*Y.S.,* III.13) – through these three phases of *dharma, lakṣaṇa* and *avasthā* my consciousness got cultured and transformed from its potential state *(dharma)* towards its further refinement *(lakṣaṇa)* and the zenith of refinement *(avasthā).* In this way, the transformation of the elements, senses and mind, which took place in me, helped me a great deal.

I used my intelligence and consciousness to qualify my *sādhanā* for further refinement. Until the refinement reached an un-oscillating state in body, senses of action and perception, mind, intelligence and the feel of consciousness neither I waned nor waxed in my *sādhanā.*

In my own *sādhanā* I covered the journey from *prakṛti* to *puruṣa* in seven stages of *sapta prajñā.* They revealed to me, the integration of the body, senses, energy, mind, intellect, intelligence and consciousness. The practice of eight aspects with this integration made me look into each *sūtra* with self awareness.

Without practice *(sādhanā)* any commentary on the Yoga Sūtra would be far too difficult a task, far beyond a normal person's capability. It is entirely due to my determined and devoted practice, and the sensitive reflection and re-reflection that took place on its account that I was finally able to approach and surmount the hurdles of such an undertaking.

I.12. – What is *yoganidrā*

Only Lord Vishnu, the sustainer of the universe, can be in *yoganidrā.*[1] God is a sinless actor *(niṣkāma karmin).* Therefore, He alone could do illuminative *yoganidrā.*

---

[1] *Yoganidrā* (yoga sleep). According to Hindu mythology, when everything perishes at the end of each *yuga* (age), there comes the deluge and the Universe remains desolate and void. A *yuga* is 124 years of Brahmā. In that deep eternal silence, Lord Viṣṇu sleeps on a banyan leaf on the surface of waters. This state of sleep of Mahāviṣṇu is called *yoga nidrā,* and the Universe remains temporarily dissolved until God reawakens. That will be the beginning of the next great age. In this state of *yoga nidrā,* Mahāviṣṇu is called Bālamukunda, and some believe that He is called Nārāyana as He rests on the waters *(nāra).* The term *yoga nidrā* is used to designate a yoga pose (see the author's *Light on Yoga,* plate n. 391). In contemporary yoga it is often used to name a state of deep relaxation along with visualisation, observation of breath and eventually a silent recitation of *mantra.*

Lord Krishna says in the *Bhagavad Gītā*: *Matsthāni sarvabhūtāni na chāhaṁ te ṣvavasthitaḥ* – "All beings abide in Me, but I do not abide in them" (*B.G.*, IX.4). In the third chapter of *Bhagavad Gītā*, He emphatically declares: "O Pārtha! For me there is nothing in all the three worlds which ought to be done, nor is there anything unacquired that ought to be acquired. Yet, I go on working. If I do not work, O Pārtha, men will follow me" (*B.G.*, III.22-23). God is constantly working. He works but He does not get involved in it. He is the Ultimate Consciousness or omniscient. He is the creator, controller, organiser and maker of this universe, including attachments, non-attachments or selfish or selfless motives. He appears to be doing nothing, yet He does everything. This is His *yoganidrā*.

Yoganidrā came into vogue recently. Some schools of yoga made this word popular and everyone started calling *Śavāsana* in a sitting *āsana* as *Yoganidrā*. Covering the head with a cloth and guiding the suspension of the activities of the mind as in *Śavāsana* is called *Yoganidrā*. For me, it is inert meditation.

Haṭhayoga Pradīpikā (I.32) mentions the suspension of thoughts in *Śavāsana* (*śava* = dead body) and *Gheraṇḍa Saṁhitā* (II.19) calls it corpse pose *(Mṛtāsana)*. *Śavāsana* is a way of simulating death so that one experiences the feel of death in such a way that the fear of death is faced. It enlivens one with new life, new hope and new light. *Śavāsana* makes one to be away from the world of joys, attachments, sorrows and sufferings and be free from mental botheration and afflictions. *Śavāsana* helps to crucify worldly tendencies and resurrect spiritual aspects. We make students do *Śavāsana* to simulate the feel of the non-existing state as in death but do not like to name it *Yoganidrā*.

Yoganidrā is the cultivation of non-attachment to worldly life. To learn non-attachment, one has to silence the body and emotions, control the movements of breath and acquire clarity in intelligence and consciousness.

Years back, in the early 60's, a prisoner, convicted of murder, from Pune Yerwada Jail was to be hanged. He wrote me a letter that was censored by the authorities. He wanted to do some *āsana* and *prāṇāyāma* so that he could die peacefully. At that time my book *Light on Yoga* was not yet ready. I wrote instructing him on what to do and sent the books like *Bhagavad Gītā* and *Rāmāyaṇa* to read. I wrote to him, how lucky he was! He knew his death whereas we do not know when death approaches us. Since he was sure of his death, I advised him to surrender peacefully to the Lord. After he was hanged, his mother wrote to me saying that her son changed after reading the letter that was written by me and was quite relaxed and peaceful with his mind on God. I say this was *Yoganidrā* for him.

In the first stages of practice of *Śavāsana* one adjusts the physical position and begins to relax the physical body. You have been taught the positioning of the body evenly from the centre of the spine, and the way of relaxing flesh, muscles, joints, limbs and torso to remain at ease in their places. At the same time you are guided to have an overall look intellectually towards each part of the body to be in close affectionate contact with the Mother Earth. It is *yoganidrā*.

In the beginning, it acts as a recuperative state to recover from voluntary as well as non-voluntary tensions. Often students fall asleep and snore in *Śavāsana*. As teachers, we do not disturb those who sleep in *Śavāsana*. Almost all can enjoy *Śavāsana* if it is done as said above. It is relaxing and recuperative.

Sleep is a mental modification. It is one of the five *vṛtti* in which there is a feel of non-deliberate restraining of the thought-waves. It is an inert state of consciousness where one does not feel the sense of its existence. During sleep, one feels free from worries, tensions and problems. In *Śavāsana,* one deliberately and passively stills all modifications as they arise and hence this state may be called *yoganidrā*. True *Śavāsana* or *Yoganidrā* occurs when the *sādhaka* connects this quiet mind to his intelligence, intelligence to the consciousness and consciousness to the self. This is taught in sitting position as *yoganidrā*.

In *Śavāsana* one has to be passively aware and remain as a witness or a spectator. Then he experiences the serene state of quietness in the consciousness with a passive alertness.

We advise deep breaths after they are made to relax the physical body and mind, and introduce them to soft and deep breaths with the right adjustment of the diaphragm and ribs, as though the breath is the string and the ribs are the pearls. As the beads are moved in *praṇava japa,* the mind and intelligence are made to move towards the self. After a while, as consciousness becomes sublime and lives in awareness, the breath gets quietened. This felt state is true *Śavāsana*. From this quietness, one experiences *manōlaya*. *Manas* is mind and *laya* is immersion. The mind dissolves along with its objects and makes one to experience equipoise as well as fullness in the consciousness.

In *dhyāna* this state of *manōlaya* or *śūnyāvasthā* (empty state of mind) is transformed and transmitted into a full moon state called *amanaskatva* or *aśūnyāvasthā* state. In *dhyāna* the conscious awareness is filtered and purified for it to trace its source, the Self or the core.

The first phase of *Śavāsana* takes one towards a sleepy state *(nidrā* or *suṣuptyāvasthā)*. The second phase takes towards a wakeful state *(jagratāvasthā)*. Oscillation between *rajoguṇa* and *tamoguṇa* is *svapnāvasthā*. There is oscillation between *suṣupti* and *jāgṛt* states and lastly without oscillation, consciousness rests in the abode of its father – the Self. Here, one remains wakefully wakeful without involvement.

Thus, *Śavāsana* leads gradually towards stillness and from stillness to silence and from silence towards spiritual bliss *(satcidānanda)*.

The coconut has a shell and within the shell is the pulp and water. Quietening the mind with *Śavāsana* is like removing the outer shell of the coconut. Our body is like the shell of a coconut. The pulp inside is *buddhi*. The sweet water is the essence of knowledge and wisdom. So let us tame the body with *dhāraṇā* through *āsana* and *prāṇāyāma*, intelligence with *dhyāna*, and savour the flavour *(rasa)* through *samādhi*. Then the Self rests in its own state. This is *yoganidrā*.

First sow the seed of yoga *(yoga bīja)* and then think of experiencing *yoganidrā (samādhi)*. First the field (body) has to be tilled for the tree of yoga to grow well in the *sādhaka*.

As *Śavāsana* strikes a perfect balance between worldly life and spiritual life, it teaches one how to be in society and yet to be away and aloof. *Śavāsana* is quite deep, as it leads one from the oscillating mundane life towards the sparkling light of divine life.

SECTION II

ON PATAÑJALI AND YOGA

SECTION II – ON PATAÑJALI AND YOGA

II.1. – When yoga came into existence and who is Patañjali

Yoga is as old as civilisation. The savage and savant both were on this earth together though they remained opposite in their thoughts to each other as day and night. The day cannot see the night and night cannot see the day. Yoga was presented for mankind (whether savant or savage) to progress from the uncivilised state of mind to a civilised state of mind.

According to *Yoga-Yājñavalkya-Smṛti,* Hiraṇyagarbha, who is none other than Nārāyaṇa, is the creator of yoga. The *Upaniṣad* say that as the golden foetus was opened, the world came into existence with all its content, including yoga.

According to some scholars, Hiraṇyagarbha was a *ṛṣi* prior to Patañjali. Some say that Kapila, the originator of *sāṁkhya,* was recognised by this name.

The essence of the *Veda* was distilled by the great seers *(ṛṣi).* Its doctrines are known as *darśana.* The six Indian schools of thought *(darśana)* were presented to us by six *ṛṣi;* Kapila presented *sāṁkhya;* Patañjali, *yoga*; Gautama, *nyāya;* Kaṇāda, *vaiśeṣikā;* Jaimani, *pūrva mīmāṁsā;* and Bādarāyaṇa *uttara mīmāṁsā.*

The philosophy and the practical method of yoga can be traced in the *Ṛgveda, Sāmaveda, Yajurveda* and *Atharvaveda.* Apart from the *Veda* references are found in the *Upaniṣad* like *Śvetaśvatara, Garbha, Bṛhadāraṇyaka, Maitrāyaṇi* and *Kauṣītaki* as well as *Ahirbudhnya Saṁhitā* (a work of *Pāñcarātra* school). Several other *Upaniṣad* like; *Yogaśikha, Śāṇḍilya, Yoga cintāmaṇi, Varāha, Yoga kuṇḍalinī* have elaborated on yoga.

The credit of collating, systematising and codifying the entire philosophy of yoga in the form of aphorisms goes to Patañjali.

There is an adage that one should not try to trace the source – family lineage and ancestry – of a *ṛṣi* or a river. The great seers never gave the source of their origin. A biography of Patañjali is available in *Patañjali's Life (Patañjali-caritam),* by Rāmabhadra Dīkṣita, a questionable biography written in the 18th century.

The name Patañjali consists of two words - *pata* and *añjali*. *Pata* means fallen; *añjali* means a gesture *(mudrā)*, where the hands are folded in offering oblation to God. An aged yogini named Goṇikā offered her prayers to the Sun God standing near a river bank before giving up her mortal body. She took a handful of water in her hand and closed her eyes to offer her yogic knowledge to God who was her witness in her *sādhanā*. When she opened her eyes, she saw to her surprise a tiny worm in her hands, which at once took a human form and prostrated to her and requested her to accept him as her pupil. She at once accepted him and named him Patañjali - the one who fell into her hands.

Nevertheless, we have *ācārya* on yoga like Ṣaṭhakopan, Madhura Kavi, Nāthamuni. and Shankarāchārya who also wrote a treatise on yoga *(Yogatārāvali)*. They left their works for us to understand the subject of yoga, filled with spiritual wisdom. The most important commentaries on the *Yoga Sūtra* can be found in Vyāsa's *Vyāsa Bhāṣya* and Vācaspati Miśra's gloss *Tattva Vaiśāradī*; also there are Bhojarāja's *Rāja Mārttaṇda Vṛtti* (XIth century), the *Pātañjala-bhaśya-vārttika* by Vijñāna Bhikṣu as *Yoga Vārttika*, and *Yoga-bhaṣya-vivaraṇa* by Śankara Bhagavatpāda. Modern commentaries like Bhāvagaṇesa Dīkṣita (a chief disciple of Vijñāna Bhikṣu), *Bṛhatī (Chāyā)* and *Laghvī*, by Nāgojī Bhaṭṭa (Nāgeśa), *Maṇi prabhā* by Rāmānanda Yati, *Sūtrārtha bodhinī* and *Yoga-siddhānta-candrikā* by Nārāyaṇa Tīrtha as well as *Bhāsvatī* by Hariharānanda Āraṇya.

The symbolism contained in the idol of Patañjali has full and rich significance. Patañjali, being the incarnation of Ādiśeṣa, is half man and half serpent, with hands folded in *Ātmāñjali* or *Namaskāra mudrā*. He holds the disc *(cakra)* in the right hand as well as the conch *(śankha)* in the left hand. A sword *(asi)* is tied to His waist and kept in a scabbard. I found the picture in a book called *Religion on Earth*. There is also a temple of the Śeṣāvatāra in Koregaon, Maharashtra, in which the idol is similar to Lord Patañjali.

In the idol the three coils below the navel stand for the three *guṇa* of *prakṛti*, namely *sattva*, *rajas* and *tamas* and the state of *guṇātītan* or *nistraiguṇyatā* asking the *sādhaka* to become a *guṇātītan* through *guṇavaitṛṣṇyam*: *tatparaṁ puruṣakhyāteḥ guṇavaitṛṣṇyam (Y.S.,* I.16) - the ultimate renunciation is when one transcends the qualities of nature and perceives the soul. *Puruṣārtha śūnyānāṁ guṇānāṁ pratiprasavaḥ kaivalyaṁsvarūpapratiṣṭhā vā citiśaktiḥ iti* (*Y.S.*, IV.34) - *kaivalya*, liberation comes when the yogi has fulfilled the puruṣārtha, the fourfold aims of life, and has transcended the guṇa. Aims and guṇa return to their source, and the Self *(puruṣa)* is established in its own natural purity.

The three coils indicate the *praṇava āuṁ*, a symbol conveying the concept of GOD as omnipresent, omnipotent and omniscient. The symbol 'ॐ' *(āuṁ)* is composed of three syllables

A, U and M with a crescent and dot on the top. The three circular coils symbolise the three syllables and the coil that is half represents the crescent.

Lord Patañjali with his three coiled body invites our attention towards the three types of afflictions (*tāpa*) namely, *ādhyātmika, ādhibhautika* and *ādhidaivika* which are to be conquered by following the path of yoga.

These three coils indicate that he was considered a master of *āyurveda*, grammar and yoga. He who wrote the *Caraka Saṁhitā* on *āyurveda, Mahābhāṣya* on grammar and *Yoga Sūtra* on yoga.

The half coil indicates the culminating state of yoga, namely *kaivalya,* where one accomplishes the purification of body, speech and consciousness *(śarīra śuddhi, vāk śuddhi* and *citta śuddhi).*

The conch in the left hand signifies the state of alertness, attentiveness and readiness to face obstacles and afflictions, which are inevitable in one's pursuit for reaching the ultimate end. It is considered as a symbol of spiritual wisdom *(jñāna).* In olden days, the conch was blown as a warning to get ready to face a disaster or calamity as it is done nowadays with sirens.

The disc in the right hand, which is a symbol of protection, signifies the immediate destruction of the onslaughts with supreme efforts.

The sword tucked to the waist indicates the vanquishing of *avidyā,* cutting away the hood of the ego, pride or sense of "I" which are the main obstacles covering the pure being.

These three weapons indicate the restraint of the mental fluctuations, the removal of obstacles and the eradication of afflictions through the method of yoga.

The hood above the head assures protection provided we surrender to the Lord. The folded hands together in *namaskāra (ātmāñjali mudrā),* signifies humility in the art of learning.

Lord Patañjali's raised hood indicates that he is our protector. His holding the sword then signifies the destruction of ignorance *(avidyā),* of yoga is to destroy the hidden evils through yogic *sādhanā* so that one begins to surrender oneself to God (*Īśvara*).

The thousand-headed cobra (*sahasra śirasaṁ śvetaṁ*) indicates that Patañjali guides us in a thousand ways by showing a number of methods of practice to find the Self *(puruṣa).*

The snake indicates the motion of the reptile i.e. continuity of *sādhanā.* It cannot end until one reaches the goal. Being half man, it indicates the individuality of man, since he has been endowed with intelligence to reach the end goal or spiritual goal in life. This representation of Lord Patañjali as a snake is an indirect guide for us to move fast in the path of yoga and be a tīvrasaṁvegin (I.21).

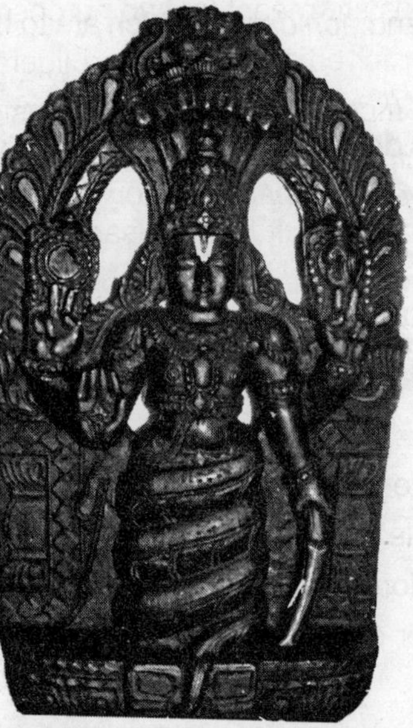

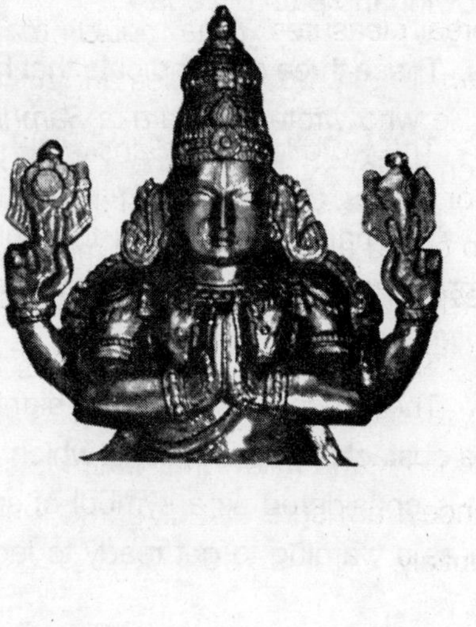

Plate n. 2 – Weapons of Lord Patañjali

In yoga texts the symbol of a serpent appears frequently. At the beginning of the third chapter, the *Haṭhayoga Pradīpikā* declares that the Lord of Serpents (Ananta or Ādiśeṣa) is the supporter of the Earth and *Kuṇḍalinī* the supporter of yoga practices. It further says that the effort and aim in the practice of yoga is to awaken this serpent Goddess. It is only through this source of the serpent Goddess, which is nothing but nature's abundant flow of energy *(prakṛti śakti),* that one enters the doorway of the absolute.

Patañjali, upright, with a coiled serpent as his supporting base and the combined head and heart conveys an image to us of one who has harnessed the potentials of nature for emancipation *(apavarga).* Here it also indicates that he resides in the state of completion and poised potential, head and heart integrated and with hands folded in a gesture of surrender to the absolute.

This is the significance of Patañjali. With prayers let us develop similar intellectual calibre with devotional efforts *(anuṣṭhāna)* and savour the wisdom of yoga.

Patañjali, with crystal clarity presents us the purpose of our life: *prakāśa kriyā sthiti śīlaṁ bhūtendriyātmakaṁ bhogāpavargārtham dṛśyam* (*Y.S.*, II.18) – nature and its evolutes, namely: the elements and their counterparts, mind, senses of perception and organs of action, and its three qualities *(sattva, rajas* and *tamas),* intelligence, consciousness and *mahat* exist to serve man, for cosmic consciousness or enjoyment or emancipation.

We know that our bodies, minds and senses are meant for two purposes; one for the enjoyment of pleasures of the world and the other for emancipation and liberation from the corporeal pleasures. Yoga moulds man to shape, modify, modulate and transform the seen *(dṛśyam),* i.e., the body, senses and mind for emancipation, which stands for the value of man.

The word 'man' in *Sanskṛt* is *mānava* or *manuṣya.* It has the same root as the word mind or *manas.* One who masters the mind is known as *manīśa,* which became *manuśya.* He is also called a *mānava. Māna* means honour, respect and dignity. One who lives in honour and respect is a *mānava* or *manuśya* or a man.

Therefore, the need of man's day-to-day life is that he needs to maintain physical health, mental peace, poise and will over matter for its conquest. Yoga leaves the decision to man to think and follow that which is stable and permanent in health, happiness, justice and prudence. I am sure that all agree that *Pātañjala yoga* suits all in today's life, if we practise reverentialy.

II.2. - Is *Aṣṭāṅga yoga* different from *Kriyā yoga*

The means and end are the same in yoga. Patañjali defines yoga as *yogaḥ cittavṛtti nirodhaḥ (Y.S.,* I.2). In the *Sādhana Pāda* he elaborates the cessation of movements in the consciousness through zeal, study and surrender to God as *kriyā yoga,* showing the ways and means to achieve this: *tapaḥ svādhyāya Īśvarapraṇidhānāni kriyāyogaḥ (Y.S.,* II.1).

First Patañjali defines yoga and then the ways and means of how to go towards it. It is a practical method but it is not a discursive subject. Hence, it is called *anuśāsanam. Anuśāsanam* is hidden in *kriyā yoga.*

Patañjali explains this threefold method of yoga as *kriyā yoga,* covering *karma mārga, jñāna mārga* and *bhakti mārga.* The burning zeal in practice is *tapas.* Self study, either through study of one's own self or by the study of the scriptures, is *svādhyāya.* Surrender of oneself to God is *Īśvara praṇidhāna.* He coins the term *kriyā yoga* for the threefold action *(tapas, svādhyāya* and *Īśvara praṇidhāna)*, for the means for the active involvement of *aṣṭāṅga yoga*. Hence there is no difference between *kriyā yoga* and *aṣṭāṅga yoga*.

Patañjali explains the action *(kriyā)* of *aṣṭāṅga yoga* up to the beginning of the third chapter to reach *nirbīja samādhi*.

Vyāsa is recognised as the foremost commentator on Patañjali. In his commentary on *Yoga Sūtra*, he says that the *Samādhi Pāda* is meant for those of *samāhita citta* or stable and cultured consciousness, and *Sādhana Pāda* for those who are caught in *vyutthāna citta* or outgoing or wandering mind.

Vyāsa categorises *citta* on five levels namely, dull *(mūḍha)*, distracted *(kṣipta)*, agitated or scattered *(vikṣipta)*, one-pointed attention *(ekāgra)* and restrained *(niruddha)*. Among these five categories of *citta*, the first three are commonly cognisable in us. So, we have to build up, cultivate and acquire consciousness to reach the divine state. But this achievement and fruition depends to some extent on the *sādhanā* of our previous births *(saṁskāra)*.

The last two categories of *citta*, namely one-pointed attention and restraint are meant for the *samāhita cittan*. The *Sādhana Pāda* takes pupils like us with *muḍha*, *kṣipta* and *vikṣipta citta* in a practical way to develop the power of attention and concentration. Patañjali cautions such practitioners who are blessed with *ekāgra* and *niruddha citta* to take the support of *Sādhana Pāda* in case of degradation or regression which may take place in their states of consciousness.

He says, *abhyāsa vairāgyābhyāṁ tannirodhaḥ* (*Y.S.*, I.11) – the restraint is possible by practice and detachment. *Abhyāsa* means *kriyā* for actions that are undertaken in the execution of practice, and *vairāgya* is not just dispassion or detachment but subjugation of diseases and passions. *Abhyāsa* means significant practice that is needed not only to reach the end but even after, as practice is needed even after surrendering oneself to God.

Patañjali lists nine impediments (*Y.S.*, I.30), four symptoms (*Y.S.*, I.31), five mental oscillations (*Y.S.*, I.6) and five afflictions (*Y.S.*, II.3) that disturb and pollute the consciousness. For this reason one needs constant attention to filter these mental oscillations and afflictions to keep the consciousness pure. Therefore one has to follow all aspects of *aṣṭāṅga yoga* on the plane of *kriyāyoga*. *Aṣṭāṅga yoga* is like an eight-faceted diamond set into the triangle shaped pendent – *kriyāyoga*.

He also shows various ways through yogic discipline of counteracting the impediments and obstacles that come in the way of *sādhanā* by applying single-minded effort to prevent them (*Y.S.*, I.32). Then he speaks of surrendering oneself to God (*Y.S.*, I.28); cleanliness in body and mind (*Y.S.*, II.43) and for establishing a stable mind (*Y.S.*, I.17; II.44).[1]

Thus *kriyā yoga* as *aṣṭāṅga yoga* brings purification of the body *(kāya-śuddhi);* purification of mind *(manas-śuddhi);* and purification of the self *(ātma-śuddhi).*

Before concluding, let me tell you that yoga changes conative and cognitive action into supramental action leading towards reflective and meditative states.

Do not differentiate yoga as *kriyā yoga, aṣṭāṅga yoga, cittavṛttinirodha yoga* and so on. These days, yoga is compartmentalised as *dhyāna yoga, samādhi yoga, kuṇḍalinī yoga, tāraka yoga, sahaja yoga* and so forth. Yoga is yoga; so don't get confused with brands.

a) – *Aṣṭāṅga yoga* (the eight aspects of yoga)

As I said earlier, inherent in the triangular *kriyā yoga* is the eight aspects of yoga as: *yama, niyama, āsana, prāṇāyāma, pratyāhāra, dhāraṇā, dhyāna* and *samādhi.*

Yama and *niyama* convey what to do and what not to do. These come under the ethical and moral disciplines. These two are the great eternal vows *(mahāvrata),* serviceable to mankind from the time when civilisation began. Actually these two convey what man's religion is and as such they are applicable to all as universal laws.

Then comes *āsana* to keep and maintain each and every part of the body in a healthy state. Next is *prāṇāyāma* in which the hidden atmospheric energy from the air is drawn in, absorbed and utilised into the system. *Pratyāhāra* is to stabilise the senses of perception and mind, so that the *sādhaka* proceeds towards *dhāraṇā* and *dhyāna* as pure intelligence surfaces to discriminate and reflect.

These five aspects of yoga have to be practised by everyone to enter the evolutory state of involution through the subtle aspects of yoga, namely: *dhāraṇā, dhyāna* and *samādhi.* The first five are universal aspects whereas the later three are dependent on individual's interest.

As body is visible and tangible, it can be easily identified. It is the cover or the garment of the self. Hence the importance to *āsana* is given to watch the body thoroughly so that the practitioner moves gradually to trace the inner sheaths of the self and touches directly the core of the Self.

---

[1] For all the *sūtra* and meanings listed here, please see the author's *Light on the Yoga Sūtras of Patañjali* – Harper Collins, London.

b) – Can these eight aspects be practised compartmentally

Practice of yoga is not an academic education. For instance Patañjali says, *ahiṁsāpratiṣṭhāyām tatsannidhau vairatyāgaḥ* (*Y.S.,* II.35) – when non-violence in speech, thought and action is established, one's aggressive nature is relinquished and others abandon hostility in his presence. So, who has to go and judge whether those who are antipathetic to each other have abandoned their hostility? A practitioner is supposed to know what results come by following *ahiṁsā.* There are *siddhi* or powers that come to a practitioner in a natural way. There is not any process of judgement through academic success or achievement. Only dispassionate practice is needed.

The eight aspects of yoga are from mundane knowledge to esoteric knowledge. We often take for granted that the water of the ocean is salty; the jewels are hidden in its depths. Similarly the esoterics of yoga are hidden inside where one needs to dive deep for it to reveal and unfold its own depth.

Though one has to journey from *yama* to *samādhi, yama* cannot be forgotten nor omitted even in *samādhi.* All the eight petals are all interlinked and interwoven as one. If one aspect of yoga is explicit, the other aspects are certainly implicit. Hence all aspects go hand in hand and not one after the other.

c) – If it is not compartmental, then how to approach it

By now you must have understood that Patañjali's eight aspects of yoga *(aṣṭāṅga yoga)* are within the purport of *tapas, svādhyāya* and *Īśvara praṇidhāna.* Action is involved in all these; hence it is also called *kriyāyoga. Tapas* stands for *karma* to gain physical strength and endurance *(śakti), svādhyāya* stands for *jñāna* and it means skill to act *(yukti)* and *Īśvara praṇidhāna* stands for surrender of oneself to the Supreme *(bhakti).* From this surrender comes freedom from bondage *(mukti).* Each aspect has its own rule and role of action. Action on *tapas* develops one to endure pains and makes one to get parched, burnt and tempered with hardships. By *tapas* the impurities get burnt in order to develop physical prowess *(śakti).* In this process, one's inner awareness surfaces and begins with self-inquiry leading him towards *svādhyāya. Svādhyāya* helps one to know his own weaknesses on emotional as well as intellectual levels. Through *tapas* and *svādhyāya,* the dirt and dust covering the intelligence get cleansed and there develops a right-skill *(yukti)* to build up righteous and virtuous quality in order to trace the core of the being. All wrong thinking and actions get eradicated and one proceeds towards *Īśvara praṇidhāna* – threshold of devotion *(śaraṇāgati).* Repeated practice of *āsana* brings *kāyaśuddhi* and *indriyaśuddhi* as well as *karmaśuddhi: kāya indriya siddhiḥ aśuddhikṣayāt tapasaḥ* (*Y.S.,* II.43) –

self-discipline *(tapas)* eradicates the impurities of the body and mind and kindles the sparks of divinity.

Then, one is introduced to *prāṇāyāma* to look and feel within; this is the threshold of *svādhyāya*. Here, the practice is clearer as the *sādhaka* is qualitatively made to look into the subtle things which makes him communicate with the individual self – *jīvātman: svādhyāyāt Iśṭadevatā saṁprayogaḥ* (*Y.S.*, II.44) – self-knowledge *(svādhyāya)*, understanding of oneself leads towards God-realisation.

By this, *jñānaśuddhi* takes place. From *jñānaśuddhi* comes *dhyāna* – the beginning of *Īśvara praṇidhāna* for the purification of *citta (bhāvanaśuddhi): samādhisiddhiḥ Īśvarapraṇidhānāt* (*Y.S.*, II.45) – surrender to God brings perfection in *samādhi*.

Āsana, prāṇāyāma and *dhyāna* aspects of *aṣṭāṅga yoga* explicitly represent *tapas, svādhyāya* and *Īśvara praṇidhāna*, but know that *yama, niyama, pratyāhāra* and *dhāraṇā* have to work concurrently and are implicitly involved in *tapas, svādhyāya* and *Īśvara praṇidhāna*; while *samādhi* leads one to God.

So, *aṣṭāṅga yoga* begins with *karma*, continues with *jñāna* and finally ends up in *bhakti*.

From *bhakti*, the *sādhaka* reaches the state of *kaivalya*, wherein he establishes himself in the pure state of consciousness: *puruṣārtha śūnyānāṁ guṇānāṁ pratiprasavaḥ kaivalyaṁ svarūpapratiṣṭhā vā citiśaktiḥ iti* (*Y.S.*, IV.34).

II.3. – *Citta vṛtti nirodha*

Yoga is *anuśāsanam* – governed disciplined action. *Citta vṛtti nirodha* (restraint of consciousness) cannot happen out of the blue. The evolution occurs gradually. If we could restrain the *citta* as per our wish or will, it would have been easy.

Anuśāsanam means to lay down the rules, to govern, to guide or give a code of conduct. The word *anu* is used as prefix, which indicates the previous link. The word *śāsanam* comes from the verb *śās* meaning to govern. So *anuśāsanam* means governance. Yoga was practised and explained by our predecessors and was later codified by Patañjali.

Patañjali uses the word *anuśāsanam* since our *ṛṣi, muni, yogi* followed from time immemorial the yogic path to discipline all levels namely the physical, moral, mental, psychological, emotional, intellectual and spiritual.

In order to reach *citta vṛtti nirodha,* we need to have *guṇa vṛtti nirodha, indriya vṛtti nirodha, snāyu vṛtti nirodha, prāṇa vṛtti nirodha, manō vṛtti nirodha, buddhi vṛtti nirodha, ahaṁkāra vṛtti nirodha* and finally *citta vṛtti nirodha.* For each of these restraints Patañjali gave *aṣṭāṅga yoga,* namely *yama, niyama, āsana, prāṇāyāma, pratyāhāra, dhāraṇā, dhyāna* and *samādhi.*

For instance, to bring stability in the organs of action and senses of perception, *yama* and *niyama* are introduced. Our actions, behaviour and flow of mental current are full of *hiṁsā, asatya, steya, abrahmacarya* and *parigraha.* These are caused by lust, anger, greed, infatuation, pride and envy. In order to go against violence, non-truth, non-covetousness, non-chastity, and possessiveness we need to practise the principles of *yama.*

Śauca, santoṣa, tapas, svādhyāya, Īśvara praṇidhāna are the *niyama. Śauca* means cleanliness. *Santoṣa* means happiness. *Tapas* means working for purity or maintaining the zeal or inspiration. If one wants to do *tapas,* he has to keep the essence of this word to inspire his mind throughout life. To be in touch from the body to the self or vice-versa is *svādhyāya.* After reaching *svādhyāya,* the art of learning humbleness becomes *Īśvara praṇidhāna.* First, the senses of perception and organs of action are to be educated by cultivating good habits. According to Patañjali these external gates, that feeds the mind, are to be controlled by *yama* and *niyama.* These two are meant for *guṇa vṛtti nirodha* and *karma vṛtti nirodha.* Our *karma vṛtti* depend upon the *guṇa vṛtti,* as one does *karma* according to one's natural instincts.

Then comes *āsana,* in which the movement of mind is controlled by the movements of the body. The body, the muscles, the sinews are controlled by *āsana.* This is why *āsana* is done for *snāyu vṛtti nirodha.*

We are made up of five elements (earth, water, fire, air and ether). Any industry needs a foundation. The element of earth is the foundation for this human body. Distribution is what we call supply and demand and demand and supply. Demand and supply depend on ether, the space we create in the body by expansion, extension, contraction and distribution. All these are done by the element of ether.

As one has a powerhouse for the production and distribution of electricity, lungs are our powerhouse; they are controlled by the air element. Then the remaining elements are water and fire. Out of these five elements, the earth, air and ether are not antagonistic. They support each other. The fire and water are the antagonistic elements in our system. Electricity is produced by heat and water. The electrical energy in our body is produced through the process of the in-breath and the out-breath. Through this respiratory motion there is a fusion created in our system between the fire element and water element to fuse and to produce a new energy known as *prāṇa* or bio-energy. To produce and store the production of energy we take deep breaths. Stagnated water has no current. Running water has the current. That is how we transform the stagnating breath into life currents through *prāṇāyāma*.

The *yogi*, realising the value of these two elements, introduced various types of inhalation, exhalation and retention in the form of *prāṇāyāma*. Through *prāṇāyāma*, the energy that is drawn is not like the stagnated water but made to flow rhythmically in the system supplying energy to the remote centres of the air cells of the lungs. Thus the lungs act as a producing machine as well as a storehouse in the various plexi *(cakra)* in the system. This is called *prāṇa vṛtti nirodha* through *prāṇāyāma*.

Having controlled the organs of action and senses of perception through *yama* and *niyama* and distributing of the energy accurately through *āsana* and *prāṇāyāma*, the next step is stilling the mind through *pratyāhāra*. *Pratyāhāra* is to study the movement of the mind within oneself. By studying the movement of the mind, one can restrain it. So *pratyāhāra* is meant for *manōvṛtti nirodha*. *Dhāraṇā* comes when the mind is controlled. *Dhāraṇā* is not just controlling the mind, as mind is already controlled by *pratyāhāra*. Here, one has to stabilise the intelligence that has a discriminative power but does not act. In *dhāraṇā* it is made to surface by stilling the intellect so that it does not create confusion. Hence, *dhāraṇā* is meant to still and stabilise the intelligence. It is *buddhi vṛtti nirodha*. When the mind and intelligence are stabilised by *pratyāhāra* and *dhāraṇā*, the next stage is meditation *(dhyāna)*, where the intelligence and consciousness are stilled and silenced. This takes one to the source from which sprouts the 'I' or 'me'. Here the diffusion of intelligence (*buddhi prasādana*) and diffusion of consciousness (*citta prasādana*) take place. Without churning the body, mind, consciousness and intelligence, meditation cannot come. In *dhyāna* if one maintains the silent state of consciousness for a long time without interruptions, it becomes *citta vṛtti nirodha*. After *citta vṛtti nirodha* comes *samādhi*. *Sama* means to see the life force (*ātman*) diffusing everywhere evenly in the body. *Dhi* means *buddhi* which has to remain even everywhere tuning towards *samādhi*. In *samādhi*, diffusion of the soul takes place *(adhyātma prasādana)*. Thus all the aspects of yoga are meant to experience this perspicacity of the self clearly *(adhyātma prasādana)*.

Unless the intelligence and self are evolved, one cannot understand what involution is. In the evolutory process one cleanses each and every aspect progressively in an involutory process, taking the cleansed aspects to its origin. This origin is nothing but the indestructible seer – Soul. *Dhyāna* practice is as we start *āsana* practice. *Japa* too is a practice. Hence, all aspects of *aṣṭāṅga yoga* come under practice.

Pātañjala yoga is like how we train our children. We guide them with what to do and what not to do in life. We tell them what they should do and what they should not do. "Don't do" comes under *yama*, and "do's" come under *niyama*. Then we send children to go and play.

Similarly, Patañjali wants us to do *āsana*. When the child devotes time to play, as parents we will often say, "Now stop playing and do your school homework and study". After education we advise them to do some service to society or do something good in life. If they don't do good to anyone and become selfish, we say, "he is educated but unfortunately not civilised, as he expresses pride in his status". Patañjali warns that after developing intelligence, he does not want us to become selfish and proud, but control pride and learn to become humble. For this he introduces meditation. Here the educated person understands what is matured *jñāna*. *Nirvicāra vaiśāradye adhyātmaprasādaḥ* (*Y.S.*, I.47) – from proficiency in *nirvicāra samāpatti* comes purity. *Sattva* or luminosity flows undisturbed, kindling the spiritual light of the self.

From this unalloyed wisdom, one reaches the state of unalloyed blissfulness. This is the means and end of yoga.

II.4. – Is ego *(ahaṁkāra)*, a friend or a foe

While explaining in section 6, on *citta vṛtti nirodha*, I had explained on *ahaṁkāra vṛtti nirodha*, which has to be achieved through *dhyāna*. Patañjali in *sūtra* II.3, explains *asmitā* as one of the afflictions. In spiritual terminology *asmitā* means pure "am-ness". Due to want of understanding this pure "am-ness" impersonates as *ahaṁkāra*, or 'I', 'me' or 'mine' before 'am', and becomes proud through an expression 'I-am', instead of the neutral 'am'. Due to ignorance in one, the pure 'am' gets converted to 'I-am' and vibrates as ego *(ahaṁkāra)*, imposing itself in the form of the true self. The 'I' begins to attach itself with all its belongings and begins to treat them as his possessions. It forgets its 'am-ness' and embraces 'mine-ness'. What one needs to do is to eradicate the 'me' and 'mine-ness'.

The word *ahaṁkāra* itself conveys that when *aham*, 'am', takes a form or shape *(ākara)*, 'am' becomes 'I am'. Here 'I' is the form.

I-ness is a needed principle in *sādhanā* but 'mine-ness' needs to be eradicated. *Citta* has three composites – *manas, buddhi* and *ahaṁkāra*. Among these composites *ahaṁkāra* is close to the pure I-consciousness. We need to have this I-consciousness, which wills us to choose the path of emancipation so that 'am-ness' exists and not 'I' or 'me'.

Asmitā appears at five places in the *Yoga Sūtra*.

In *Samādhi Pāda*[1] the word *asmitā rūpa anugamāt* conveys the comprehending state of being one with oneself. Here, *asmitā* is illuminative *(sāttvic)* state of the inner consciousness.

It appears twice, in *Sādhana Pāda, sūtra* II.3[2] and *sūtra* II.6.[3] *Asmitā* has been explained as ego or pride. The practitioner, being non-illuminative, identifies himself without the knowledge or understanding that something beyond "me" exists.

In the *Vibhūti Pāda,*[4] *asmitā* is said to be the offshoot of the first principle of nature, *mahat.* One relinquishes the pride or the ego by sublimating it and then integrating that same 'I' with the seer. The senses of perception have a natural inclination towards worldly objects and send imprints to the mind. *Buddhi,* one of the facets of *citta,* plays a big role in controlling and taming the senses and mind, while *asmitā* acts as a friend in building up the *sādhaka* constructively towards the final goal of life.

Finally, *asmitā* of *Kaivalya Pāda* is a refined quality of 'I'. We all move in the web of our emotions, moods, thoughts and actions according to our inbuilt tendencies, known as *nirmita citta.* This *nirmita citta* in each one of us has its characteristics. Hence, we think that we will not be able to change this state of ours. But the accurate yogic practices bring changes to undergo transformation on *citta* for it to develop maturity *(nirmāṇa citta).* This *nirmāṇa citta* springs from *sāttvic* consciousness. The *asmitā* mentioned in *Vibhūti Pāda* is of *sattva dharma* by nature but as *indriyajaya* is yet to take shape towards *sattva,* a tinge of *rajoguṇa* will be there. The *asmitā* of *Kaivalya Pāda* is charged by *sattva guṇa* leading *citta* towards *nirmāṇa citta; nirmāṇacittāni asmitāmātrāt* (*Y.S.,* IV.4). Thus *asmitā saṁprajñāta samādhi* of *Samādhi Pāda* and *asmitā* of *nirmāṇa citta* are the same. Being totally *sāttvic* by nature, it is called *sāsmita.*

The ego or *asmitā* explained in the second chapter is the mistaken identity of *sāttvic* 'I', and undoubtedly acts as a foe. Patañjali explains pride as *kleśa; dṛk darśanaśktyoḥ ekātmatā iva asmitā* – identification of the seer with the instrumental power of seeing is ego. The *ahaṁkāra* of the third chapter is the ego of *mahat.* This ego comes with *nirmāṇa citta.* If fissures occur in *nirmāṇa citta, chidra citta* forms; *tat cchidreṣu pratyayāntarāṇi saṁskārebhyaḥ* (*Y.S.,* IV.27) – In

---

[1] *Vitarka vicāra ānanda asmitārūpa anugamāt saṁprajñātaḥ* (*Y. S.,* I.17) – practice and renunciation develop four types of awareness in the consciousness. These are *vitarka, vicāra, ānanda and asmitā.*

[2] *avidyā asmitā rāga dveṣa abhiniveśāḥ kleśāḥ (Y. S.,* II.3) – the five afflictions which disturb the equilibrium of consciousness are: ignorance or lack of wisdom, ego, pride of the ego or the sense of 'I', attachment to pleasure, aversion to pain, fear of death and clinging to life.

[3] *dṛk darśanaśaktyoḥ ekātmatā iva asmitā* (*Y. S.,* II.6) – assuming that the ego as the seer, is pride.

[4] *grahaṇa svarūpa asmitā anvaya arthavattva saṁyamāt indriyajayaḥ (Y.S.,* III.48) – through *saṁyama* upon the purpose of the conjunction of the process of knowing, the ego and nature, there is mastery over the senses. See the author's *Light on the Yoga Sūtras of Patañjali,* Harper Collins, London.

spite of this progress, if one is careless during the interval, fissures arise due to the latent hidden impressions, that start creating divisions between the consciousness and the seer. Even claiming the famous *Upaniṣadic* dictum, *Ahaṁ brahmāsmi* – I am *brahman,* is a sort of *ahaṁkāra,* as it carries a tinge of ego. The God men claiming that they are the incarnation of God is also a state of *ahaṁkāra.*

In the last *sūtra* Patañjali explains the state of pure existence and termination of *ahaṁkāra* as the aims and pursuits end and the *guṇa* involutes towards nature; *puruṣārtha śūnyānāṁ guṇānāṁ pratiprasavaḥ kaivalyaṁ svarūpapratiṣṭhā vā citiśaktiḥ iti* (*Y.S.,* IV.34) – *kaivalya,* liberation, comes when the yogi has fulfilled the *puruṣārtha,* the fourfold aims of life, and has transcended the *guṇa.* Aims and *guṇa* return to their source, and consciousness is established in its own natural purity. Here *asmitā* becomes a friend.

I would like to bring to each one's attention the words of Lord Krishna, where he shows ways of distinguishing the difference between *asmitā* and *ahaṁkāra*:

Dhūmenā 'vriyate vahnir yathā 'darśo malena ca I
yatho 'lbena 'vṛto garbhas tathā tene 'damāvṛtam II *(B.G.,* III.38)

As a flame is covered by smoke, a mirror by dirt or dust and an embryo enveloped by the womb, *asmitā* (the pure consciousness or the Self) is covered by the conception of 'I-am-ness' or haughty individuality.

II.5. – On *śraddhā* (faith)

There is no equivalent word in English for *śraddhā,* though it is translated as "faith".

In *Samādhi Pāda* Patañjali refers to the word *śraddhā* at a precise stage for the practitioner. He did not explain *śraddhā* when he speaks of *abhyāsa* or practice. Probably he did not explain it then because in *abhyāsa* one may be likely to slip or give up efforts. Patañjali advocates continuous, steadfast effort so that the subject reveals information to build up faith on its own. He says: *sa tu dīrgha kāla nairantarya satkārāsevito dṛḍhabhumiḥ* (*Y.S.,* I.14) – long, uninterrupted, alert practice is the firm foundation for restraining the fluctuations.

He advises his pupils to take to *abhyāsa* with respect, dedication and devotion. Often one may hear, saying that "I believe, but I do not practise. Faith or *śraddhā* is when unknown information reveals itself from *abhyāsa* to *sādhanā.* If *abhyāsa* means repetitive practice to learn, *sādhanā* stands to practice for accomplishing one's aspirations. The significant word *satkāra* means total involvement with respect and devotion.

In the beginning our aspirations and belief are strong. But when the aspirations begin to fade the interest diminishes. "Make believe" is not faith. Easily we believe and say that we have faith. Faith comes only after some revelation. Therefore Patañjali uses the word *śraddhā* after *samādhi,* as *samādhi* is a state of divine revelation.

In order to intensify one's *sādhanā,* Patañjali uses *śraddhā* at an appropriate time when the *sādhaka* has trust in himself to proceed and progress further. Faith is not expressive but action oriented.

Vyāsa mentions that *śraddhā* sustains the yogi like a benevolent mother and that intellectual strength is born into whomsoever pursues the discriminating knowledge *(viveka)* with *śraddhā.* Vācaspati Mīśra considers *śraddha* as "the root of yoga" and insists that it does not let the *sādhaka* fall down in the wrong path.

Patañjali is a theist, yet he does not ask anyone to believe God blindly. Otherwise he would not have demanded efforts from one. His faith is an illuminative revelation of wisdom. *Bhagavad Gītā* puts it beautifully:

Sattvānurupā sarvasya śraddhā bhavati bhārata I
śraddhāmayo'yaṁ puruṣo yo yacchraddaḥ sa eva saḥ II
Yajante sāttvikā devān yakṣarakṣāṁsi rājasāḥ I
pretān bhūtagaṇāṁścā'nye yajante tāmasā janāḥ II (*B.G.,* XVII.3-4).

The faith of everyone, O Bharata, conforms with his nature. A person of faith is verily what his faith makes him.

Sattva-type men worship gods; the *rajas*-type worship gnomes and demons; and men of *tamas*-type worship ghosts and hosts of spirits.

Have you ever read Prahlāda's story in *Bhāgavata Purāṇa* (7th *skandha*)? Prahlāda was the son of a demon king called Hiraṇyakaśyapu. This demon hated Lord Nārāyaṇa or Vishnu as God. In his reign no one was allowed to utter "Nārāyaṇa" or Vishnu. But his son, being a devotee of Lord Vishnu, was always thinking and uttering the name of Nārāyaṇa as *Āuṁ namo Nārāyaṇāya.* Once his father asked him about things that he had learnt. He told: "I prostrate to Mahāvishnu, the root cause of all things seen and unseen, the sustainer of this visible universe, who is without beginning, middle and end and who is without origin, growth and decay". His father got annoyed and tortured him throwing him down from the top of a hill, leaving him alone amongst snakes and so forth. In spite of all these tortures Prahlāda kept on doing *Nārāyaṇa japa,* and remained firm in his faith that Nārāyaṇa alone is the Ultimate and there is none greater than Him. One day, the king challenged his son: "You think Nārāyaṇa is great in everything and exists everywhere." Then the demon king asked his son Prahlāda that if God exists everywhere and in everything, "Then show me whether HE is in this pillar". His son replied in full faith: "Yes, He is there." The demon king in anger struck the pillar with his sword. It broke open and Lord Vishnu in the form of Narasimha, a human body with the head of a lion appeared and killed Prahlāda's father – the demon king. This is the grace of God, the grace of the *guru* and the faith of a *bhaktan.*

Faith needs to be firm and profound. Belief is objective and faith is totally subjective. *Śraddhā* is of three factors namely, *śravaṇa* – listening to the wisdom of wise people, *manana* – reflecting on their wisdom, and *nididhyāsana* – meditating on that experienced wisdom. *Śraddhā* guides the intelligence *(buddhi)* to verify the truth. That is how knowledge dawns. Vigour and courage *(vīrya* and *śraddhā)* follow each other and cultivate right and ripe memory to move towards the real knowledge of wisdom.

II.6. – Is yoga a healing subject or a spiritual subject

No doubt yoga is a preventive, healing and a spiritual subject. But the effect of yoga is limited according to one's aim and practice. One may think on higher levels but as far as my experiences are concerned, one is still close to the body, which is nearer and dearer. Man talks about spirituality but in the depth of his heart, he thinks of the body and mundane pleasures. This is a contradiction in thought and action.

In recent years yoga has gained popularity as a curative science. People think that almost all diseases can be cured by yoga. When I speak on the principles of cure, many may feel that I am only harping on a physical level and not on a spiritual level.

The Institute is thirty-two years old, yet questions arise in the minds of the students according to the calibre of their brain at their level of practice.

Most of the members at the institute are of normal, average intelligence. As many lack maturity and wisdom it takes time to move towards spiritual life. The aim of yoga is to illuminate the body, mind and self. Yoga acts as a key to unlock man's potencies to reach that state of illumination so that he touches the seer. For this, all practitioners need patience.

At present many of us are seekers, and not seers. As seekers questions arise as they feel something lacking in their practices. When the seeker transforms into a seer, no questions arise. Factually it is the seer that acts as a seeker creating doubts and confusions for illuminating himself. Hence the seeker rubs himself with his intelligence and removes doubts and confusions to transform himself into a seer. Then intuitive intelligence and wisdom dawns; splits *(chidra)*, and makes the dualities *(dvandva)* to disappear in him.

Normally, we are caught in the day-to-day material world. We cannot cut ourselves off from the material world. We are not capable of renouncing the world, as this is very difficult to do at one stroke. We may remove the garments we wear, but can we remove the body like those garments? Renunciation is complete surrender of oneself to the Supreme God. This does not come unless one cuts of all the webs of nature's qualities.

In the majority of people the mind is closer to the body. As a healing subject naturally one begins yoga at the physical level as well as the physiological level. The mind we refer to here is the one, which is close to the body, but far away from the Self.

When Patañjali deals with *vṛtti sārupyam itaratra* he refers to the mind that is closer to the Self *(Puruṣa)*. Here, the Self sees through the mirror of its mind, which acts as a reflective mirror and becomes one with this reflective mirror – the mind. Mind takes this advantage, as if it is the Self.

The Self or the seer is the source of the mind but the mind being clever does not allow the seer to see directly. It assumes the role of the seer and takes the lead. As the mind gets caught in the web of worldly attractions, it is caught also in pains and pleasures and tempts man towards the never-ending pleasures causing the Self to become involved. Therefore, the mind needs intellectual churning to be free from them. From this, one should know how hard it is for people with average intelligence to practise spiritual yoga. This is the line of demarcation between the real seer and the imaginary seer.

Patañjali commences yoga from the seer *(puruṣa* or *dṛṣṭa)*, *tadā draṣṭuḥ svarūpe avasthānam* (*Y.S.*, I.3) – then, the seer dwells in his own true splendour – showing that it is possible for one to move from the knowledge of the body towards the knowledge of the seer.

Patañjali mentions *vyādhi* as the first obstacle. I have to go back in order to explain *vyādhi*. God created man with nine gates *(navadvāra)*,[1] two eyes, two ears, two nostrils, mouth, anus, and generative organ. As we are susceptible to the nine planets *(navagraha)*, we are

---

1 *Śvetāśvatara Upaniṣad*, III.18, *Yoga-tattva Upaniṣad* (140-142) and *Mahābhārata* (XII.203.35). *Katha Upaniṣad* (V.1) talks of eleven gates *(ekādaśa dvāram)* adding the navel and the crown of the head or *brahma randhra*. See *Aṣṭadaḷa Yogamālā*, vol. 1, pp. 120, 134; vol. 2, p. 16, and especially vol. 3, p. 314.

susceptible to *navadvāra*. The *navadvāra* hunt for pleasures which later lead to physical and mental diseases, known as *ādhyātmika, ādhibhautika* and *ādhidaivika roga* or *tāpa*. Patañjali calls these *tāpa* (*Y.S.*, II.15), as *kṛta, kārita* and *anumodita* actions of *karma* (*Y.S.*, II.34).

Kṛta means done by one, *kārita* means caused by someone to be done and *anumodita* means permitted or given consent by one to be done. In the first case of the *kṛta-karma* it is due to one indulging directly. The *ādhyātmika* diseases are invited diseases and come under this category. The *ādhibhautika* are caused by others as *kārita-karma* because of one's own weakness, but would not like to commit directly. The allergic diseases fall under this category. *Anumodita-karma* are the actions in which one gives permission to act though one does not indulge directly. The *ādhidaivika* diseases are the type that are built up by past actions and become the seed of destiny as fate. The *kṛta* and *kārita-karma* are fruition of our latent behaviours. Their effects are immediate. Therefore, they are called *sopakrama*. *Anumodita-karma* is slow in fruition, so they are called as *nirupakrama*.[1]

The diseases affect the individual because of weakness that sets in the body and mind on account of disuse, overuse or misuse, which *āyurveda* calls *prajñāparādha* (deliberate wrongs). When *navadvāra* are used rightly, they keep one free from diseases and yogic practice is meant to maintain these *navadvāra* healthy.

Śarīramādyam khalu dharma sādhanam. The body is a fountain to follow the duties of *dharma, artha, kāma* or *mokṣa*. Hence the importance is given to the body so that the body is made as a shrine, for the ever shining Self to shine. If these gates *(navadvāra)* of the body are not disciplined then they bring nine forms of diseases, like *vyādhi, styāna, saṁśaya, pramāda, ālasya, avirati, bhrāntidarśana, alabdhabhūmikatva* and *anavasthitatva*. These are known as *navāntarāya*. Hence yoga helps to check, control and then purifies the mind and diverts it towards spiritual *sādhanā*. Till then to talk of spiritual *sādhanā* is a meaningless thought.

Cleanse the body through yogic means so that it can look after itself and allow the mind to get attached to the Self. Then the mind rests on the lap of the seer. The seer being the soul and self sees through its vehicles which exist in the form of *ahaṁkāra, buddhi, manas, citta, jñānendriya* and *karmendriya*. When these vehicles are controlled and silenced, the seer starts looking directly. In a true sense this is direct perception. Thus yoga helps and teaches us

---

[1] According to sage Patañjali, every action and every mental process leaves a subliminal imprint or *saṁskāra*. These imprints later create on their turn actions or mental activities for which they are responsible. Any action or mental activity for which a *saṁskāra* is responsible is called the *vipāka* of that *saṁskāra* (*Y.S.*, I.24, II.13, IV.8). In his commentary under III.22, Vyāsa explains that the actions whose fruition appears in the same life period are of two types: *sopakrama* (with intense activity) and *nirupakrama* (without intense activity). *Sopakrama* has a quick *vipāka* and shows its results soon, whereas *nirupakrama* has a slow *vipāka* and its fruition is slow.

to see not through the reflections of the mirror, but through the seer directly. This is the spiritual level of *sādhanā.*

As we need a bridge to move from one bank to the other, we need to build a yogic bridge so that we cross over from the body to the Self.

As Gangā, Jamunā and Saraswati get united to join the ocean, yoga unites *śarīra, manas, ahaṁkāra* and *buddhi* and unites them to join the sea – the Seer.

a) – On supernatural powers

If one has to go to the other bank of the river, he has to cross over using a boat or a bridge. It is the same in yoga. Often one attains powers through yoga which one has to abandon if one wants to reach the shore of the spiritual bank.

One may cross over the physical obstacles. But to abandon the so-called super natural powers needs a strong will power. Then only the gates of the spiritual kingdom open to the *sādhaka.*

All movements in the Universe are the manifestations of *śakti* (power). We have *śarīra śakti, prāṇa śakti, nāḍī śakti, manô śakti, buddhi śakti, citta śakti* and *ātma śakti.*

For example if I show strong intellectual power with physical power you listen and surrender. In olden days a king's ambition was to conquer kings, subjugating them to remain under his control and thus become an emperor. Through the practice of yoga, if one conquers the evolutes of the *prakṛti,* namely, the elemental body with its characteristics, senses, mind, intelligence, the five *vāyu,* the 'I'-consciousness and conscience *(antaḥkaraṇa),* yield their power and strength *(siddhi)* to the yogi and that *siddha* becomes the Lord of *prakṛti.*

Patañjali has spoken about powers in *Vibhūti Pāda*, which happen through yoga *sādhanā.* These powers come to a *sādhaka* as a guide to indicate that the *sādhanā* is on the right path. Some *sādhaka* get imprisoned by them and lose sight of the ultimate goal of experiencing the true essence of yoga. Patañjali mentions in clear terms that these powers appear supernatural or supernormal to others whereas for the *siddha* they are normal and natural but act as hindrances to *dhyāna* and *samādhi: te samādhau upasargāḥ vyutthāne siddhayaḥ* (*Y.S.,* III.38) – means that attainments are impediments to *samādhi* although they appear as powers to others. Here one can understand the value of *sūtra* 20 of *Samādhi Pāda.*

People around us influence our body, mind, intelligence and surroundings by sweet words. *Prakṛti* too, of which we are constituted, influences us a great deal. The supernormal powers also influence one who has conquered and subjugated *prakṛti.* A *siddha,* whose aim is for the sight of the Self, does not give any value to them. If by chance he is caught in these powers, he becomes worse than normal people in his behaviour.

These *siddhi* come to tempt those who are near the zenith on the ladder of yoga, i.e., *kaivalya.* We have read that eminent yogis and saints fell to the enticement of celestial beings. *sthānyupanimantraṇe saṅgasmayākaraṇaṁ punaraniṣṭa prasaṅgāt* (*Y.S.,* III.52) - when approached by celestial beings, there should be neither attachment nor surprise, for undesirable connections can occur again. So, be careful and remember Patañjali's advice: A sādhaka strives to be free from afflictions. The yogi, with super powers, has to handle these judiciously to extinguish them" - *hanam eṣāṁ kleśavat uktam* (Y.S., IV.28).

Let the foremost aim of *sādhanā* be enlightenment (the *ātmadarśana*) and not power *(siddhi).* As Patañjali says, we may become *videhin* or *prakṛtilayin* but not a *kṛtārthan* (exalted one).

II.7. - The four aims *(puruṣārtha)* and *citiśakti* through yoga

The *puruṣārtha (dharmabhūmi)* are the aims of man's life. Body is the abode of action *(karmabhūmi)* for emancipation *(mokṣa).* As man has freedom of will to act, he is called a *karma-puruṣa.* The body which is basically of five elements *(pārthiva śarīra)* unites after death with the mother earth. In life, *karmendriya* and *jñānendriya* are there to serve the mind. The actions of *karmendriya* and *jñānendriya* distract the mind. But man is gifted with intelligence and can think judiciously to have a grip over the senses and mind. The 'I' provides the energy for will-power.

The four *puruṣārtha* provide guidelines as to how one should lead a righteous life *(dharma)* to reach the virtuous life *(śīlatā).*

The four aims *(puruṣārtha)* of life are: right sense of duty *(dharma),* wealth or life's requirements *(artha),* desire for progeny and accomplishments *(kāma),* and lastly emancipation *(mokṣa),* where one becomes free from the cycles of birth and death.

These aims are ideals for all of us to work out direction and approach in life with a logical, balanced thinking process. But man being a mixture of good and bad, strong and weak, virtue and vice, will either be good-natured *(sat-śīlata)* or bad-natured *(duḥ-śīlata). Śīla* means disposition towards virtue.

The qualities *(guṇa)* play a major role in moulding man in a right way, or a wrong way, or with the mixture of both. Patañjali says that a yogi's actions are neither white, nor black nor grey, and for others the three follow. See *Y.S.,* IV.7 – *karma aśukla akṛṣṇaṁ yoginaḥ trividham itareṣam.*

The first aim in life is the sense of duty *(dharma).* The foundation of *yama* and *niyama* given in *aṣṭāṅga yoga* helps man to follow the ethical path, or the path of the sense of duty. Desires have no end. Desires induce greed and make man pursue and get satisfaction which has no bounds. The more the gratification, the more the wants increase and an indiscreet way of living sets in. So, forbearance and tolerance have to be cultivated through the principles of *niyama. Āsana* and *prāṇāyāma* help in building up endurance and patience, and controlling indiscreet actions. Wants and lust gradually get diminished and faith *(śraddhā)* and steadfastness *(samādhāna)* set in. This discipline helps in building up the means to fulfil the meaningful desires. Thus, these aspects of yoga play to experience the aims of *artha* and *kāma.*

From here, one is inclined to move towards *mokṣa.* In *sūtra* IV.26, Patañjali calls it *kaivalya prāgbhāram* (gravitational pull on account of *kaivalya),* as *citta* has learnt to gravitate towards the Self from the land of the worldly pleasures.

In short, *yama* and *niyama* act as a background for discipline. *Āsana* and *prāṇāyāma* work as a means channelling and directing one to acquire *samādhāna citta* (composed mind). *Pratyāhāra* and *dhāraṇā* guide for control, the third aim – *kāma,* and help one to cross over from the sensual pleasures towards spiritual bliss. *Dhyāna* and *samādhi* put us on the threshold of *mokṣa.*

The aims *(dharma, artha, kāma* and *mokṣa)* are framed for us to act with right attitudes. These right attitudes are covered in the *aṣṭadaḷa yoga* of which we have to follow with intensity *(tīvra saṁvega).* See what Patañjali says: *sattva puruṣayoḥ śuddhi sāmye kaivalyam iti* (*Y. S.,* III.56) – when the purity of intelligence equals the purity of soul, the yogi has reached *kaivalya,* perfection in yoga.

Then one experiences an untinged, untainted and untouched state of life, the end aim, liberation *(kaivalya).*

That is how Patañjali ends the achievement of yoga in the last *sūtra* of the last chapter where he says, "As you experience the POWER OF THE SELF *(citiśakti),* I have no more to explain!!!"

a) – *Citiśakti*

Citi is *ātmā*, the Self. The power of the Self *(citiśakti)* is the very source of our existence. It is the seed for transforming the power of consciousness *(cittaśakti)* towards absolute consciousness.

Puruṣa, citi, ātman, dṛṣṭan, are synonymous words for the seer or the Self. *Puruṣa* means man. *Puruṣa* means *(puri śete iti puruṣaḥ)* that one who dwells in the body. The Self in the body is the king and the body in which He dwells is His empire. Patañjali uses *citi* on *sūtra* IV.22, but here in the last *sūtra*, he uses the word *citiśakti: puruṣārtha śūnyānām guṇānām pratiprasavaḥ kaivalyam svarūpapratiṣṭhā vā citiśaktiḥ iti* (*Y.S.*, IV.34) – from this state on, the yogi is devoid of all aims of life. As Seer, he is free from the qualities of nature and lives in the state of emancipation, with his consciousness established in his own natural purity.

Patañjali arranges the words in this *sūtra* in an ascending order as far as the *sādhanā* is concerned. The first word *puruṣārtha śūnyānām* means devoid of fourfold aims of man. *Puruṣa* means the Self and *artha* means to strive and achieve these four noble ambitions. These fourfold aims of *puruṣa* are *dharma, artha, kāma* and *mokśa*, which mean performance of one's duty, acquisition of wealth, gratification of desires and liberation from worldly life. These aims and objects are meant for us to attain the state that is beyond the fourfold aims.

The next word is *guṇānām pratiprasavaḥ*. This word indicates the inter-relation between *puruṣa* and *prakṛti*. The *guṇa* or qualities of nature are *sattva, rajas* and *tamas*. Evolution of *prakṛti* takes place when these *guṇa* vibrate. In the involutionary process the *guṇa* return and dissolve in the root nature *(mūla prakṛti)*. *Prati* means to go against and *prasava* means procreation. Hence, *pratiprasava* means involution. The organs of action, senses of perception, mind, intelligence, I-ness and consciousness serve and fulfil *puruṣa* and finally withdraw and merge in the root nature. In this state, the *guṇa* do not function. So the *sādhaka* becomes *triguṇarahitan* – devoid of *triguṇa (guṇātitan)*.

When the involution of *prakṛti* reaches the source, the seer or *puruṣa* stands alone and this is *kaivalya*. This extinction of the conjunction of the seer with nature is *kaivalya*, a state of aloneness or being one with the Supreme Self.

Patañjali conveys this state as *svarūpa pratiṣṭhā* establishing oneself in one's own nature. Here the seer shines in his pure pristine and untainted original state.

Finally, the word *citiśakti* is significant to us, as the text ends with the word *citiśaktiriti*. *Citiśakti* is the power of the Self. *Puruṣa*, the Self, is the *ātman* and *puruṣaviśeṣa* is *paramātman* (*Y.S.*, I.24). Patañjali indicates that when the Seer or the soul dwells in its own place, that place is nothing but the place of the Universal Soul. Hence *citi* means the soul and *śakti* means the power of the soul, i.e.; *Paramātman* or God. *Iti* means the end.

Vyāsa, in his commentary on the *sūtra; yogaḥ citta vṛtti nirodhaḥ* (*Y.S.*, I.2), refers to *citiśakti* or the power of the soul. The characteristics of soul are narrated by him as changeless *(apariṇāmi)*, non-movable *(apratisaṁkramāyāḥ)*, a seer who sees the objects shown to him *(darśita-viṣaya)*, pure *(śuddha)* and infinite *(ananta)*. Though the characteristics of *puruṣa* and *viśeṣa puruṣa* appear to be the same, the difference is that self *(jīva puruṣa)* acquires through *sādhanā* that state, while *Īśvara* is totally free from conflicts, unaffected by actions and untouched by cause and effect. He is not only the unexcelled seed of all knowledge but also the seed of all seers. Hence, God is *citiśakti* or the source of souls.

Patañjali uses the word *dṛṣṭā* for seer and *dṛśya* for consciousness. Again, he uses the word *puruṣa* and *prakṛti* for soul and consciousness. He attributes source of vision to the soul as *dṛkśakti* and *citta* or consciousness as instrumental power of seeing as *darśanaśakti*. The *puruṣa* being the master, he is recognised as *svāmiśakti* and *prakṛti* being owned by the Lord as *svaśakti*. He mentions individual soul also as *pratyakcetanā*,[1] whereas the universal soul as *parākcetanā*.

He mentions God – the Universal Soul – as the seed of all knowledge, *sarvajñabījam* (*Y.S.*, I.25) and to reach that seed he guides the consciousness of the *sādhaka* to move towards *nirbīja* state.

Man is a *karma puruṣa* as he is under the bondage of *karma* and continues to rotate with the wheel of birth and death. The word *puruṣārtha śūnyānām* indicates that the *karma puruṣa* is liberated from this bondage and transforms himself as *dharma-puruṣa*. *Guṇānām pratiprasavaḥ* indicates how this *puruṣa* is liberated from bondage. He is a *kevala puruṣa* as he exists purely as soul, without any denomination. The word *kaivalya* indicates that the *puruṣa* is imperishable and eternal as others are perishable. He is transformed from *karma puruṣa* to *kevala puruṣa*, or the *jīvātman* becomes a *muktātman*.

Patañjali recognises the soul as *puruṣa* and God *(Īśvara)* as *puruṣaviśeṣa*, distinct from *puruṣa*. Therefore, to know *citiśakti* you have to know all the entities of *svaśakti* or *prakṛti*. Consciousness is *citta* and the seer is *citi*. *Citiśakti* is the power of soul. That power of the soul is nothing but Universal Soul or *Īśvara*. Thus, yoga integrates *prakṛti*, *puruṣa* and *Īśvara*.

---

[1] *Tataḥ pratyakcetana adhigamaḥ api antarāya abhāvaḥ ca* – Meditation on God with the repetition of āuṁ removes obstacles to the mastery of the inner self (*Y.S.*, I.29). *Pratyak*: inwards; *cetanā*: consciousness.

II.8. - Does a Yogi need to be *bhaktan*

Patañjali being a devotee of God *(bhaktan)* starts with *bhakti mārga: Īśvara praṇidhānāt vā* (*Y.S.*, I.23) - surrender to God. Naturally he wants the yoga *sādhaka* to be a devotee of God. But before that he wants one to do the *karma* to purify himself. It is only through *karma* that one gets *jñāna*. By *karma-śuddhi*, he gains *jñāna-śuddhi* and through this he earns *citta-śuddhi* and becomes a *bhaktan* or a *paramaikāntikabhaktan*.[1]

In the second chapter Patañjali speaks of actual *sādhanā*. He addresses the neophyte in this *pāda*. His answer for a beginner is *kriyā yoga*. *Kriyā yoga* is not different from *aṣṭāṅga yoga*. *Kriyā yoga* is a capsule covering all aspects of *aṣṭāṅga yoga*. *Kriyā yoga* is just a mental preparation or theoretical foundation for *aṣṭāṅga yoga*.

Watch the sequential order that Patañjali gives - first *tapas*, then *svādhyāya* and finally *Īśvara praṇidhāna*. The beginner has to practise yoga action-wise, and then there has to be mental preparation to gain the knowledge - both material and spiritual - so that he finally surrenders to God *(Īśvara)* with devotion.

In the first chapter, Patañjali explains *bhakti mārga* in *sūtra: tajjapaḥ tadarthabhāvanam* (*Y.S.*, I.28). This chapter is meant for the advanced *sādhaka (tīvra saṁvegin)*. That is why it is known as *Samādhi Pāda*. On account of *karma śuddhi* the practitioner begins *sādhanā* for *citta śuddhi*. When *citta śuddhi* occurs, it is possible to reach *kaivalya* as well as *Īśvara praṇidhāna*. If that is not possible for a *sādhaka*, then he has to get *citta prasādanam*. See the sequential order of aphorisms from I.23 to I.29, which are about the path of *bhakti*. When a *bhaktan* with *Īśvara praṇidhāna* does *japa* with *artha bhāvanam*, the obstacles are removed and mastery is gained for him to be close to the Soul. But if the practitioner is immature then the obstacles come in his way, for this he needs to start the *sādhanā* to acquire *citta prasādanam*, i.e.; extension and expansion of the consciousness. For this he has to go back and practise from the base of the *aṣṭāṅga yoga* which are enfolded in *kriyā yoga*. Patañjali expresses it as *ekatattvabhyāsaḥ*. In this way *Īśvara praṇidhāna* continues as explained in *niyama*. Therefore one has to love and live in the practice first. One has to be a *bhaktan* to the subject and then it is possible to switch over to God or *Īśvara*.

In the fourth chapter he may not be using the word *Īśvara praṇidhāna* but if one observes the sequential order of *sūtra* from IV.25 onwards it indicates the final stage of *citta śuddhi* leading towards *kaivalya* or *citiśakti* - the *Īśvara*.

---

[1] *Parama* means ultimate, *eka* means one, *antika* means last - end. The one who is a *bhaktan* whose goal is to reach the ultimate end - God - is called *paramaikāntikabhaktan*.

When the *sādhaka* becomes distinctly a seer he distinguishes the difference between consciousness and soul (*citta* and *citi*). In this situation the *citta* of the *sādhaka* gravitates towards *kaivalya*. Many a time the *sādhaka* experiences fissures created by latent impressions. In order to extinguish them, he has to intensify the thought of *Īśvara praṇidhāna* through *japa* and *artha bhāvanam*. Then he reaches the highest state of *samādhi* wherein he is freed from *kleśa karma; tataḥ kleśa karma nivṛttiḥ* (*Y.S.*, IV.30) – it means that the end of afflictive actions takes place and the mind moves towards the Soul – IV.30. This is how *Īśvara praṇidhāna* rescues the *sādhaka*. In the beginning of the *sādhanā* itself he sows the seed of *bhakti*. However he clearly brings the stages of maturity in the path of *bhakti*. He defines *Īśvara* very distinctly and explains the *bhakti* clearly and concisely. *Samādhi* cannot happen without *bhakti*. Hence, the ultimate *samādhi* and the summit of *bhakti* are one and the same. That is why Patañjali declares that *samādhi* is possible by *Īśvara praṇidhāna: samādhisiddhiḥ Īśvarapraṇidhānāt* (*Y.S.*, II.45) – surrender to God brings perfection in *samādhi*.

II.9. – The Importance of *Īśvara praṇidhāna* – Devotion to God

Īśvara means God, the Supreme One. The word comes from the root *Īśa*, and it means the one who commands and rules over 'EVERYTHING'. He is the one to whom the whole universe belongs, yet he is not attached to everything. The word indicates the supremacy of God. The concept of *Īśvara* is conceived as the only one who has unsurpassed knowledge *(jñāna)*, strength *(bala)*, unrivalled sovereignty *(aiśvarya)*, valour *(vīrya)*, potency *(śakti)*, and luminosity *(tej)*. He establishes His supremacy unchallenged in all these six aspects.

Patañjali specifically defines God with very special words: *kleśa karma vipāka āśayaiḥ aparāmṛṣṭaḥ puruṣaviśeṣaḥ Īśvaraḥ* (*Y.S.*, I.24) – *Īśvara* is the one who neither gets afflicted by any action nor enjoys the effects of those actions. He is untouched by afflictions, reactions of actions or their effects. He remains neutral to all actions, reactions, pains and pleasures, therefore, He is *puruṣa viśeṣa*. *Puruṣa* means a human and also the soul *(ātman)*. *Viśeṣa* means distinct to human souls. Hence, Patañjali points to *puruṣa viśeṣa* as the Supreme Universal Soul. He is the seed of knowledge *(sarvajña bījam)* (*Y.S.*, I.25), the origin of illumination. He is omnipotent, omnipresent or omniscient, yet He appears in form as the *guru* of all *gurus* (*Y.S.*, I.26).

It is true that among the six schools of Indian philosophy only yoga defines God. Patañjali defines yoga as *cittavṛtti nirodha* and says that due to the restraint of mental modifications the *ātman* abides in his own grandeur. He does not refer to God in his preamble but introduces *Īśvara* at a chosen time and at a right place, only when one experiences *samādhi.*

However to know the importance of God we need to understand three technical words: *virāma pratyaya, bhava pratyaya* and *upāya pratyaya.*

Virāma means rest or pause and *pratyaya* means going towards. It means to have faith and firm conviction. Between the *sabīja* and *nirbīja samādhi,* there is a state where one finds a resting place or a plateau or a state where there is no progress or regress. It is neither a negative nor a positive state. *Virāma pratyaya* is a kind of a threshold between *sabīja* and *nirbīja samādhi.* At this stage, the *sādhaka* easily gets attracted towards *siddhi* or lands upon *bhava pratyaya,* where he is either a *videhin* or *prakṛtilayan.*

The word *bhava* comes from the root *bhu,* which means to be or being in. The word indicates the original state of being or existence and *pratyaya* means going according to that conviction. The *videhin* remains in a bodiless state and not in a *svarūpāvasthā* state. Similarly, the *prakṛtilayin* remains merged in the elements of nature. Landing on the plateau or threshold, he follows either *bhava pratyaya* or *upāya pratyaya,* according to his respective target: *prakṛti* or *puruṣa* or *puruṣa viśeṣa.* In *upāya pratyaya,* he does not stagnate at a dead end like a *bhava pratyayan.* This *upāya pratyaya* stands for those who have reached *sabīja samādhi* state but pursue the *sādhanā* with faith, vigour, memory and intense contemplation.

Upāya means to come near, to approach, to have proper application of means, to go towards the target. At this juncture the *saṁskāra* or subliminal impressions play a great role. These *saṁskāra* lead the *sādhaka* from *virāma pratyaya* either to go in the way of *bhava pratyaya* or in the way of *upāya pratyaya.* It depends upon the aim of the *sādhaka.* The former one merges through involution into *prakṛti* and the latter one takes one to reach the *puruṣa.* One has to be clear to know the importance of *virāma pratyaya, bhava pratyaya* and *upāya pratyaya, Īśvara* and *Īśvara praṇidhāna.*

Upāya pratyaya is a long practice to reach the goal. In *bhava pratyaya,* it just happens that due to the wrong notion of the *sādhaka* he unknowingly ends the *sādhanā* in *prakṛti,* whereas in *upāya pratyaya* he is alerted to proceed with strong faith, firm conviction, endless vigour, unfailing memory and the awareness to reach the highest state of *samādhi.*

There are four grades of *sādhaka* – mild *(mṛdu),* medium *(madhya),* average *(adhimātra)* and intense *(tīvra).* The destination of *nirbīja samādhi* will be reached by the *sādhaka* according to his *saṁvega* (intense in speedy alertness). *Vega* means speed. *Saṁvega* is a technical word. It is a qualitative speed in performance without any deficiency or dearth. If the *sādhaka* is matured enough to maintain all the four legs of yoga namely, *śraddhā, vīrya, smṛti* and *samādhi-*

prajñā constantly at the highest level with full confidence and without any tinge of doubt, he proves himself to be a *tīvra saṁvegin.* He is the one who reaches the destination quickly. *Mṛdu* or *madhyama saṁvegin,* being deficient and slow in action and qualitative thinking, will reach destination bound by time. Above all these four categories of a *sādhaka* there is a fifth one with a topmost grade, a true *bhaktan,* who does not think of anything except God *(Īśvara praṇidhānin).* He is the fastest, quickest and the first to reach the *nirbīja samādhi.* He will be in the state of *svarūpa pratiṣṭhā.* Here Patañjali's emphasis is on *bhakti mārga.*

As all cannot be *Īśvara praṇidhānin* overnight, he has given alternative ways to reach that level. Hence, Patañjali's indication is that one has to stick to *upāya pratyaya* to mould and shape himself to become a *bhaktan.* Therefore Patañjali orchestrates *sādhaka* from the very beginning. The word he uses is *kriyā yoga.* He advises a neophyte to adhere to *sādhanā* with ascetic devotion, constant reflection and profound faith in God. His advice is based action-wise on *tapas, svādhyāya* and *Īśvara praṇidhāna.* As a beginner, one has to get focused in practice and study with reflection what to do, so that he removes the blemishes and finally surrenders the fruit to God.

He classifies *Īśvara praṇidhāna* as part of *niyama.* With *tapas* the impurities begin to get burnt gradually and self-discipline settles in. The body, senses and mind begin to be pure and attain a new status. *Svādhyāya* or self-study begins to clear the mind and bring the *sādhaka* closer to his *Iṣṭa devatā,* the desired deity and that is the soul. Surrender to God takes him closer to *samādhi.*

When one decides to adopt yoga as a daily routine, whether it is *āsana* or *prāṇāyāma* or *dhyāna,* the element of *niyama* is involved in it. At this stage one may not be sure about the concept of *Īśvara* or the role of *Īśvara praṇidhāna,* but the very notion of *Īśvara praṇidhāna* gives unknowingly or unexpectedly a kind of relief and a moral support to the *sādhaka* for *sādhanā.* Obviously the *saṁskāra* of *Īśvara praṇidhāna* is carried gradually to further one's practice. This helps him when he lands at *virāma pratyaya* and is likely to miss the bus for the finality of *Īśvara praṇidhāna. Upāya pratyaya* helps the *sādhaka* to reach the aim of surrendering totally to *Īśvara (Īśvara praṇidhāna).* As *bhakti mārga* is not possible for all, Patañjali, through *aṣṭāṅga yoga,* helps one to reach the state of *samādhi,* which leads towards surrender to the Supreme. This is how Patañjali shows alternative ways to all to reach the same destination. In case the *sādhaka* develops pride in his success, he cautions that a fall may occur: *hānam eṣāṁ kleśavat uktam* (*Y.S.,* IV.28) – the *yogi* has to relinquish all powers. Otherwise, he will be caught in the web of afflictions again.

In a way the *sādhaka* is compelled to gravitate towards the *jīvātman* and later *jīvātman* towards *paramātman.*

Therefore my advice is: Do the *sādhanā*, understand the *prakṛti, puruṣa* and *puruṣa viśeṣa.* At right time the importance of *Īśvara* and *Īśvara praṇidhāna* is revealed on its own. To realise *Īśvara* one needs *sādhanā.* To understand *Īśvara* one needs maturity. To reach *Īśvara* one needs love and devotion.

To tread the path of yoga one needs all the three paths of action, namely: *karma, jñāna* and *bhakti.* Often, we are caught in *abhāva pratyaya.* In sleep there is a feeling of non-beingness or non-existence. This is *abhāva pratyaya.* But when we come out of sleep we do not deny our existence. We do not say that we died in sleep and now we are alive after sleep. If we have not seen or experienced God, it does not mean that God is absent or nonexistent. We are *abhāva pratyayin* so we don't witness His existence due to our ignorance. We have back bodies. We cannot see the back, but we can feel it. To feel the back, the senses, mind and intelligence have to move inwards. They get introverted. If this looking in is intensified one can feel the back. If carried further, one day one may be able to sight the soul and Universal Soul.

In sleep our belongings exist though we are unaware of our bedroom. Our consciousness is narrowed in sleep. Our consciousness needs to get expanded to know God. In wakeful state the consciousness is full of the other four modifications except the notion of God and sleep. This is nothing but ignorance. To know God, to feel His presence, to realise His existence, one needs to be in a *wakefully* wakeful state *(jāgṛtajāgṛtāvasthā).* It is called *turyāvasthā.*

Ignorance narrows the *citta* and knowledge expands it. To know *Īśvara,* the *citta* has to expand to its optimal level. The expansion of *citta* itself is *jāgṛtajāgṛtāvasthā.* One cannot see God in a sleepy state. *Nidrāvasthā* being an *avidyā* state shuns God. At least begin to dream God. One needs *bhāvana* of *Īśvara pranidhāna* to dream God. That is why Patañjali insists on *citta prasādanam.* By dispositioning the *citta* on God in a *wakefully* wakeful state, the *citta* is made to flow in same thought both in dreamy and sleepy states.

Then the journey takes us from *ātma pratyaya* to *paramātma pratyaya.*

II.10. – Does yoga suggest *saguṇa bhakti* or *nirguṇa bhakti*

Sabīja means with support and *nirbīja* means without support. As there is *sabīja* and *nirbīja prāṇāyāma* and *sabīja* and *nirbīja samādhi, bhakti* too is of two types, one is *saguṇa bhakti* and the other is *nirguṇa bhakti.*

Saguṇa bhakti means *sadguṇa vṛtti. Saguṇa* and *sadguṇa* stands for righteous and virtuous properties and qualities, whereas *nirguṇa bhakti* is beyond the expression of qualities.

God is with form as well as without form. As humans we find it easier to conceive of God with form than without form. We have a form and as such we imagine and think of God not only in a human form but also as *saguṇa* or *sadguṇa Brahma.* By nature we have the mixed qualities of *sadguṇa* and *durguṇa.*

If *sadguṇa* is of righteous and virtuous character, *durguṇa* is a non-righteous and non-virtuous quality. Hence we attribute God in *saguṇa* or *sadguṇa* form as well as with *kalyāṇa guṇa* (auspicious character).

It is hard for a man to imagine God without form. So men in their inquisitive innovation make God look like man for worship, as *citta* needs a support to think or worship Lord. Hence, we worship God in form and pray with devotion. Thus came *saguṇa Īśvara.* Patañjali covers not only *saguṇa bhakti* but also the *nirguṇa bhakti,* which conveys the qualities beyond possibilities.

Patañjali defines God as; *kleśa karma vipāka āśayaiḥ aparāmṛṣṭaḥ puruṣviśeṣaḥ Īśvaraḥ* (*Y.S.,* I.24) – He is the Supreme Being, totally free from conflicts, unaffected by actions and re-actions, and untouched by cause and effect. Here he explains God in *nirguṇa* form saying that He is above all *puruṣa,* the soul, hence He is the Supreme Soul. In this sense, He is termed as *puruṣaviśeṣa.* God is the seed of all knowledge. All knowledge sprouts from his unexcelled seed of knowledge. God is a *jñāni,* a *karmi,* yet unsurpassed by anyone and unaffected by anyone or anything indicating *nirguṇa Īśvara* as Brahman. *Tatra niratiśayaṁ sarvajñabījam* (*Y.S.,* I.25) – He is the unexcelled seed of all knowledge.

In the succeeding two *sūtra* he speaks of him in *saguṇa* form: *sa eṣaḥ pūrveṣām api guruḥ kālena anavacchedāt* (*Y.S.,* I.26) – In the personal form of God; He is the first, foremost and absolute guru, unconditioned by time; and *tasya vācakaḥ praṇavaḥ* (*Y.S.,* I.27) – He is identified with the sacred syllable *āuṁ,* called *praṇava.* This explanation suggests *saguṇa Īśvara* and *saguṇa Brahma. Citta* catches the word *guru* as a personified God. The first and foremost *Guru* is timeless. Patañjali's concept of *Īśvara* takes, suddenly, a shape or a form, as *guru,* and becomes *saguṇa* so that the *sādhaka* can worship God in *saguṇa* form. Patañjali explains God in *saguṇa* form with the sacred syllable *āuṁ* called *praṇava,* which represents

God in a number of ways; as *vācaka* conveys connotation and denotation of God in *āuṁ.* Then he explains the method of worship: *tajjapaḥ tadarthabhāvanam* (*Y.S.,* I.28) – the *mantra āuṁ* is to be repeated constantly, with feeling, realising its full significance.

Patañjali begins with the concrete practice called *japasādhanā. Japa* means repeating the name of God. He advises one to repeat the *mantra āuṁ* with *arthabhāvanam. Artha* means the 'meaning' and *bhāvana* means the 'feeling'. *Artha* is connected with the head and *bhāvana* is connected with the heart. The meaning of *āuṁ* is realised by the brain and felt in the heart, and the confluence of head and heart reveals the direct perception of God. This kind of *japasādhanā* is *saguṇa bhakti.* Again he has referred in *niyama* as a means*: svādhyāyāt iṣṭa devatā saṁprayogaḥ* (*Y.S.,* II.44) – Self-study leads towards the realisation of God or communion with one's desired deity.

Iṣṭadevatā means one's desired deity. Here, Patañjali definitely indicates God with form. A neophyte cannot worship a formless God. He has to worship God with form only. So *svādhyāya* of *niyama* indicates *saguṇa bhakti.*

Patañjali has introduced worship in both ways so that the *sādhaka* can progress gradually with proper physical, psychological and mental approaches. The *bhakti* aspect is hidden in all the eight petals of yoga and it evolves gradually to develop the emotional aspect required for devotion. In *yama* also there is an indirect suggestion to gravitate mentally towards *Īśvara praṇidhāna* as mentioned in *niyama.* He says *āsana* leads one towards *ananta-samāpatti,* and *prāṇāyāma* towards *dhyāna* gravitating the *citta* towards God. *Dhyāna* helps to subjugate the ego, a big obstacle in devotion, and *samādhi* to get absorbed in *Īśvara* with *bhakti.*

In the last *sūtra,* Patañjali highlights the glorious knowledge *(viveka khyāti)* to return to the source of consciousness with its own natural purity (*Y.S.,* IV.34). This is nothing but *parajñāna* and *paravairāgya,* and therefore without elaborating the path towards God-realisation, he ends the *sūtra.* As it becomes a natural tendency for anyone to move towards God, from here he leaves the readers to infer *kaivalya (paramabhakti),* as its end is excellence in devotion *(śaraṇāgati yoga).*

SECTION III

ON *AṢṬĀṆGA* YOGA

SECTION III – ON *AṢṬĀṄGA YOGA*

III.1. - *Yama*

III.1.1. – On practice of *yama*

The principles of *yama* are: non-violence, truthfulness, non-stealing, controlled celibacy, and to be non-covetous. These principles are the main life force foe living for us as humans, but we often act in the opposite direction. Our way of living is an admixture of good and bad actions that are constructed upon desires, greed, anger, hatred, infatuation, pride, jealousy and animosity.

Like the coin having two sides, our mind too has two sides. One side of the mind represents good actions with good imprints and the other side of the coin acts quite the opposite. The imprints of good actions help one to be contented, happy, helpful, soft, noble and peaceful. That mind remains harmless, friendly, forgiving, compassionate, moderate in approaches, lovable, steady, straightforward, non-possessive, generous and charitable.

The ocean is the abode of water, yet in it are crocodiles, fish, whales, tortoises, pearls, corals, serpents, conches, shells, and so forth. In the same way, our consciousness with its content of emotions, desires, intellectual ambitions and pride is the abode of both good and bad thoughts.

We have to learn to watch our own nature in this vast ocean of consciousness to find out what kind of person we, as individuals, are. Our actions and thoughts depend upon our ways of behaviour as we often act according to our ways of thinking. When we are diseased, we need a treatment for cure. As the quality of the tree depends on the quality of the seed, the consciousness needs the treatment of 'right deliberation' and 'right action' which comes through yogic practices.

The principles of *yama* cannot easily be followed, but we have to adopt them and learn to eradicate the defects of our nature by right knowledge.

The *sūtra* composed by Patañjali, shows what happens when one goes with the current of thoughts or against their current; If he goes with the current of thought the seer identifies with the fluctuating consciousness. *Vṛtti sārūpyam itaratra* (*Y.S.*, I.4). If he goes against the current the seer dwells in his own true splendour; *tadā draṣṭuḥ svarūpe avasthānam* (*Y.S.*, I.3). *Vitarkabādhane pratipakṣabhāvanam* (*Y.S.*, II.33) – principles which run contrary to *yama* and *niyama* are to be countered with the knowledge of discrimination.

Most of us know that violence, untruth, tendency to steal, uncontrolled sexuality and possessiveness are inherent in human nature. Patañjali, as a psychologist, elegantly suggests their opposites, instead of naming them directly.

He puts them in an abridged and aphoristic form. Those aphorisms are: *ahiṁsā satya asteya brahmacarya aparigrahaḥ yamaḥ* (*Y.S.*, II.30) – non-violence, truth, abstention from stealing, continence, and absence of greed as the five pillars of *yama,* and at the same time he wants us to understand *vitarkaḥ hiṁsādayaḥ kṛta kārita anumoditāḥ lobha krodha moha pūrvakaḥ mṛdu madhya adhimātraḥ duḥkha ajñāna anantaphalāḥ iti pratipakṣabhāvanam* (*Y.S.*, II.34) – uncertain knowledge giving rise to violence, whether done directly or indirectly, or condoned, caused by greed, anger or delusion in mild, moderate or intense degree results in endless pain and ignorance. He wants us to practise *yama* through introspection and insight to eradicate the pain and ignorance.

Each *sādhaka* needs to watch his thoughts and actions moment to moment and think why and how he does an action, and the intention behind such action. His intentions might be good but the application may be wrong. Hence, he has to verify and discriminate to build up the principles of *yama*.

When children, adolescents and youngsters have to concentrate on their studies, or health, hobbies, or occupational aims, they naturally flirt in love making or gossiping, deviating from their studies. When a person gets married, it is obvious that he is no more a celibate; but the celibacy needs to be followed even in marital life. Yet there is a difference between youngsters and adults. Youngsters demand and stimulation comes mostly through their body. They do not calculate with their minds. Whereas the demands for the grown-ups are more from the head and mind. Either way, the basic problem of dissatisfaction and enhanced desire leads towards *abrahmacarya.*

People hanker after money, name and fame and do not feel ashamed about these. What is kleptomania? Why does the tendency of stealing exists in some? Knowing this inner tendency of men, Patañjali wants one to become a non-stealer *(asteyin).*

It is interesting to note that the instigators for actions are senses of perception and mind. For this, Patañjali advises us to use discretion in using the peripheral organs of the body (hands, legs, larynx, generative and excretory organs) through the five principles for *yama* for their cleanliness *(karmendriya-śuci).*

Basically, the principles of *yama* are at the source points of senses of perception and mind. In order to balance the intelligence and emotions, and thoughts and actions perfectly, one has to prudently discriminate while selecting what to do and what not to do with a composed reflective mind in judging actions and thoughts.

There is a beautiful way that we can see the inter-linking effects of the *aṣṭaṅga yoga,* of the *Yoga Sūtra.* In order to adopt *yama* we have to follow the principles of *niyama. Āsana* and *prāṇāyāma* bring the required bio-physical and chemical changes in order to make us adept in *yama* and *niyama.*

a) – On *ahiṁsā* and *satya*

I have dealt with *ahiṁsā* and *satya* on several occasions in the volumes of *Aṣṭadaḷa Yogamālā.* Hence, I am not elaborating them here.

But so much I would like to say is that Mahatma Gandhi and Martin Luther King are examples for us to know where *ahiṁsā* and *satya* lead us.

In *ahiṁsā* we have to develop words of peace, good will and love in thoughts and actions whether one is in a sleepy state, a dreamy state or in a wakeful state.

The effect of non-violence is that one abandons hostility and develops friendliness and tolerance.

Similarly, by sticking to *satya* (truth), one's words become so potent that whatever is said, happens.

b) – On *asteya*

Desire *(vāsanā)* is eternal. Due to its eternality we are caught in the cycles of birth, afflictions and death. Actions and thoughts go hand in hand. Each action leaves its imprint on the mind, like "you think and so you do". These thoughts and actions build up memories and leave impressions *(saṁskāra),* as imprints *(smṛti-saṁskāra).* This is like a tri-pod. Each action and thought has a cause or a motive, which is known as its *hetu. Hetu* means purpose. There is a purpose behind each action and thought, which yields its fruit *(phala)*. This fruit becomes the seed for the succeeding thoughts and actions. As the seed is, so is the harvest. As the desires are, so is the course of action to get the desired fruit. Hence, yoga wants us to follow the principles of *yama* for *guṇa vṛtti nirodha*. Honestly, desires *(vāsanā)* do not fulfil the real interest of man.

A person might be poor, hungry, uneducated and jobless. It can lead him to steal or rob. He will take chances to fulfil his desire. But if it becomes a habit, then he may end up as a full-time robber or a dacoit. This becomes his *guṇa vṛtti*. White collared people in society may steal important things in their own way. Emotional blackmailing and intellectual theft are forms of robbery. Getting the work done by the labourers without giving proper returns is also robbery. The trend of giving and receiving bribes is no less than robbery.

When one establishes himself in *asteya*, his desire will be between the banks of *dharma* and *mokṣa*, i.e., the rivers of *artha* and *kāma*. Those who follow the straightforward, simple life will have much more satisfaction than those who cheat or play double games.

Of one whose mind is well established in non-stealing, Patañjali says, that precious jewels come to him on their own, without expectations; *asteyapratiṣṭāyāṁ sarva ratnopasthānam (Y.S.,* II.37) – honesty pays its dues in the form of *asteya*.

Asteya itself is the most precious jewel. It contains the merit of justice and restraint. It creates the sense of duty and faith. It balances well between courage and patience. *Asteya* is the best gem, which comes when one is well established. Stealing is done for a momentary satisfaction but non-stealing gives the wealth of virtue, the noblest of wealth.

In the 47th *śloka* of chapter II of the *Bhagavad Gītā*, Lord Krishna advises: *karmaṇyeva adhikāraste mā phaleṣu kadācana*. Do your duty, do not expect the fruits. One's rights are only for actions and not for their fruits. So virtue in the form of precious gems comes for him unexpectedly. This is the fruit of *asteya*.

c) – On *brahmacarya*

The word celibacy is not the correct translation to convey the meaning of *brahmacarya*. It means religious studentship, it is religious self-restraint. Brahma is the supreme principle of creation. To know the Supreme Brahma a disciplined and thoughtful approach is needed. This is *brahmacarya*. Another meaning for *brahmacarya* is control of sexual impulses and desires. This impulse is biological, instinctive and emotional. When it is a mental tendency for the sake of joy and satisfaction, it is unholy, and makes one a maniac. When it is from the heart, that action fulfils the needs of a human being.

Patañjali does not explain what *brahmacarya* is, but gives the benefits of it. He says, *brahmacarya pratiṣṭhāyāṁ vīryalābhaḥ (Y.S.*, II.38). The word *vīrya* means semen, physical and mental vigour, strength, power, intellectual maturity, heroism, prowess, valour, fortitude, courage and so forth. It is suggestive of the energy at the physical, mental, emotional, intellectual and spiritual levels required to be earned and stored to reach the Supreme. The first step is on the physical level which demands the control over the organs of action. A man who is impotent and lacks sexual desire cannot be called a celibate. By preserving that energy, one gains valour. A man, having potency, and not allowing his mind to waver, is a celibate. His mind does not get affected whether he looks at a girl of sixteen or a woman of sixty. He is free from attraction. He does not search or reach for anyone or anything outside of him to fulfil his wants. He is complete and full within himself. This is celibacy. The other stage of *brahmacarya* is when one moves in word, thought and action totally towards God.

Viṣayavatī vā pravṛttiḥ utpannā manasaḥ sthiti nibandhanī (Y.S., I.35) – or by contemplating on an object that helps to maintain steadiness of mind and consciousness brings about direct perception of its essence.

This direct perception with absorption is perceived and conceived In practice, which in turn develops awareness and sensitivity towards the inflow of life to such a degree that he may gain insight into phenomena as well as the nature of the seer.

In the *aṣṭaṅga yoga* of Patañjali, the process of involvement and absorption into that which is perceived or conceived begins in *āsana* and *prāṇāyāma*. It is a training that is continuous from *āsana* to *dhyāna*, increasing in subtlety and penetration with each progressive stage. If established at the beginning with *āsana* as its working base a momentum and power *(vīrya)* is built up in the practitioner that propels him to move closer to that Self.

Āsana and *prāṇāyāma* help to sustain *brahmacarya* as thoughts and actions gets inverted and makes the practitioner to move towards the soul *(Brahman).*

The long practice of *Halāsana* pacifies the generative organs. *Baddha Koṇāsana* and *Upaviṣṭha Koṇāsana* reduce the urge for sex while *Śīrṣāsana* and *Sarvāṅgāsana* pacify the mind over undue desires. The inversions help to balance hormones and mind. Practice of *prāṇāyāma* like *Ujjājī*, *Viloma* and *Pratiloma* help to arrest the mental desire and transforms the sexual energy into spiritual energy. *Recaka kuṁbhaka* would be of great help whereas *pūraka kuṁbhaka* or backbends increase and tempts for the physical demand.

The one who always moves his energy of body, senses, intelligence and consciousness conscientiously towards *brahma* (the Supreme), he is a *brahmacārī; brahmeṇa carati iti brahmacārī* – This is celibacy of body, mind and self.

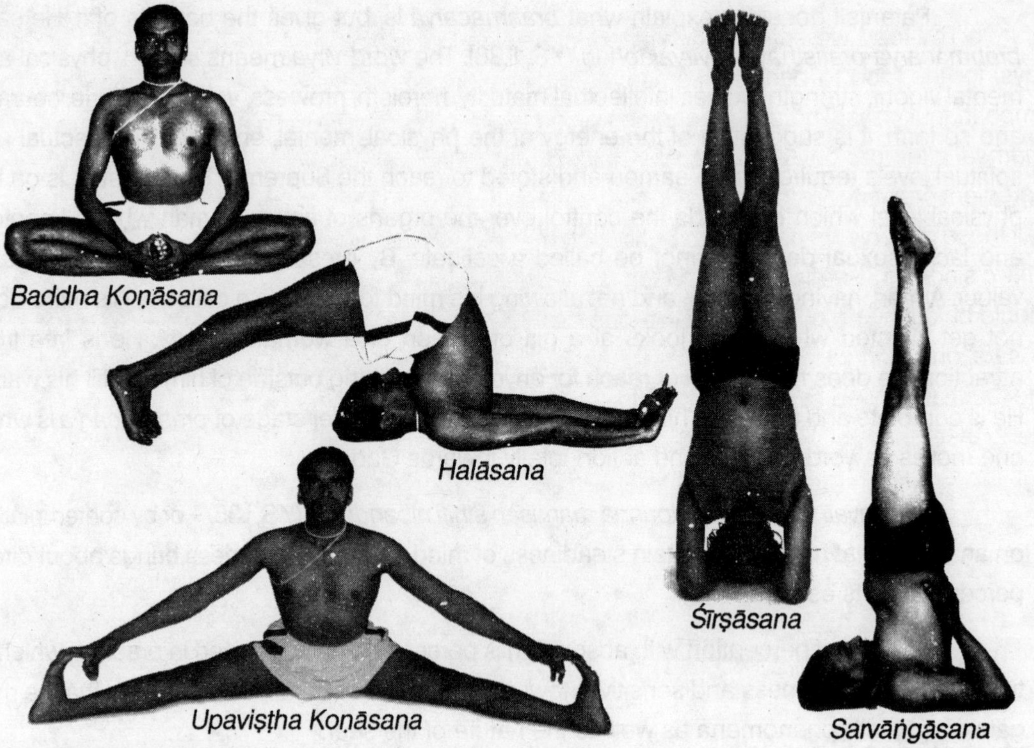

Baddha Koṇāsana

Halāsana

Śīrṣāsana

Upaviṣṭha Koṇāsana

Sarvāṅgāsana

Plate n. 3 – *Āsana* for celibacy

EFFECT OF CELIBACY

Brahmacarya pratiṣṭhāyāṁ vīryalābhaḥ. Patañjali says it means that when the *sādhaka* firmly establishes continence in him, knowledge, vigour, valour and energy flow profusely in him.

The *prakṛti* has *triguṇa* – the three qualities – *sattva, rajas* and *tamas.* Each human being is born with these *guṇa* according to his past *karma.* In man *Jñāna* and *karma* go together. According to one's *jñāna* he does *karma* and according to the quality of his *karma* he develops *jñāna.* He gets knowledge by action and earns knowledge through action. The aim of all of us is to reach the illuminative *sāttvic* state. This also is a quality of *brahmacarya.*

The *triguṇa* and *tridoṣa* get imbibed from the parents, as they are the seed for our birth. Their constitutions get injected into us.

Knowing our weaknesses we turn to build up our personality with our efforts through good qualities and reform ourselves for the better. Here the seven ingredients *(saptadhātu)* play a great role in developing vigour and valour. *Āyurveda* explains that these *dhātu* hold, support and sustain human beings – *dhāraṇāt dhātavaḥ.*

The food we eat gets converted into seven ingredients. It takes one lunar month (28 days) for the food to become semen. After digestion the food becomes *rasa* – the chyle or lymph in four days. The chyle becomes blood in the next four days. The blood becomes flesh *(māṁsa)* after four days. It takes four days for the metabolic function of the body to get each ingredient converted into the next ingredient. This way the full cycle gets completed in 28 days. If all these ingredients have to be purified by the body, then the food should be pure, clean and *sāttvic* since its essence has to reach up to the semen *(śukra)*. While eating our mental state should be calm and quiet. Half of the food that we take is absorbed by the body to sustain itself as *sāra*; one fourth is thrown out as roughage and wastage known as *kitta* and the remaining one fourth is utilised by our mental body as *sattva*. So this *sattva* part builds our mind, memory, intelligence, consciousness, straightforwardness, steadiness and forgiveness. If the food is *sāttvic*, then its *sāra*, *kitta* and *sattva* will be *sāttvic*. If it is *rājasic*, the three will be *rājasic*, and if *tāmasic*, these are covered by *tāmasic* nature. If we have to change radically, then the drastic step has to be taken in our food intake, lifestyle, way of thinking and perception.

The word *vīrya* indicates valour, vigour and courage. If a person is of *sāttvic* nature, the seven ingredients (*saptadhātu*) remain in a balanced state. In him the semen, being the final essence of the ingredients *(dhātu)*, remains with potency and gives tremendous vigour and power on physical, moral, intellectual and spiritual levels. If one has to be well established in *brahmacarya* then not only the food for the body has to be *sāttvic*, but the food for the senses, food for the mind, food for the intelligence too has to be *sāttvic*. The mind should not pick up emotional sensualities for their gratification. The organ of speech has to avoid discussions on sensual desires. The intelligence should guide the mind and senses to see good, hear good, taste good, speak good and feel good. *Āyurveda* says that the semen will be full of *ojas*. Semen can give birth to a new life as a progeny or it can transform one to a new-life on moral, intellectual and spiritual levels. The clarity and purity gained on these levels is called *tejas* or *ojas*. That is its *vīrya*. If *āyurveda* refers to it as semen *(śukra)*, yoga refers to it as *vīrya*.

Vasiṣṭha was a *brahmarṣī* – the one who has realised *brahman*. He was the *guru* of Rāma. His hundred children were of a calibre of the highest standard. Vasiṣṭha calls himself a *brahmacārī* since his intellectual and spiritual energy flow was towards *brahman*. Lord Hanumān was a *brahmacārī* yet his sweat had vigour – *vīrya*. He met Rāvaṇa who had kidnapped Sītā. When Rāvaṇa set fire to Hanumān's tail he burnt Lankā. After burning Lankā, he went to the ocean to extinguish his burning tail. At that time a few drops of his perspiration were swallowed by a crocodile and it gave birth to Makardhvaja as a son of Hanumān. Sweat in *āyurveda* is considered as impurity *(mala)* to be thrown out. Hanumān's sweat had this potency. Compare this sweat to the sweat of sick and diseased people. Then one will know why the body has to be pure.

Bhīṣmācārya too was a *brahmacārī* as he had taken oath and promised his stepmother that he would not marry or have a child to claim the throne. With his strong will-power he lived the life of a *brahmacārī* until the end. This grandsire of Kaurava and Pāṇḍava was filled with physical and mental vigour as well as strong will-power. Even death could not approach him until he wished for it.

These are the examples of *brahmacarya* and that is how celibacy and valour are related. Patañjali puts it short as *ṛtam* – seasoned intelligence and matured wisdom.

d) – On *aparigraha* (non-possessiveness)

Parigraha among *yama, abhiniveśa* among *kleśa* and *smṛti* among *vṛtti* are very closely related and dependent on each other. These put us in the endless chain of life with the interruption of birth and death, as they have some kind of attachment to the individual 'I'.

Parigraha means possessiveness. Greed is hidden in this possessiveness. Man asks for everything and accepts everything. In the end he will not hesitate even to grab.

Even a wise and learned man is not free from *abhiniveśa. Abhiniveśa* means attachment to life. But people like Vasiṣṭha and Vyāsa were liberated souls and hence were free from the fear of death.

Though we know that death comes only once, the taste of death mingles with us as an instinctive memory that strikes from the previous life. We witness death everyday as we see people dying. Knowing that our parents and grand parents have left, we too know that we will follow the same route. Yet we think that we are going to be permanent on this earth. The ego or I-consciousness sustains and supports this feel of permanency, though the inner intelligence knows that life is perishable, transient and non-eternal. This is basically an instinctive defect.

Smṛti or memory is so strong that it stores all our experiences, imprints and thoughts; it recollects our attachments, possessive nature, aversion, anger and animosity. *Smṛti* collects physical, intellectual and emotional experiences as well as the feel of sensitivity. It is a storehouse of wanted, unwanted, wished and unwished memories. This is the reason why we are in the clutches of *abhiniveśa.*

The roots of *parigraha* are; desire, anger, greed, infatuation, pride and jealousy. *Abhiniveśa* is the stored desires and attachments *(vāsanā).* The memory *(smṛti)* being the storehouse of imprints *(saṁskāra)* fuels them further. The principles of *yama* and *niyama* help to sublimate these mental upheavals.

On the sublimation of *parigraha*, knowledge of past and future lives unfolds when freed from greed or possession; *aparigrahasthairye janmakathaṁtā saṁbodhaḥ* (*Y.S.*, II.39). About *abhiniveśa* Patañjali says, *svarasavahī viduṣaḥ api tatha ārūḍhaḥ abhiniveśaḥ* (*Y.S.*, II.9) – self-preservation or attachment to life is the subtlest of all afflictions. It is found even in wise men. About *smṛti* he says, *anubhūta viṣaya asaṁpramoṣaḥ smṛtiḥ* (*Y.S.*, I.11) – memory is the unmodified recollection of words and experiences.

Birth is the result of *vāsanā*. Śankarācārya says, *punarapi jananam punarapi maraṇam punarapi jananī jaṭhare śayanam:* as long as we are caught in the *vāsanā*, the process of birth and death continues, and we will be entering into the womb of a mother again and again. It is important for us as *yoga sādhaka* to think of *aparigraha*. How many of us find excuses for avoiding the practice of *āsana* and *prāṇāyāma*. First we say we have no time as we have to look after our work, our business and so on. The seeds of these excuses are hidden in possessiveness. I am not saying that one should avoid his responsibilities. One needs to look after his family and business, but at the same time he has to give time for himself through yogic practice to keep aloof from the thoughts of the world. Avoid those activities where one spends time and energy for no reason. Start with small good things so that the attitude gets changed. Yogic practice is one that makes us to live without fear. It takes a long time to live not with desires but to live with a purpose. Then we know how this affliction is reduced through yoga making them weak for fading out so they do not affect us much.

Smṛti means memory where impressions from each and every experienced action and knowledge are stored in a part of the brain. Thoughts, imaginations, emotions and sensitivities are stored in memory. Memory is honest in itself. Whatever has been experienced is stored by it. But it gets coloured in expressions and tilts the original imprint. Memory can remain pure through *aṣṭaṅga yoga*.

The knowledge stored in memory gets filtered by *viveka* as *jñāna* gets filtered through the practice of yoga and experienced knowledge filters *jñāna* into *viveka* (wisdom). While speaking of *nirvitarka samāpatti*, Patañjali uses the expression *smṛti pariśuddhi* (fully purified memory). We practise *āsana*, *prāṇāyāma* and *dhyāna* to train the memory to be clean for it to guide us towards intellectual progression.

In *Vibhūti Pāda* Patañjali speaks of latent impressions, *saṁskāra sākṣātkaraṇāt pūrvajātijñānam* (*Y.S.*, III.18) – through direct perception of subliminal impressions, the yogi gains knowledge of his previous lives.

In *Kaivalya Pāda* Patañjali again says, *jāti deśa kāla vyavahitānām api ānantaryaṁ smṛti saṁskārayoḥ ekarūpatvāt* (*Y.S.*, IV.9) – though life is interrupted by changes in species and lineage, place and time, memory and impressions exist uninterruptedly to connect them to the present life. Memory and subliminal impressions do not perish easily. There might be gaps between one life and the next, or one may be born in different species altogether, yet memory and impressions carry these desires *(vāsanā)* which are eternal. The eternality of *vāsanā* expires only by knowing the eternal entity within. In the same chapter Patañjali says that when the *yogi* sees that *citta* and *ātman* are distinct, pores in the *citta* may still appear, hidden impressions may still surface: *tat cchidreṣu pratyayāntarāṇi saṁskārebhyaḥ (Y.S.,* IV.27).

Therefore, in order to know the cause, one needs to trace the hidden *vāsanā*, in the form of fear of death, memory, latent imprints, cleansing of memory and the eternal principle behind all these factors. This so-called eternal *vāsanā* ends only when *yoga-sādhanā* changes our attitude to conquer fear and bring restraints on thoughts and actions. Then *karmaśuddhi*, *jñānaśuddhi* and *cittaśuddhi* take place.

The psychology of *aparigraha* connects us with the lives of the past. When we use the words 'destiny' or 'fate' we do not try to inquire or penetrate. The destiny reveals to a yogi who works through non-attachment, sacrifice, satisfaction and contentment.

III.2 - *Niyama*

III.2.1. – Control on the senses of perception

The five principles of *yama* play a great role in bringing the organs of action under control; *niyama* helps in cleansing the senses of perception *(jñānendriya śuci)*. When the organs of action and the senses of perception are controlled and cleansed, the mind gets non-attached and becomes free from them. This makes the mind to move in a new channel to get attached to the core of the Self.

The principles of *niyama* are meant to discipline and cleanse the senses of perception in order to use them for right means. This is the basic step to keep the senses away from being drawn easily towards the outer objects or things in life. Suppose one engages the eyes for reading good books, seeing good things, ears for listening to educative talks like *Bhagavad Gītā*, *Brahmasūtra*, the attitude changes. Let the nostrils breathe the fragrance of fresh air. Let the tongue taste good *sāttvic* food. Let the skin feel the divine touch through *āsana*. This way one can learn to develop divine sensory perception.

The first basic principle of *niyama* is *śauca*. It means cleanliness. The very word represents the cleansing of the senses of perception and their disengagement from the objects of temptations.

Santoṣa is contentment. This contentment comes if one correctly measures the scale of need with greed, as greed leads to various types of motivations. To have contentment, we need *tapas*. *Tapas* is a burning zeal that helps to purify the organs of action, senses of perception and the mind. Then comes *svādhyāya*. *Svādhyāya* is to study our own existence from the skin to the innermost Self. *Svādhyāya* helps the outgoing mind to focus on the core. When we are close to our self, we then become fit instruments to surrender to God.

Patañjali begins *niyama* with the cleanliness of the body, then the mind and thereafter with the knowledge of the self. Only after knowing the self, one reflects upon it and becomes fit enough to surrender to God. Rāmānuja reverses the process. He says that due to the past *karma* or sin, or *vāsanā*, one's nature shows always a strong inclination towards doing something wrong or bad. Hence he says that focus on God may help in not doing wrong things.

The principles of *niyama* enable the energy of the senses to reach the Ultimate, as it helps in controlling and disciplining them.

III.2.2. – On *Īśvara praṇidhāna*

Patañjali explains *Īśvara praṇidhāna* in a single *sūtra*, *tajjapaḥ tadartha bhāvanam* (*Y.S.*, I.28). The *sūtra* has three words and conveys every aspect of worship. *Tat* means that; that is *praṇava* – *āuṁ*. *Japa* means repetition of it and *arthabhāvanam* means the feeling from understanding and digesting the meaning of it. Though *arthabhāvanam* is taken as a single word, it has two aspects; *artha* means value of the word, and when repeated one gets the feel of it as *bhāvanam*. The tongue may repeat *āuṁ* but the meaning has to touch the heart with felt feelings. Therefore *tat* means *āuṁ* and that has to be conceived. The feel of devotion, dedication, respect and surrendering cannot be taught, forced or induced. One has to get involved from the conscience *(antaḥkaraṇa)*.

I have taken this *sūtra* literally in my practice of *āsana* and *prāṇāyāma*. For me *tat* means *āsana*. *Āsana* are my prayers. I search in each *āsana* to find right means *(artha)*, and digest the entire action of the *āsana* to feel the bliss *(ānanda)*. Similarly, I savour the breath, with my soul spreading in the body through inhalation, holding it steadily in retention and watching it recede towards its source in exhalation.

Niyama works on *trikaraṇa śuddhi* or the purification in *kāya, vāca, and manasa* (body, speech and mind).

Karaṇa means instrument. We have external instruments *(bāhya karaṇa)*, namely the body, senses of perception, mind, intelligence, I-ness, consciousness *(citta)* and conscience *(antaḥkaraṇa)*. All these need to be educated to experience the content of the above *sūtra*. This is exactly what I did and am still doing through *āsana* and *prāṇāyāma*.

Repeating the name of God is *japa*, which is a kind of *tapas*. *Artha* is to know the meaning of the word. It indicates resources. *Artha* being *svādhyāya*, one has to know the meaning of the name of God by study and one has to learn through the source books like *veda*.

Bhāvanam is to feel in the heart of what is understood. *Tajjapaḥ tadarthabhāvanam* (*Y.S.*, I.28) and *tapaḥ svādhyāya Īśvarapraṇidhānāni kriyāyogaḥ* (*Y.S.*, II.1)[1] are understood through the flow of intelligence of the head and heart on God. *Kriyā yoga* contains the composites of *śakti* through *tapas*, *yukti* through *jñāna*, and *bhakti* through *Īśvara praṇidhāna*. Similarly *japa*, *artha* and *bhāvanam* contain respectively the composites of *karma, jñāna* and *bhakti*.

The *praṇava āuṁ*, which denotes *Īśvara*, has to be repeated with the organs of speech, mouth, tongue and larynx *(bāhyakaraṇa)*. The meaning has to be understood through the intellect of the brain *(jñāna)* and the feel of it *(bhāvanam)* from the intelligence of the heart *(antaḥkaraṇa)*. All three are required to experience it. *Japa* or repetition of *āuṁ* should be followed as a *karma* or *kṛti* so that the body, organs of action and senses of perception get not only cleansed but accomplished for further progress in yogic endeavour.

Kāya indriya siddhiḥ aśuddhikṣayāt tapasaḥ (*Y.S.*, II.43) – self-discipline *(tapas)* burns away impurities of the body and senses and kindles the sparks of divinity.

By understanding the meaning of *āuṁ*, which connotes *Īśvara* through *svādhyāya*, the *jñāna* flourishes and the communion with the desired deity is established.

Svādhyāyāt iṣṭadevatā saṁprayogaḥ (*Y.S.*, II.44)

---

[1] See the author's *Light on the Yoga Sūtras of Patañjali* (Harper Collins, London)

Self-knowledge *(svādhyāya),* understanding of oneself leads towards God-realisation. *Yathābhimata dhyānāt va* (*Y.S.,* I.39). *Āuṁ* has to be pleasing to the mind to use it for meditation. When *āuṁ* becomes pleasing, the *sādhaka* begins to hold it for it to set in the heart, and understanding of the self gets materialised. When intelligence is fully matured, then it leads him towards *samādhi.*

Samādhisiddhiḥ Īśvarapraṇidhānāt (*Y.S.,* II.45). This *sūtra* conveys that either *samādhi* leads one towards God *(Īśvara praṇidhāna)* or *Īśvara praṇidhāna* causes *samādhi.*

In *Śrīmad Bhāgavatam* Prahlāda enumerates the nine aspects of worshipping Lord.

Śravaṇaṁ kīrtanaṁ vishṇu smaraṇaṁ pādasevanaṁ I
Arcanaṁ vandanaṁ dāsyaṁ sakhyaṁ ātmanivedanaṁ II (*Śrīmad Bhāgavatam* VII.5)

Hearing the names and glory of God Vishnu *(śravaṇam),* chanting His names and glory *(kīrtanam),* remembering His name *(smaraṇam),* rendering service unto Him *(pādasevanam),* worshipping *(arcana),* paying obeisance *(vandanam),* dedicating one's actions *(dāsyam),* to be friendly *(sakhya),* and offering oneself for His service and care *(ātma nivedanam)* are the nine types of worship hidden in *kriyāyoga* of Patañjali.

The *japa, artha* and *bhāvanam* are implicit in these nine aspects of *bhakti.* In fact the body, senses of perception, organs of action, mind, intelligence, I-ness, consciousness and conscience are all made to be in tune with the three paths of *karma, jñāna* and *bhakti.*

It is also interesting to know that the principles of *niyama* in a nut shell insulates all the other aspects of yoga, namely; *āsana, prāṇāyāma* and *pratyāhāra* in *tapas*; *dhāraṇā and dhyāna in svādhyāyā* and *samādhi* or *kaivalya* in *Īśvara praṇidhāna.*

III.3. - *Āsana*

III.3.1. – What is an *āsana*

Āsana means a seat as well as a posture. The word *āsana* comes from the root *āsa,* which means to sit or to lay down. It means to assume and assert a particular position bringing both description and definition in the position. It also means to exist, to present, to dwell-in, to abide. *Āsana* is a state where one arranges and assumes a particular position or form and re-forms it for a right configuration with study *(svādhyāya)*. Positioning the body for posing means action. Re-posing means reflective action. So after action one has to observe, re-think and re-reflect on parts of the body that work and parts of the body that are not working. Similarly, one has to observe which part of the body, the mind is penetrating and which part is not penetrating. Again, one has to look and see along with the body's extension, expansion and contraction, whether the mind and intelligence concurrently and evenly occupies the entire body in its extension, expansion and contraction. This is reflective re-posing.

While performing the *āsana* this action, reflection and reaction makes the practitioner to re-adjust his intelligence sensitively and accurately to cover each limb from end to end. If one learns to extend equally this intellectual sensitivity to all parts of the body along with the self, the *āsana* transforms into contemplative or meditative *āsana*. This must be the aim of each *sādhaka*, to reach the ultimate descriptive and definitive condition in all the *āsana*. Then his practice turns divine.

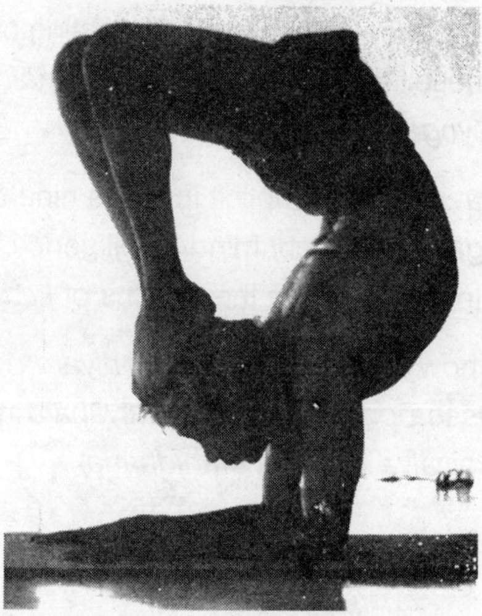

Plate n. 4 – Extend intellectual sensitivity equally, along with the self

The 12th and 13th *sūtra* of the *Vibhūti Pāda* is interesting and should be noted by all practitioners. *Sūtra* 12 defines and explains what is concentration *(ekāgra citta): tataḥ punaḥ śānta uditau tulya pratyayau cittasya ekāgratāpariṇāmaḥ* – where study of the rising and falling thought processes are kept in balance, so that a steady uninterrupted flow of intensive attention takes place in the *citta*. This is concentration (*ekāgra citta*). Then the 13th *sūtra* explains with: *etena bhūtendriyeṣu dharma lakṣaṇa avasthā pariṇāmā vyākhyātāḥ* – it means that the cultured potential *citta (dharma),* transforms for further refinement (*lakṣaṇa*), to reach the zenith of the assumed state or position. This definition is enough for us to know what perfect *āsana* means.

Dharma is sense of duty, *lakṣaṇa* is qualified sense of duty and *avasthā* is stability in body, mind, intelligence and consciousness. In this state, no further oscillations or alternations takes place. In this perfect presentation of the *āsana*, one reaches from one pointedness to no pointedness.

Again, one can trace what an *āsana* means from: *tasya vācakaḥ praṇavaḥ* (*Y.S.*, I.27), and *tajjapaḥ tadarthabhāvanam* (*Y.S.*, I.28).

For me, *āsana* represents God. He is represented in *praṇava – āuṁ*. Their repeated attempt is *japa*. Assuming the *āsana* is *ā*. After assuming the *āsana*, reflecting on the *āsana*, its purpose, usage and significance are the means, wealth *(artha)*. This stands for *u*. After reflection and reposing the *āsana* and experiencing the right feel in the form of exhilaration and bliss represents *bhāvanā* and *ṁ* in *āuṁ*.

Here one reaches from one pointed state to a no-pointed state, expressing an undisturbed state in body, senses, mind, intelligence and self.

This is what an *āsana* is and only in this state of presentation: *sthira sukham āsanam* (II.46), fits in precisely and accurately.

III.3.2. – Effect of *āsana*

The body is inert *(tāmasic)*, mind is dynamic *(rājasic)* and soul is illuminative and quiet *(sāttvic)*. The practice of *āsana* is to extinguish differences of these *guṇa* between body, mind and self (see *sūtra* IV., 32, 33, 34).[1]

Āsana practice keeps the organic, cellular, circulatory, digestive, respiratory, reproductory and glandular systems of the body, in a healthy balanced state. *Āsana* are done for maintaining

---

1 *tataḥ kṛtārthānāṁ pariṇāmakrama samāptiḥ guṇānām* (IV.32) – when a virtuous state of consciousness is attained, qualities of nature *(guṇa)* come to rest. Having fulfilled their purpose, their sequence of successive mutations is at an end.

Kṣaṇa pratiyogī pariṇāma aparānta nirgrāhyaḥ kramaḥ (IV.33) – as the mutation of the *guṇa* cease to function, the movements of moments and time come to a stand-still. This deconstruction of the flow of time is comprehensible only at the stage of emancipation.

Puruṣārtha śūnyānāṁ guṇānāṁ pratiprasavaḥ kaivalyaṁ svarūpapratiṣṭhā vā citiśaktiḥ iti (IV., 34) – *Kaivalya*, liberation, comes when the yogi has fulfilled the *puruṣārtha*, the fourfold aims of life, and has transcended the *guṇa*. Aims and *guṇa* return to their source, and consciousness is established in its own natural purity.

control on all these systems including muscles, fibres, tendons and the nervous system *(snāyu vṛtti nirodha)*.

Praśnōpaniṣad explains that if consciousness is the elder brother, *prāṇa* is the younger brother, the youngster is more energetic than his elder. The younger brother, in the form of energy, works faster in all the yogic movements than its elder brother, the consciousness. While practising *āsana*, the consciousness as the elder brother has to guide the younger brother *prāṇa*, to flow and function with rhythm.

We have been gifted with *prajñā* and *prāṇa*. If *prāna* is energy, *prajñā* is consciousness. These two are life's twins. In the normal walk of life they never function with equal potency. Through *āsana* and *prāṇāyāma*, they are made to move together to co-operate and co-ordinate the body with perfect understanding between them. The main aim of *āsana* is to awaken and bring the latent energy and consciousness that is hidden in the body to surface and act in unison. Here, the intelligence is made to act dynamically to connect the outer body with the inner body and the outer mind with the inner mind. This union of the outer body the inner body with the mind helps the consciousness to be in one with the entire human system. This is the value of the *āsana*.

Āsana awakens the *prāṇa* and develops *prajñā*. I call it *prāṇa jāgṛti* and *prajñā jāgṛti*. First the practitioner needs to bring energy and consciousness to the level of the body. Then *prāṇa jāgṛti* and *prajñā jāgṛti* are brought to function evenly in *prāṇāyāma* to enrich that *prāṇic* energy. This process continues until *samādhi*.

Patañjali says that to avoid failure in his endeavour the *sādhaka* must develop four aspects in his yogic discipline, namely: faith, vigour, memory, and power of absolute absorption *(śraddhā vīrya smṛti samādhiprajñā)*. If faith is *prajñā*, vigour is *prāṇa*. Memory is strengthened with *prāṇa* and utilised by *prajñā*. With this the matured state of awareness *(samādhi prajñā)* is achieved. Thus, *āsana-sādhanā* helps the *sādhaka* in awakening *prāṇa* in order to develop *prajñā*.

III.3.3. – Can the practitioners of *āsana* in the circus become yogis and yoginis

As this question was posed to me on several occasions, I think here is the right place to cover it. If I were a circus performer and studied my state of mind at those times I could have answered with ease whether he/she becomes a yogi or yogini or not.

It may be possible that they do not churn their intelligence on yogic discipline. Probably they may not involve their intelligence as much as a yoga practitioner does. Yet their daily practice keeps them mobile and active, though they often suffer injuries in the early part of their life.

Elasticity of the body is not always a God given gift. But the after-effects of movements presented with mobile and flexible bodies are quite different to that of a yogi's presentation of *āsana*. Those who engage in them are not interested to know whether their limbs of the body are aligned or their minds are involved with their bodies or not. In case they get involved totally, co-ordinating their minds with the body and in paying attention on interweaving the body and mind with the self, then who knows, they may become good yogis or yoginis.

In our class, we find often some supple bodies. They do not respond to challenges, nor balance evenly with counter challenges. But as a yoga teacher I explain the difference between a healthy suppleness and a non-healthy suppleness. I point out how elastic persons use the parts of body that bend without any co-ordination from the other parts and mind. I teach how to resist and make those parts stiff which bend without any response. I bring awareness in their intelligence to hold the muscles and limbs of the body firm in their movements. This brings a tremendous difference in their presentation where their intelligence is brought to function with the feel of each fibre and tendon to be alive. This way I advise them that each of their movements has to be challenged and equally counter-challenged when encountering the suppleness. The fibres, spindles should communicate and talk to each other in their hidden inexplicable language.

If those who perform in circuses follow these guidelines, who knows they may turn out as yogis or yoginis.

III.3.4. – Are *āsana* contortions

Āsana are not contortions of the body. Patañjali says that the effect of *āsana* leads one to get perfection in body, graceful form, loveliness and beauty, physical, mental and intellectual vigour, firmness and hardness and the brilliance of a diamond, and it brings softness in his heart due to purity of intelligence that equals the purity of the soul.

This study gave me the idea that such exalted wisdom in the yogis, said by Kalidasa: "A person's nature is as hard and brilliant as a diamond and at the same time as soft as a flower": *vajrädapi kaṭhorāṇi mṛduni kusumādapi.* Each *āsana* has a beautiful shape, grace and elegance that bestows power and makes the practitioner as strong as a diamond and at the same time as soft as flower.

While performing *āsana,* there should be no contortion, distortion or refraction. It should not happen even in infinitesimal particle of the muscle tissue. This is the definition of *sthira sukham āsanam* (*Y.S.,* II.46), as well as *rūpa lāvaṇya bala vajra saṁhananatvāni kāyasaṁpat,* (*Y.S.,* III.47).

Thank God, since two decades the words contortion and contortionist are disappearing from the vocabulary as far as *āsana* are concerned. *Āsana* are not contortions, but the art of positioning the body in different shapes without altering its anatomical structure. As each and every part of a vehicle has to be lubricated for smooth running and durability, *āsana* does that for the vehicle, the body, of the Soul. For healthy dynamic positive life, not only do the joints, muscles, fibres, tendons and cells get auto-massaged but total attention is paid to explore the unexplored areas within the body. These seemingly impossible positions, as per our knowledge, are of great value.

How does one value art? Has music or painting any value as gold or currency? Art is meant for art's sake. Its value is self-satisfaction, contentment, happiness and elation. Moreover, its spiritual value cannot be measured or gauged. *Yogāsana* are not an entertainment *(bhogāsana),* into twists and bends of strange and unnatural positions, but a part of an inward journey.

III.3.5. – Can *āsana* evolve the practitioner

Bees go to drink the hidden nectar of the flower. The flower does not go to the bees asking them to suck its essence. We, as bees, have to go to the *āsana* to savour their essence. *Āsana* do not come to us asking us to savour their flavour.

Does the *āsana* evolve or do we evolve? *Āsana* are adopted by us. As we involve ourselves more in their practice, we evolve. Obviously the quality of presentation of *āsana* improves as we proceed. Though we often use the word "perfection", it is not easy to reach. We have to experiment through performance and experience. The body, mind and self have to be brought to co-ordinate without any sense of relationship (subjective-objective) between them.

Then it is possible to experience perfection. But this being a practical experience cannot be explained or defined. My practice has made me to live in the unison of body, mind and soul.

Practice towards perfection is a step of the ladder that one goes on climbing to reach the subtlest of the subtle and firmest of the firm. Know this as perfection.

When we start to practise *āsana*, *prāṇāyāma* and *dhyāna*, they act as objects and we act as subjects. We have to use these objective aspects to evolve ourselves so that we move towards subtler and finer aspects, and experience soon the loss of separate identities of object and subject as they become one. This is the state that Patañjali explains in the first chapter – *kṣīṇavṛtteḥ abhijātasya iva maṇeḥ grahītṛ grahaṇa grāhyeṣu tatstha tadañjanatā samāpattiḥ* (I.41) – the yogi experiences that the knower, the instrument of knowing and the known are one and the same – the seer. Like a pure transparent jewel, he lives in this unsullied purity.

III.3.6. – Why basic *āsana* differ in different schools

If Patañjali had described the *āsana* in detail with sequential form everything in his treatise, then probably differences would not have been there. Patañjali's *Sūtra* is practical, with a philosophical background. Hence, his book is in the form of aphorisms. His explanations on *āsana* and *prāṇāyāma* are concise. Whereas the *Haṭhayoga Pradīpikā* is a technical book with stanzas, and deals on *āsana* a little more. The *sādhaka* has to trace the *āsana* and *prāṇāyāma* through other yoga text-books to understand the subject on *āsana* of Patañjali.

I cannot find an answer regarding different schools prescribing variations in the basic *āsana*. Speaking for myself, I have worked myself for years and years to explore this field. For example, when I wrote *Light on Yoga*, I gave a five and half year course and I forgot to mention that it was intended for highly intense students to master within that time. But today, with my vast experience, I say that the same course cannot be perfected in those five and half years. It takes more time than what I anticipated then. At that time I did not think of mild or medium practitioners but measured the readers according to my keen practice and my mental trend.

Over the years not only the anatomy of human beings surfaced with clear thoughts and depth of the anatomical structure, but also the anatomical structure of the *āsana*. I codified the *āsana* and showed their stages. If I had not studied the living anatomy of human beings and anatomical structure of each *āsana*, I would have probably given whatever method was available to follow. I began watching thousands and thousands of bodies with their mobility as well as their rigidity of the muscles and joints. It gave me a fund of knowledge to study the basic of the basics of each *āsana* and I say it is not possible to learn in six years as I mentioned in *Light on Yoga* but it may take a life time.

When young I found that *Trikoṇāsana* was easy and *Pārśvakoṇāsana* difficult. Hence, I introduced *Trikoṇāsana* in the book. Today I see that many do with ease *Pārśvakoṇāsana* and not *Trikoṇāsana*. Many have the confidence to do this *āsana* with bent knee with comfort, rather than *Trikoṇāsana* with straight legs. Such observation opened my eyes to simplify and present *āsana* from the base of the basic foundation. This way of study helped me to evolve in sequencing *āsana* that would not be difficult for many. If teachers teach basic *āsana* according to their own body's mobility, they are not going to be good teachers.

A teacher has to see the presentation of hundreds of people and change his teachings as per their needs and find out how they react. This helps him to adopt and adapt the ways of planning to teach.

If one goes to different doctors, each one prescribes different medicine for the same ailment, according to his understanding. It is same with yoga. It is possible to iron out these differences and agree on a mutual programme if all yogis could meet. Unfortunately, many of today's yoga masters may not be true practitioners. Short courses are held everywhere and teaching certificates are issued.

Once I was called to attend and prepare a syllabus of yoga for children. They all wanted meditation to be introduced, but I protested and told them that children know only two things: either to be totally active or go to sleep at once. As they do not have emotional disturbances they need no meditation. Why make children intellectually impotent at that age was beyond my comprehension. I wanted them to focus their intelligence and develop attentiveness. But my views were not taken into consideration and they formed a syllabus as a pilot plan for schools with no background of experience. Teachers and members who serve such committees ought to be practical and broad-minded.

If we sit together and work out a system, probably we may present a syllabus minimising the difference and is beneficial to everyone. This I have undertaken and many do follow.

Probably the ego in yoga teachers is the cause of presenting the *āsana* differently in different schools.

III.3.7. – Are *āsana* new or old

Actually there are no demarcations in *āsana* like old and new. The yoga texts proclaim eight and half million *āsana*. As such why worry about new and old?

We came to know only a few decades ago that nuclear energy can destroy the whole world. When we did not know about it before, did not the nuclear energy exist? It was there, but we were not aware of that. Similarly, everything that exists in the world is real, but we don't know. Only if someone rediscovers something, they term it as new. I haven't created but re-discovered. I might have modified or connected the loose links. All these *āsana* were practised and were in vogue as we see them in temple carvings. These carvings on temple walls are enough proof for us to believe that innumerable *āsana* were there in existence. As God is the creator of this world, His creation has no end and whatever was created will be there. Hence, there is nothing new or nothing old.

III.3.8. – *Āsana* on mental health and stability

Body is a gross form of the mind and mind is the gross form of the soul. As such one should not read too much on differences between body and mind as mind and soul are encased in the body. Therefore they cannot be separated. If one gets pricked, does it not affect his mind and self? In case one is in sorrow and misery, does it not affect his body? This is enough proof to point out that the body and mind are inter-connected and inter-woven. Only we have to learn to inter-relate them through *āsana* and *prāṇāyāma*. It is not fair to say that physical diseases are different from psychological diseases as one causes the other to suffer or elate. Any psychological tension, whether stress, strain or pressure, depends upon the physical non-well-beingness. If one is upset physically, it affects the mind and the mind broods on it. Therefore, whatever forms of suffering are there, they are termed as psycho-somatic disease, or somato-psycho disease. Similarly the psychological pressure or the physical disease has a bearing on physiological organs such as the liver, spleen, pancreas, intestines, heart and lungs.

When one speaks of the physical body he has to correlate always that the physical and physiological bodies have a bearing on the psychological and intellectual bodies. One cannot control an afflicted organ by the mind, but he has to act co-ordinating his body and mind to work on that afflicted organ. Body has to be used by the mind in a right way to get well again. Mind is the instrument of consciousness (all pervading power). The consciousness has to discipline the mind by making it to work on the body for it to function well in order to keep it healthy. The soul enlightens the consciousness, to guide the intelligence. The intelligence in turn guides the mind to work on the body for it to function healthily.

Patañjali defines *āsana* and *prāṇāyāma* without giving names. Through their practice, one begins to concentrate first on the physical and organic body. When they are kept healthy, he moves toward the soul. The moment the mind turns towards its source, it loses its identity and remains beyond peace and sorrow. This is how *āsana* frees one from the physical frame of mind and leads one towards the healthy spiritual frame of mind. This is how the values of *āsana* affect the mind.

MENTAL STABILITY

As body and mind are naturally integrated, they influence one another. Hence, the *āsana* practice not only affects the body but affects the mind and in turn both affect the self. The mind being very mercurial gets caught in sorrows, pleasures, emotions and moods. *Āsana* has the power to work in such a manner that they change the attitude of our body, mind, intelligence and ego confidently to undergo a stream of change by making them ecstatically happy and exultant so that they move together in unison and meet the soul.

The varieties of *āsana* help our musculo-skeletal body to undergo changes with the help of our mind. For example, if the shoulder blades are out, one will have a hunch back, the slight structural defect is enough to change our mood and attitude. The caved in chest does not allow one to breathe correctly. The protruded abdomen restricts the movements and makes one lazy. Therefore, varieties of *āsana* are necessary if needed to change the structure of the body.

Similarly, if one of our inner organs suffers with some problem, it affects our mind. For instance, take glandular system. If the thyroid has less iodine, there will be more secretion of hormones and on account of this obviously one suffers from mental imbalances. The hypo and hyper thyroidism affects both body and mind. Adrenals change the personality of man. High blood pressure causes anxiety and fear. For this reason innumerable *āsana* were discovered and propounded by ancient yogis, in order to gain permanent over-all physical and mental health and harmony,

If a person is depressed or moody, talking on philosophy is meaningless. Instead he or she has to build up the courage with the help of seasoned masters with loads of experience to solve practically his or her problems and eradicate confusion.

There are specific *āsana* such as *Śīrṣāsana*, *Sarvāṅgāsana*, *Viparīta Daṇḍāsana*, which build up courage.

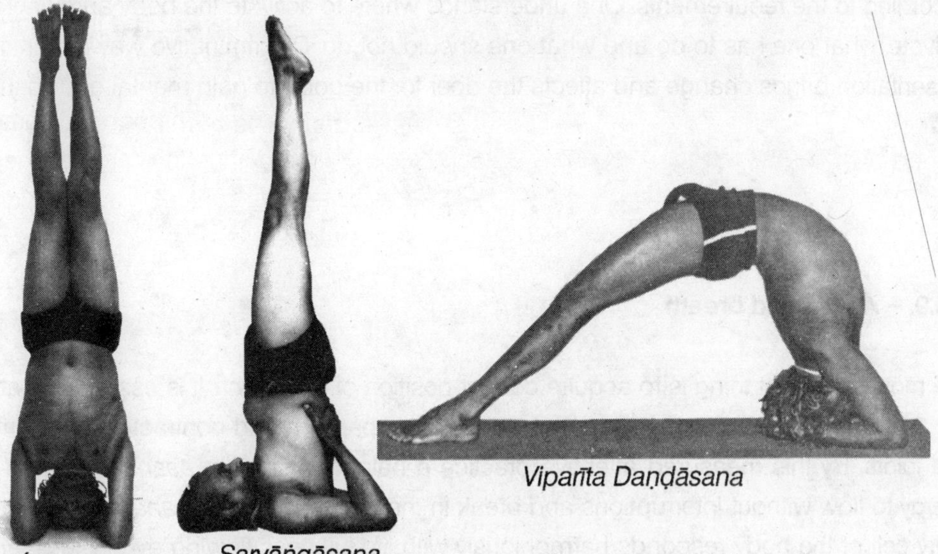

Śīrṣāsana *Sarvāṅgāsana* *Viparīta Daṇḍāsana*

Plate n. 5 – *Āsana* to build courage and bring intellectual clarity

A person might be highly intellectual but gets caught in emotional problems. Mental health needs both intellectual as well as emotional stability.

The intelligence in a person has two branches. One branch moves towards the brain while the other towards the heart. When one is depressed, the upward flow of energy facing the brain gets retarded. The retarded energy makes one to brood and it sinks the mental heart. Some *āsana* work on emotional quietness by stabilising the emotional centre. Some *āsana* help one in developing intellectual sharpness, alertness, smartness and power to endure any type of physical load whereas some other *āsana* makes the mind move inwards to penetrate the interior mind. Particularly, the inverted *āsana* not only bring intellectual clarity but also emotional stability. In these inverted *āsana* the head is subdued and heart is energised. The life-energy flows in these regions creating joy without any disturbances.

As the mind of everyone does not act in the same manner, to mention specific *āsana* is difficult. An old man may not be able to perform all the *āsana* meant for depression, as a youngster can. Therefore, the variety of *āsana* is required to be known. One has to see, who can perform what? What is the capacity to bring the required change? So one has to work personally within himself as well as with the patients. Techniques of yoga have to be co-ordinated through experimentation and study of one's own problems.

The practice of *āsana* stimulates deep bio-chemical changes. The brain and the glandular system undergo transformation. The metabolism of the body is adjusted and corrected according to the requirements. One understands where to activate the body and where not to activate, what one has to do and what one should not do. Discriminative way of thinking and presentation brings change and affects the doer for the good to gain mental equilibrium.

III.3.9. – *Āsana* and breath

The most important thing is to acquire correct position of the *āsana*. It is essential to attend to the *āsana* with a measured freedom of extension, expansion and contraction in the muscles and joints. By this measured attentive practice a balanced state in *āsana* is earned for the energy to flow without interruptions and break in the body. Accurate *āsana* is when each and every cell of the body responds harmoniously with life-full-ness flowing evenly and smoothly. This accurate presentation of *āsana* helps the intelligence to adjust the flow of the breath according to the extension or contraction of the lungs, without disturbing the position of the body in the *āsana*.

Compartmental attention and practice of *āsana* not only makes the breath go zigzag but also disturbs the mind . As ants move on a single path without losing the line, the self has to move in line with the *āsana*. Like a spider moving in its web, the consciousness, intelligence, mind, senses of perception and organs of action, along with the breath, must move in line to the self and close to each other in the *āsana* without disturbing the flow of energy or the touch of self with the body.

Each and every cell, fibre, sinew of the body is to be attentive. This is *ekāgratā citta* in *āsana*. When *āsana is* performed with this one-pointed attention, one experiences their wholeness.

Holding of the breath is not the aim in *āsana*. Each breath has four blades – inhalation, inhalation-retention, exhalation and exhalation-retention. They have to be used according to the need of the body in *asana*, as each *āsana* has its own breathing pattern.

First learn to be attentive to the wholeness of an *āsana* and watch the breath. Take each breath in such a way that the position of the *āsana* is held in a disturbed state without swinging but steadily maintaining throughout the course of the *āsana*.

Through this practice of taking each breath in each *āsana*, one realises why yogic texts insist on mastery of *āsana* before *prāṇāyāmic* breathing.

See how all the great scientists work day and night in their laboratories to find out even a little bit of fact. Is it not their total absorption that is nothing but the quality of meditation. It is the same in *āsana sādhanā*, where one has to look and enter the unthought parts in the frontier of the body and reach those parts so that he experiences the fact of what Ultimate Truth is!!

Meditation is enhancement, expansion and enlightenment of the intelligence. Through the practice of *āsana* and *prāṇāyāma* one mends, sharpens and moulds the intelligence, and stays in the *āsana* as if he is in a state of meditation.

Let me remind the *sādhaka* to the aphorisms of Patañjali: *prayatna śaithilya ananta samāpattibhyām* (II.46), and *tataḥ dvandvaḥ anabhighātaḥ* (II.48) – when perfection in *āsana* is achieved, the infinite being that is within is reached. Then on, the pairs of opposite do not exist.

This way of practice of *āsana* takes one to be steadfast in the body and makes him to experience the Self dwelling in its own true splendour. This is the hidden wisdom of *sthira sukham āsanam (Y.S.,* II.46).

III.3.10. – Body and mind in *āsana*

Yoga is meant to yoke and unite not only the limbs of the body, but also the mind and the self.

If the vessels are of different shapes, the occupying water takes those shapes touching the jar everywhere evenly. In the same way one has to practise *āsana* for the mind, intelligence and consciousness to touch and occupy evenly every nook and corner of the inner surface of the body without leaving any room. Even the lobes of the brain are to be placed harmoniously and balanced with the centre of the spine. This is how one has to practise all the *āsana* and reach that natural state experiencing serenity and oneness from the skin to the self in *āsana*.

While practising *āsana* bring a hairline stretch as fibres are like an extended thread. As one combs the hair, the practitioner has to comb the fibres in *āsana*. With a clear picture of the *āsana,* he has to measure the flesh on either side of that hairline to test the evenness, and make the energy to percolate without void and make the mind to touch evenly all sides of the body as if it is saying, "I am touching the minutest parts of the body." While doing the *āsana,* the intellectual flow has to convey its presence to the self. This state in practice is called *tanmayatā*. *Tanmayatā* is a state of engrossment or absorption.

I would like to give *Tāḍāsana* as an example to think and act in all *āsana*. When one stands in *Tāḍāsana*, the intelligence flows on the outer heel of one foot and on the inner heel of the other. The moment one feels that the intelligence is not even on the feet, he has to act to align the muscles (the jar), so that the intelligence finds its level on the inner and the outer frontiers of the feet, giving a correct shape to the legs for the accurate presentation of the *āsana*.

Treat the inner, the outer, the front and the back skin as banks of the intellectual river and see whether the flow of the river touches the four banks of the body in each *āsana*, without deviation. See in the *āsana* or *prāṇāyāma* practice that the intelligence flows like a river and not like a brook. If the intelligence moves like a brook it is a violent practise. A brook deviates and breaks its banks in its flow but a river flows within its banks. The water of the brook flows aggressively gouging the banks, while the flow of water in a river is smooth, quiet and serene. Hence, follow the analogy of the flow of the river in *asana* and *prāṇāyāma* practice.

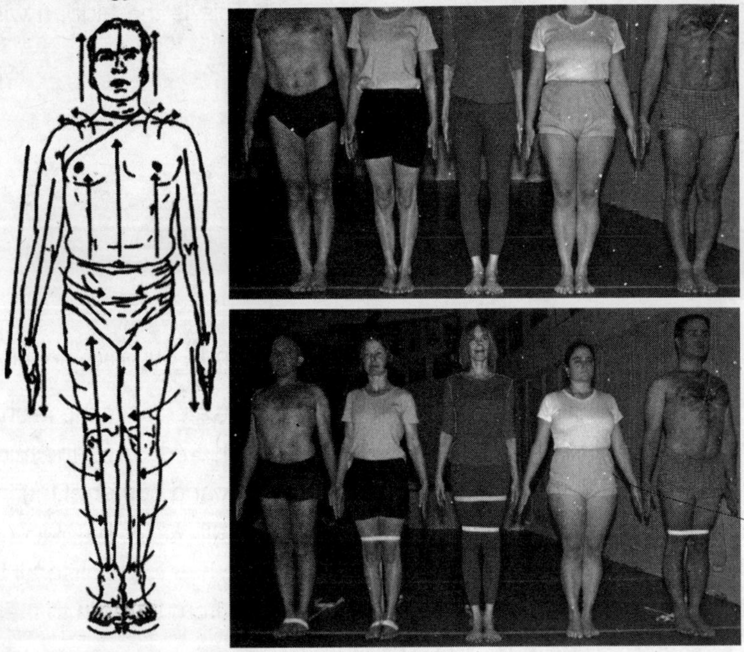

Plate n. 6 – Standing in *Tāḍāsana*

We have a river of intelligence, river of consciousness, river of attention, river of awareness. This attention and awareness has to flow steadily and smoothly to seep into the frontiers of the body. This is the right practice of *āsana*, or the *summum bonum* of the *āsana* practice.

III.3.11. – Importance of Inversions

Nothing in yoga is nadir or zenith. Hence, a *sādhaka* has to respect and consider that all things are important.

Inversions are not only good but also effective as the venous blood is made to flow back without strain for recharge. Standing on the head is not all yoga. It is a leaf of the tree of *āsana*. *Āsana* are like the countless leaves of a tree where each leaf does its function to preserve the branches, the trunk and the root. The brain draws one quarter of arterial blood for oxygenation. Inverted *āsana* does this, with less strain and without stress on the arteries. Freshness in thinking is the attractive effect of the inversions.

Inversions are not the starting point in yoga. One has to learn to stand on the legs before trying to stand on the head. So one is taught to do *Tāḍāsana* and many other *āsana* before *Śīrṣāsana*. The body has to get used to inversions, otherwise fear complexes set in and a beginner says good-bye to practice. Beginner's are trained in sequential order starting with standing positions to forward extensions. Then they are taught to stand on the shoulders. This way they are taught step by step sequentially and once he learns shoulder stand *(Sarvāṅgāsana)*, then head balance *(Śīrṣāsana)* is taught. That is how the uninitiated is initiated towards *Śīrṣāsana* as inversions prove heaven to the brain.

III.3.12. – *Āsana* and metabolism

The metabolic clock sets the functioning of millions of cells in the body which integrate and disintegrate (catabolism-anabolism) for health or otherwise. Yoga practices ensure the full functioning of the life cycle of a cell. But no one uses this potential metabolism of the cell fully.

The cells are affected easily not only by the faulty physical and physiological functioning but also by the psychological and emotional state under duress. The practice of yoga affects the whole of man from the physical, moral, mental and spiritual levels, and as a result the cell-metabolism will be found totally on a different level.

Though modern medicine is a boon, unfortunately it has its limitations. The practice of yoga deals with a living anatomy. I can certainly say that the cellular life is prolonged as the cells are nourished through *āsana* and *prāṇāyāma*. Often with these practices the inner clock of metabolism becomes adjustable. You can slow down or make the metabolism to act fast according to the need of the system. Only one needs to have a good subjective knowledge of yoga, which depends upon repeated practice that filters the experiences also.

III.3.13. – Escapism in *sādhanā*

About thirty years ago I had two severe accidents. I had lost both control and balance as the injury were excruciating. I could not sit or stand. I could not lift my shoulders or move them up or back. Even stretching or bending the knees was painful. If I had gone to a doctor, it would have meant I lacked faith in my yoga. As I had practised yoga for years I decided to endeavour with determination and courage. I began my practice from scratch and it took me years to recover to a great deal. But some *āsana* still elude me, which is pointless to worry about. Due to the age factor, I have to make a lot of effort to maintain the practices even now. So I am happy in what I am doing, accepting the present situation rather than not trying at all.

I now do *āsana* that were impossible, after years of accidents. Even at the Barbican demonstration, in London, 1984, I could not move well, and friends asked me how I would put up with the pain whilst demonstrating. I said I will take care of the pain later but let me finish the demonstration. I did it and the entire audience stood up and clapped for minutes in appreciation of the presentation.

After ten years of accident, I could do a better *Vṛścikāsana*. I was observing carefully even a hairline movement of the body while doing *āsana*. These injuries made me a humble disciple of yoga, a better teacher and an encouraging performer. I hope this is sufficient encouragement for anyone to stick to the *sādhanā*. One need not be dissatisfied, or contented either. Even if one is lazy and dull, my advice would be to do what one can according to the situation and be happy even for a stretch of a hair's breadth. With this attitude, one can practise and not escape on some pretext or the other.

Many drop out, due to lack of enthusiasm. Treat this escapism as well as laziness as a friend and not as a foe. Take these things as encouragements to try and act again. They teach us to be patient and tolerant. Negativity is like a thick black cloud. The black clouds ultimately rain. If escapism, laziness and indiscipline are black clouds, know that it will rain when the practitioner's make up their mind to do. Then the heavy head gets light and one becomes alert and active, and attracted towards furthering the *sādhanā*. As each cloud has a silver lining, each impediment has a silver lining in one's *sādhanā*. Accept this and pursue the *sādhanā*.

III.3.14. – Is a *tīvra saṁvegin* an *ati-yogi*, or a vehement *sādhaka* a fanatic yogi

Recently, my method of practice has been coined as Iyengar Yoga. Only recently I came to know that one of the magazines on yoga (*Yoga and Life*) criticised me mentioning that I am an *ati-yogi* along with some other yogis. The article says that B.K.S. Iyengar, being the pupil of Prof. T. Krishnamacharya, is an *ati-yogi* (fanatical yogi). The author of the article has categorised me and my *guru* as *ati-yogi*. The article mentions that we are all fanatic *yogi*, going beyond normalcy. In other words it means we practise excessively. At the same time, the magazine praises me for becoming popular for the way my pupils do not get exhausted practising with my approach to yoga and the dramatic way of keeping the body beautiful.

Unfortunately it is a misquotation of Patañjali and an erroneous understanding of yoga. Patañjali explains four types of practitioners, namely; feeble, moderate, keen and supremely vigorous and intense in practice. If someone practises according to the precept of vigorous practice how does he become an *ati-yogi?* If one performs with emphasis on the elegance and beauty of *āsana*, one is stigmatised for attracting popularity.

Regarding the quality of *āsana*, Patañjali says in *Vibhūti Pāda*: *rūpa lāvaṇya bala vajra samhananatvāni kāya sampat* (*Y.S.*, III.47) – the wealth of a yogi's body is to have a perfect formation in body, possessing beauty, elegance, grace and strength with a lustrous complexion like a diamond, endowed with firmness and compactness.

In *Sanskrit*, there are two words for beauty, namely: *saundarya* and *lāvaṇya*. *Saundarya* means beauty in form and *lāvaṇya* means the elegance of beauty. Patañjali did not use the word *saundarya* but uses the word *rūpa* and *lāvaṇya*. *Rūpa* expresses the structural beauty and *lāvaṇya*, the elegant beauty of each part. If I ask my pupils to place each part of the body, each cell of the body elegantly in its place to beautify it without causing contortion or distortion, do they turn out to be *ati-yogi?* Patañjali includes strength, hardness and firmness, along with grace. All these explain the importance of correct *āsana*. Therefore, bringing such qualities while doing the *āsana*, does one become an *ati-yogi?* Patañjali wants the body like a thunderbolt.

He obviously wants the practice to be intense and pure for which we have to chisel and shape each part and each organ of the body from outside as well as inside.

The *yogi* of today have taken only one way, non-violent passive practice, and stop if it pains. Patañjali clears this through *bādhana* and *bhāvana* in the *Sādhana Pāda*; *vitarkabādhane pratipakṣabhāvanam* (II.33). He counsels the practitioners to cultivate a temperament of balancing *hiṁsā* (violence) with *ahiṁsā* (non-violence and vice-versa). He wants us to re-think pains (*bādhana*) to counteract with feeling (*bhāvana*).

If one feels the pain or hurt in the parts on one side of the body, he has to question why it is not happening on the very same parts of the other side of the body. Instead of advising not to practice, I say to investigate and experiment what wrong stretches are happening for the pain to occur and what right stretches are happening in not feeling the pain on the counter-part. This is *vitarka*, or analysis. If each one of us observes and learns to balance by adjusting the over stretch or the wrong stretch and the painful stretch to that of the non-painful side, learns to place the parts with measured alignment and correct judgement, so that the wrong stretch is converted into right stretch, then the words 'violence' and 'non-violence' fade from one's thoughts.

Today's yogis do not want their pupils to do *āsana* with effort, fearing that they may lose them. For them any extension or stretch which pricks the mind is *hiṁsā*. But they forget Patañjali when he says that adherence to a single-minded effort prevents these pains. Telling people to do only what is possible as *ahiṁsā* practice is an illusory notion. Many do not know how and when to balance *ahiṁsā* with *hiṁsā* and *hiṁsā* with *ahiṁsā* or the difference between hypo-action and hyper-active action. Even in hypo-activity, or non-violent activity, *hiṁsā* or violence is implicitly involved, though one thinks that it is a non-violent action *(ahiṁsā)*. Similarly in hyper-activity or violent activity (*hiṁsā*), yet in *ahiṁsā* it is explicitly involved. Hence, the definition of *āsana* as steadiness *(sthira)* and comfortable *(sukha)* are taken in a perverse sense.

See the contradiction in their studies of the *Yoga Sūtra*. Chapter I *sūtra* 13, says, "Practice is the steadfast effort to establish steadiness in oneself." Even if disharmony is there, I like to remind you here what Patañjali says in I.32, to face and make all efforts with single minded attention to remove any disharmony or dis-alingment in body and mind. Yet, again in II.47, he emphasises to achieve perfection of *āsana* with effort, so that the effort becomes natural, all resistance to effort fades-out and one feels effortlessness and can experience the intimate being that resides within the body.

If one sits comfortably on an easy chair, why does he get up after a few minutes when it becomes uncomfortable? Why does he change the position? Why does he shift the weight? We do not question these. In no *āsana*, can you be steadily comfortable unless there is perfect effort. See: *tatra sthitau yatnaḥ abhyāsaḥ* (*Y.S.*, I.13) – practice is a repeated effort to gain steadiness. How can this be forgotten?

If one uses a part of the body and neglects the other part of it, certainly the imbalance occurs. It means there is imbalance of *hiṁsā* with *ahiṁsā* and vice-versa varying in degrees in the *āsana*. The *āsana* should be weighed as a goldsmith assays gold. One has to weigh the body, as far as the *āsana* are concerned, architecturally, iconically and holistically, presenting them with veneration. Then, the intellectual energy and consciousness flow evenly on the right and the left sides lattitudinally as well as from north and south longitudinally (head and feet), front and back (anteriorly and posteriorly), evenly without deviating the channels in the body. This right flow of *prāṇic* energy with intellectual energy along with consciousness keeps one's body and mind pure both within and without. There should not be any languor or lassitude. Attention and vigour with a specific purpose in mind without allowing the energy to get dissipated is practice. In this type of practice there will be no pains but only knowledge.

Each one has to measure and weigh the energy and save it but not allow it to go to waste. This thinking and practising is not *ati-yoga* but is a judicious, precise and enlivening yoga. In such a practice, there is no fatigue, no *ati* and no *hiṁsā*.

III.3.15. – *Ajñāna yoga* to *prajñāna yoga* (from nescience to enlightenment)

In the early days of my practice, no doubt it was on a physical level. As years went by, I developed enthusiasm, interest and zeal to move towards *tīvrasaṁvega* (intensely intense) practices.

This interest, zeal and enthusiasm blended my *sādhanā* towards intellectual keenness and made me practise with energetic intensity. Enlightenment did not come to me by my mere attempt.

Though I had to face lots of physical pains and mental disenchantments, fortunately my zeal paid no heed to those impediments. My inner voice persistently made me to continue in spite of aches and disenchantments. Now, the effect of my efforts has influenced thousands and thousands of people all over the globe. I thank Lord Patañjali for gracing me to stick to practice without distracting thoughts.

Man is made of five elements and something beyond these also. Though I practised *āsana* using these five elements, I tried to search out and trace who is behind this elemental body while doing the *āsana*.

To prepare a pot, a potter is needed. I searched for that potter within me while practising. Being sincere and deep in my approach, I began to realise the secrets of Patañjali's sayings of knowing the doer, the instrument and the force behind the aim. I tried to experience his words that the perceiver *(grahitṛ),* perceiving *(grahaṇa)* and the objects perceived *(grāhya)* are one and the same (see *Y.S.,* I.42).

When I had pain I tried to find out who is suffering with pain? I gradually realised that the capital "I" never suffers, nor has pain. Realising that the true "I" does not suffer, my vehemence and enthusiasm directed me to go beyond the known small "i" or me.

It is not just hours of practice that were important, but I utilised my *āsana sādhanā* to watch carefully moment to moment my physical and emotional reactions of my head and heart, which revealed to me that I could come out of these limitations. My adherence to yoga and sincere watchful devoted practice changed not only my destiny but also my ways of living.

I feel that I should not talk much on my successes, because one does not know what is in one's destiny. But one can certainly safeguard by remaining non-attached to successes by sticking to the *sādhanā*. I say with my hands on my heart that I am free from sorrows (*kleśa*) to a great extent.

Patañjali after explaining the *dharmegha samādhi (Y.S.,* IV.29), explains the effect of this samādhi in the succeeding sūtra: "then comes the end of affliction from actions," *tataḥ kleśa karma nivṛttiḥ (Y.S.,* IV.30) – it means the *sādhaka* becomes free from afflictions.

I can assure anyone that if he does *āsana* and *prāṇāyāma* regularly, as I did with attention and devotion, he too can experience freedom from physical and mental sorrows. For me *āsana* and *prāṇāyāma* are my *Iśṭa-devatā* by choice.

In practice, one has to ensure that he balances his body and mind evenly weighing aggressive force with non aggressive force. Effort and effortlessness should be carefully balanced in each *āsana.* While doing the *āsana* one has to watch the breath, where the breath touches, and question why it is not touching the other parts. Similarly, one has to observe with the intellectual eye whether the energy is distributed evenly and equally throughout the body. This observation is *svādhyāya.* Know that each *āsana* is a chapter *(adhyāya)* in itself. Only one has to learn to know how to read it.

Prāṇāyāma is not mere breathing or retention of the breath. Inhalations and exhalations are like the movements of the mind. Stability in the in-breath, out-breath and retention means stability in the mind. Soul is reflected in the stable mind. Hence, I watch my *pūraka, recaka* and *kumbhaka* in each cycle of *prāṇāyāma*. If practice does not lead towards knowledge and understanding, then it is *ajñāna yoga,* and if it leads towards knowledge and illumination, it is *prajñāna yoga*. Hence, observe while practicing whether it ends up in *ajñāna yoga* or *prajñāna yoga*. *Prajñāna sādhanā* leads one towards the withdrawal of the senses *(pratyāhāra)*.

In a perfect *āsana*, the consciousness tends to go inwards. It is under a centripetal state. The efforts end at this stage and awareness begins to spread all over like water spreading evenly on the floor. This is the centrifugal state of consciousness. In *āsana* one has to get glimpses of this feeling by connecting the entire frontier of the body towards the core and vice-versa. If the centripetal state is *dhāraṇā,* the centrifugal state is *dhyāna*. So diffuse the centripetal state harmoniously everywhere turning *dhāraṇā* into *dhyāna*.

It is a fact that *āsana* is only one limb of yoga, but one can feel and experience the other limbs of yoga without branding them with names. The practice of *āsana* for me is like worship. Saints worship God. In my practice I worship *āsana* as my deity. If one can understand what I am saying, then he may go beyond the realm of the physical frame with clear intelligence and clean consciousness to experience the essence of life. This essence of life is enlightenment, which is nothing but Self-realisation. From this state proceed towards God-realisation.

III.3.16. – Centre of gravity in *āsana*

I am not a scientist to speak on gravity. We are on this planet because of gravitational force. The earth is moving around the sun due to the solar gravity. The gravity changes according to the power of attraction.

As far as the *āsana* is concerned, the centre of gravity is not the same for each *āsana,* as each has a different position and hence the centre of gravity changes. If one stands on his legs and does *Tāḍāsana*, and if the weight on the legs is unequal, it means the centre of gravity has changed. In slanting the body, the gravity changes. One may not fall from the *āsana*, but one has to recycle the slant that is created by shifting to the other side so that one brings back the centre of gravity to the base.

As far as the presentation of *āsana* goes, if one adjusts the body with right presentation, he experiences the feel of lightness. In this state know that the centre of gravity has changed in that *āsana*.

The *Haṭhayoga Pradīpikā* (I.17) says that the practice of *āsana* has to be such that it should bring levity in the body and mind *(aṅgalāghvam)*. The body has to feel the lifefulness and lightness in a perfect presentation. In order to bring this lightness, one needs to work in a particular way to ensure that the body does not become heavy or sway or sink. In each *āsana*, one has to feel the sense of ascendance and upliftment in the body and intelligence. This firm presentation brings lightness and one feels the elevation in mind.

In *Utthita Trikoṇāsana*, if one overextends and brings hyperextension in the leg muscles, the heavy weight is felt on the legs but if one stretches the thigh muscles in par with the calf muscles they move up and one feels the lessening of weight on the legs. If the distance between the two legs is adjusted properly one does not feel the body sagging. From this measured adjustment one experiences where the centre of gravity should be.

In *Sālamba Śīrṣāsana* often one pushes the shoulders downwards. On account of this downward stretch pain in the neck and shoulders appears. As one drops the shoulders downwards in Tāḍāsana, he has to ascend the sagging shoulders and legs in *Śīrṣāsana* to remove congestion in the neck which causes pain.

If the body in each *asana* is properly adjusted the centre of gravity shifts and this causes emotions and intelligence to change for the better in the *āsana*.

While doing the *āsana*, if the chest sinks one feels emotional disturbance. This is particularly felt when one is depressed or in a state of loneliness. Sometimes even fear complexes sink the body's position changing the centre of gravity. The moment the chest opens in back-bends, the emotional centre opens, the body changes its shape and one feels elated. But if the chest gets collapsed, then the mind sinks and the emotional weather becomes heavy, which means that the gravitational force has changed.

If the position of the body is corrected in *āsana* emotional stability occurs, which makes one to understand the trueness of the *āsana*. If the position of the body is wrong, then the practitioner suffers body pain, which in turn disturbs his mind.

When one does *āsana* while drowsy or in a doped state, the state of body and mind changes and he injures the brain. He remains morose and blank, which means that he has disturbed his intellectual gravitational force.

The centre of gravity of the body and the mind as well as the emotional and the intellectual centres should remain aligned. Then one finds the correct centre of gravity in an *āsana*. This way one has to find the centre in each *āsana*.

When Patañjali mentions *ananta samāpatti* in *āsana*, it means that in each *āsana*, the body and mind have to gravitate towards the centre of the soul. To touch that infinite within, the finite body has to work through āsana to develop sharpness of intelligence. This is the way one has tu rectify and perfect each *āsana* in order to gravitate towards that right centre. It depends not only upon one's intellectual calibre, but also on the devotional approach in his endeavour.

The true centre of the body is the Soul or the Core of the being. Whichever may be the *āsana*, the contents of the body, right and left sides are to be measured and balanced evenly in line with the Soul or the Core.

For example *Paripūrṇa Matsyendrāsana*. If the practitioner weighs the front, back and side trunk with equidistance to the core of the being, along with parallel adjustments of the spinal muscles, shoulder-blades, muscles of the arms, grips of the wrists and legs, I say he is close to the *ananta samāpatti*, i.e., embracing the Soul evenly from all sides of the body, directing towards the Soul as if all parts of the body are completely mingled to the core.

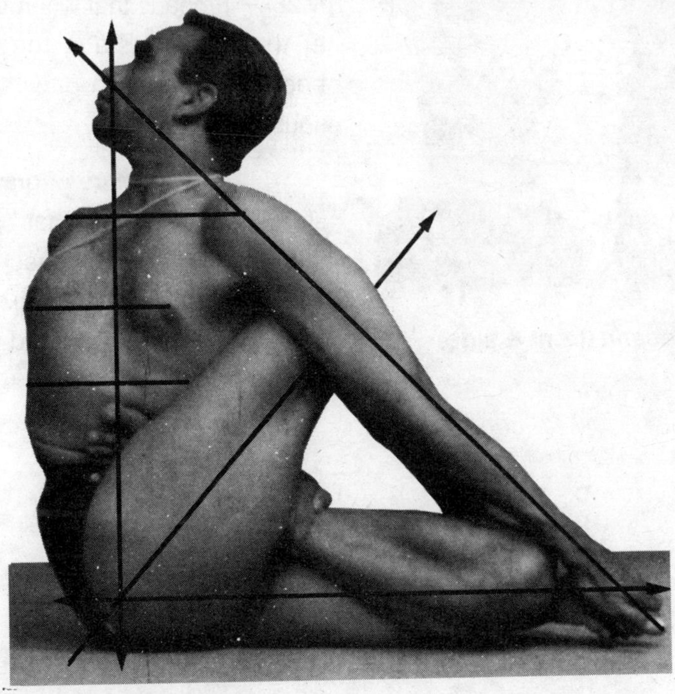

Plate n. 7 – *Paripūrṇa Matsyendrāsana*

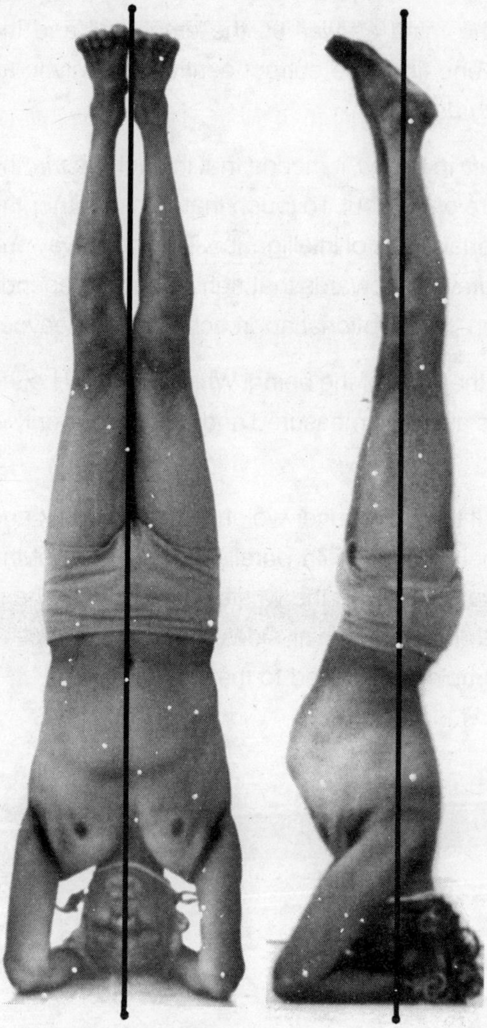

Plate n. 8 – *Sīrṣāsana* (front & side)

Let me take *Sīrṣāsana*. In this *āsana*, the sides of the body should be equi-length to the centre body and various parts of the arms and legs should be connected to the Self by maintaining the length of the body in line to the Soul, without bringing the legs forwards or backwards. The *Sīrṣāsana* must be like: *samaṁkāya śirogrīvaṁ dhārayam acalaṁ sthiraḥ* (*B.G.*, 6.13) – the crown of the head, the middle of the throat, the perineum, the middle of the knees, ankles and feet should be in a plumb line. Then this *āsana* is considered as a perfect *āsana*. This way all the *āsana* have to be practised to be in line to the core to experience the infinite that is within.

In *Kaivalya Pāda* Patañjali says: *tadā vivekanimnaṁ kaivalyaprāgbhāraṁ cittam* (*Y.S.*, IV.26) – it means that when the intelligence is at the exalted state, the consciousness becomes pure and gravitates towards the source – the Soul.

As the centre of gravity is not a fixed state in each *āsana*, what I stress is to trace the centre of gravity in each *āsana*. Be alert while doing the *āsana* so that the consciousness is gravitated towards the soul.

III.3.17. – *Śavāsana*

Śavāsana requires will-power to smooth the nerves, keep the brain restful and the flickering mind quiet.

The one who knows the art of full extension and expansion of the body and mind knows the art of total relaxation. Otherwise it is casual and compartmental.

I advise all not to do *Śavāsana* in between each *āsana* but at the end of the *āsana* as well as after a *prāṇāyāma* session.

Beginners strain a lot while learning *āsana*. They struggle to stretch their muscles to get movements in their bodies. They don't know how and where to activate and how and where to remain passive. As they are raw in their body actions, they strain their minds and intelligence creating tension in body, mind and intelligence. While learning the *āsana,* they have to direct their awareness in various directions, and hence they feel the stress. They also have to co-ordinate actions simultaneously with each and every part of the body, which exhausts them. Finally they are deeply involved with intellectual attention while doing the *āsana*. Therefore, their brain gets exhausted. At that stage *Śavāsana* acts as a boon or elixir.

Śavāsana may be done when one's brain refuses to attend, or the body does not take it and the intellect feels dull. It requires a great effort to learn the art of keeping the brain receptive. Hence each *āsana* teaches *Śavāsana* in various parts to get the right feel of relaxation, both in body and mind. Then when *Śavāsana* is done, one experiences the relaxation totally. While practising, each *āsana* creates a new life and a new energy and a perfect *āsana* does not exhaust the practitioner. An incomplete and imperfect *āsana* does exhaust. While performing *āsana*, one should not waste energy but generate it, so that they keep the body, mind and intelligence fresh, enjoying perfect *Śavāsana*.

Many students struggle to relax in *Śavāsana*. In that case *āsana* like *Uttānāsana, Paśchimottānāsana, Halāsana, Setu Bandha Sarvāṅgāsana, Viparīta Karaṇi* are good as they relax the practitioners faster than *Śavāsana*. *Uttānāsana* with legs apart and head on a stool, half *Halāsana* with legs resting on a stool relaxes the brain as well as the nerves quicker than in *Śavāsana*.

Very often in *Śavāsana* the body may relax, but the brain bubbles with thoughts jumping one after the other. At that time, it is better to devote to an *āsana* where the brain remains more restful and peaceful than in *Śavāsana*. Soon these *āsana* invigorate, which one can make use of for good, fruitful work with an attentive stable mind. When the body is rested and the mind relaxed, I do not put the pupils in *Śavāsana*.

These days, meditation is taught without studying whether one is fit or not. The moment the aspirants close their eyes, their minds begin to brood with thought waves or spend time in fear. It is better to stick to these *āsana* and enjoy restfulness instead of creating restlessness and fear in *Śavāsana*.

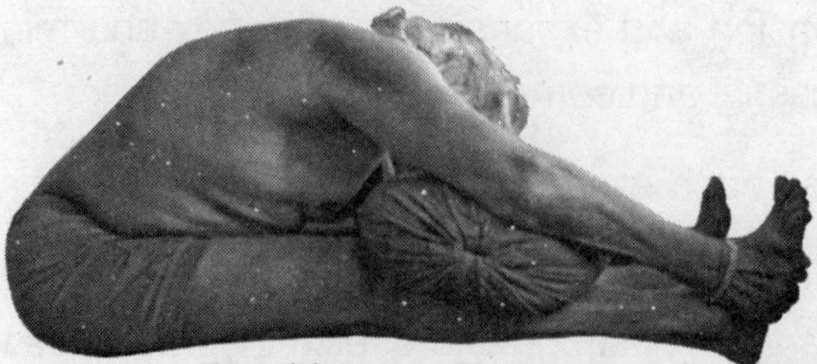

Paśchimottānāsana

Setu Bandha Sarvāṅgāsana

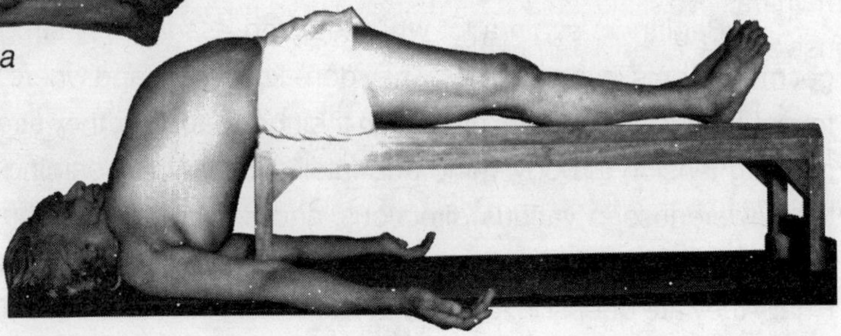

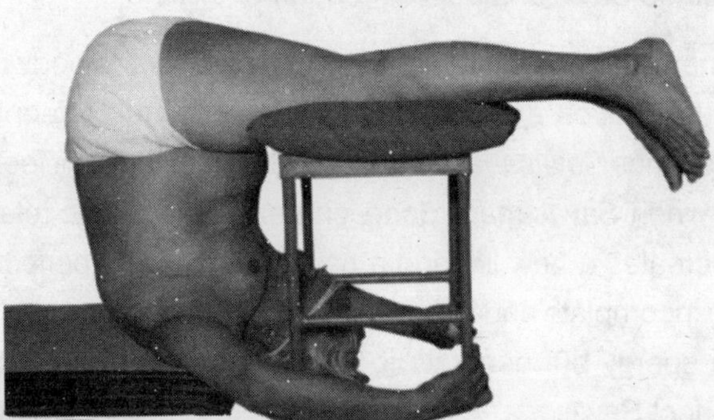

Halāsana

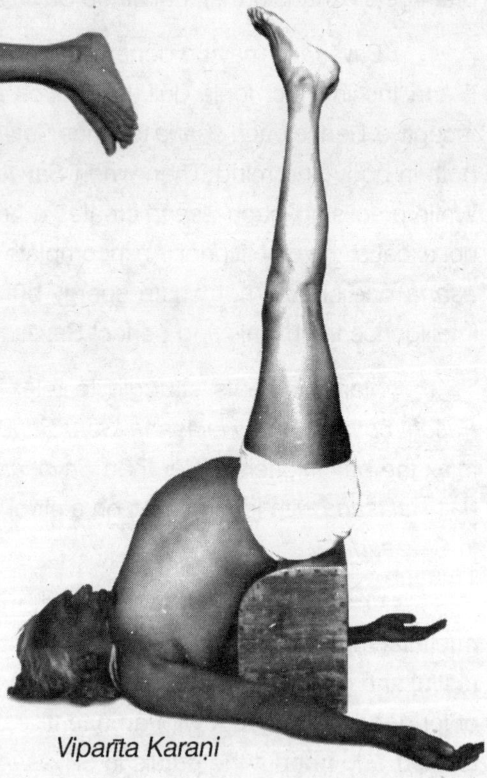

Viparīta Karaṇi

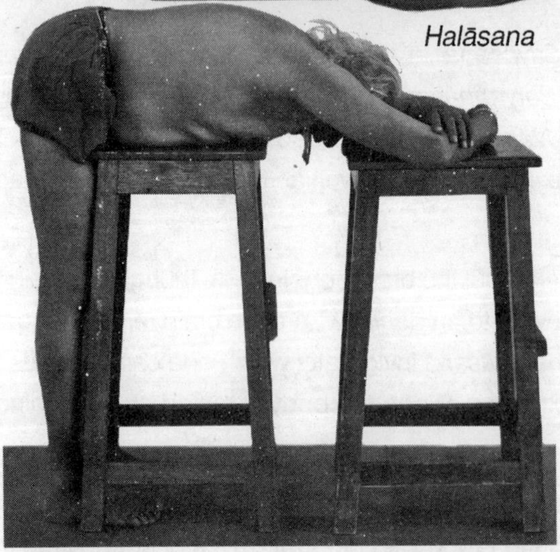

Uttānāsana with legs apart and head on a stool

Plate n. 9 – *Āsana* to relax the brain and nerves

We have the conscious front brain and the unconscious back brain. While doing *āsana*, we use the front brain and in *prāṇāyāma* we use the back brain. In *prāṇāyāma, Jālandhara Bandha* is taught so that the front brain remains quiet and the back brain observes and guides. This brings quietness in the practitioner. In *prāṇāyāma*, the active frontal brain is made to remain passive. *Śavāsana* is taught after *prāṇāyāma* for the *sādhaka* to return gradually from a pensive state towards an active state.

Practice of *Śavāsana* acts as a bridge between *āsana* and *prāṇāyāma*. If one practises *prāṇāyāma* after *āsana* he needs to do *Śavāsana* in between. After *prāṇāyāma* one needs *Śavāsana* to come back from passive state to an active state. As one cannot jump to active life immediately after *prāṇāyāma, Śavāsana* is a must. *Śavāsana* is just a pause between passive and active life. *Śavāsana* should not be done in between each *āsana*, as it not only interrupts the single flow of attention but also makes the body simultaneously dull and rigid, and the following *āsana* does not come with ease.

Since the right side is considered an auspicious side it is better to roll to the right side after *Śavāsana*. The right side is equated with *piṅgaḷā* or the active *sūrya nāḍī*. That is what one gets by turning to the right. Since the weight of the body should not fall on the heart muscle directly, it is better to roll to the right so that the heart is not strained. A pregnant women can certainly get up from the left. In case of backache he or she can roll the trunk to that side where the pain is less, and then face the floor to get up.

III.3.18. – Connection between *āsana, prāṇāyāma* and *rāja yoga*

Rāja means a king. The king of this empirical body, mind, intelligence and consciousness is the soul *(puruṣa)*. The body *(prakṛti)*, is the field *(kṣetra)* and the soul *(puruṣa)* is the knower of the field, or the fielder *(kṣetrajña)*. *Prakṛti* is meant to serve the soul *(kṣetrajñanaṇ)* as the Soul is the king of nature and its evolutes. *Sūtra* II.23 says, the purpose of the conjunction of the Soul with the body is for unfolding the inherent powers of nature and spirit for the Soul to discover its own nature.[1] Yoga being the instrument, leads each practitioner to trace the king – the soul. As the soul is the master of all, some named yoga as *rāja yoga*.

---

1 *Sva svāmiśaktyoḥ svarūpopalabdhi hetuḥ saṁyogaḥ*

As the army is trained by the king to serve him and his subjects, so too the body, mind, ego, intelligence and consciousness are trained and disciplined to serve the *ātman*. Lord Krishna says in the *Bhagavad Gītā:*

Uddhared ātmanātmānaṁ nātmānam avasādayet I
Atmaiva hyātmano bandhur ātmaiva ripur ātmanaḥ II (B.G., VI.5)

He (a man) should raise himself up through the self and never debase himself; for verily self alone is his friend, and self alone is his enemy.

We should know the self through the mind and intelligence. Lord Krishna uses the word *ātman* for the self, but it refers to one single mind.

Without knowing the mind, it is hard to know the consciousness and without knowing the consciousness, it is not easy to know the self. Without knowing the individual self it is difficult to understand the Soul. That is why *Maitrāyaṇi Upaniṣad* says, *mana eva manuṣyāṇām kāraṇam bandha moksayoḥ* (VI.34.11) – mind alone is the cause of bondage and liberation. Basically we have to train our body, senses, mind, intellect and consciousness so that they become friends of the self, hence their discipline is essential for them to be closer to their master.

The word *Raja Yoga* never appears in the *Yoga Sūtra*. Only Svātmārāma in the *Haṭhayoga Pradīpikā* says: The knowledge of *haṭha* is given solely for the attainment of *rāja yoga – kevalam rājayogāya haṭhavidyopadiśyate* (I.2), and: All these methods of *haṭha* and *laya* are but the means for the attainment of *rāja yoga,* realisation of the *ātman – sarve haṭhalayopāyāḥ rājayogasya siddhaye* (IV.103). It also says: Neither *haṭha yoga* is perfect without *rāja yoga,* nor *rāja yoga* without *haṭha yoga – haṭham vinā rājayogaṁ rājayogam vinā haṭhaḥ* (II.76).

It is a statement expressed in *Haṭhayoga Pradīpikā* that practice of *āsana* and *prāṇāyāma* acts as a means to reach the goal of knowing the individual self. From this knowing of the individual self, the aim should be to realise the Soul – the King – the *Rāja;*

Indriyāṇām mano nātho manonāthastu mārutaḥ I
Mārutasya layo nāthaḥ sa layo nādamāśritaḥ II *(IV.29).*

The mind is the lord of the organs of senses. *Prāṇa* is the lord of the mind. Absorption *(laya)* is the lord of *prāṇa* and that absorption is *nāda* – a rhythmic inner sound.

One does not know where the body ends and the mind begins; and where the mind ends and the self begins. There is no demarcation. They are interwoven. If body is one end of the thread *(sūtra),* the Soul is the other end. To reach the other unknown end of the thread (Soul), one needs to begin from the known end of the thread, the body and the mind.

To know the mind, the controller of the senses *(indriya)*, one has to study to know the functions of the organs of action and senses of perception. When one begins to control one's body, he realises that the mind, which controls it, could be its friend or foe. Hence, he begins to tame the body and mind so that they act as friends and not as foes in tracing the Soul.

The breath is the controller of the mind. Patañjali speaks of disciplining *śvāsa* and *praśvāsa*, the incoming and outgoing breaths, which are unrhythmic, shallow and hollow. This unrhythmic breath creates ripples in the consciousness *(citta)*. By attending and disciplining the breath, the flow begins to become rhythmic, subtle, deep, soft and smooth. He gets absorbed *(laya)* in it as breaths have a mystical sound *(nāda)*.

The senses, mind, intellect and ego are the vehicles of consciousness, and consciousness is the vehicle of the Soul. Similarly, body is represented through the anatomical and physiological bodies, including brain, nerves and mind. If brain is the seat of the intellect of the head, consciousness is the seat for the intelligence of the heart.

While practising *āsana* and *prāṇāyāma* we have to learn to utilise the *prāṇa* to uplift the body to the level of the *citta*.

Mind is always in doubt and suspicion. Mind is not a true discriminative power. Therefore it remains in doubt. As the mind cannot rule over its ruler *(citta)*, it tries to rule over the body, organs of action and perception. It needs discipline and here comes *āsana* and *prāṇāyāma* to discipline the mind. When Svātmārāma says: *Indriyāṇām mano nātho manonāthastu mārutaḥ*, he refers first to the mastery of *āsana* and then to *prāṇāyāma*: *Mārutasya layo nāthaḥ sa layo nādamāśritaḥ*. As the sound of breath is the master of breath, Svātmārāma says that the breath is dependent upon that mystic rhythmic sound.

Āsana makes the wind *(vāta)* to move in the body. If wind *(vāta)* moves inadequately, the body fails to remain healthy. Unless the five winds of *vāyu* do not move to their fullness, unrhythmic movements happen in the presentation of *āsana*. Adjustments and stability cannot be achieved. Rhythmic and steady movement of breath brings stability and comfort in the *āsana*. This is *sthira sukham āsanam* (*Y.S.*, II.46).

For example, in *Sālamba Śīrṣāsana* one might be physically stable, but a sudden disturbance or fear disturbs the *āsana*. Svātmārāma says: *Cale vāte calam cittam niścale niścalam bhavet* – when the breath is irregular the mind is unsteady, or when the breath is steady the mind is still and hence the body remains in stillness.

When the breath or *prāṇa* gets disturbed, *sthiratā* and *sukhatā* get disturbed and mind gets caught in the state of duality. The second part of the *śloka* points to the conquest of *prāṇāyāma. Nāda* is sound. When the breath becomes rhythmic, subtle and deep, the sound of breath becomes subtle and rhythmic and mind gets dissolved with it. Mind moves within as to the sound of the breath. It is called *ajapā japa* in the *Haṁsa Upaniṣad* (10-13). In *prāṇāyāma* the breath has its own subtle sound as *soham*. In *prāṇāyāma* this *soham japa* happens on its own. It is a *japa* without a *japa*. The sound of inhalation is *saḥ* and of exhalation is *ham*. This *soham* is the *nāda*, the inner mystical divine sound. *Saḥ* stands for God and *ham* for the individual soul - 'I' or *ahaṁ*. The existence of individual self *(jīvātman)* is in *paramātman*, the Universal Soul. This 'I' comes from 'He' – the Supreme. *Saḥ* means 'He'. The inhalation signifies the very life with a sound *saḥ* – which means, "I come from Him." The exhalation signifies the sound *ham*. It means, "I surrender to Him from whom I come." This is *soham*.[1]

While doing the *āsana*, one has to see whether these vehicles are getting disciplined or not. They have to follow the king within. For example take *Setu Bandha Sarvāṅgāsana*. While doing it, one stretches the legs far away from the self creating disparity between body and self. If he tries to draw the legs towards the Self, one begins to bring the legs and mind closer to the self. This way, if he brings the body and mind closer to the self in each *āsana*, the dualities of body, mind and self will not bother but only parity remains.

This art of right stretching is really not known to many. People criticise me as if I am interested in stretching the muscles. In that case I would have said "good-bye" to yoga long

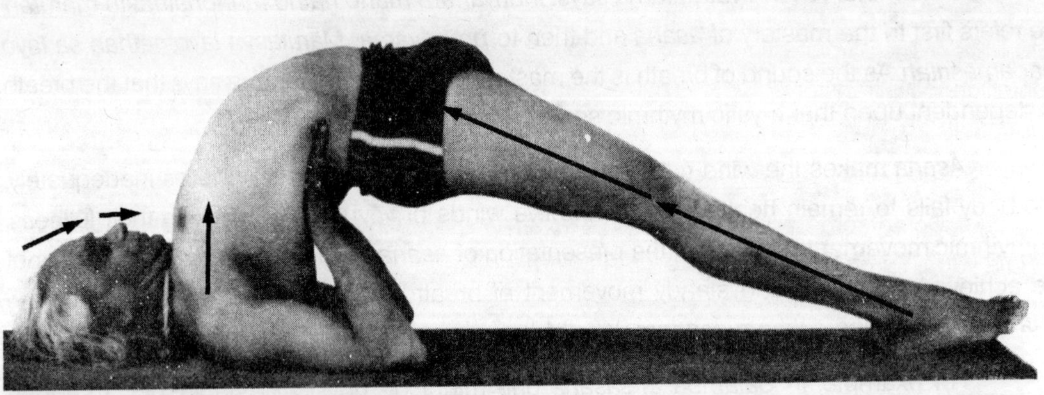

Plate n. 10 – *Setu Bandha Sarvāṅgāsana*

---

[1] According to *Gheraṇḍa Samhitā* every living being *(jīva)* performs this *japa* unconsciously, but constantly 21,600 times during 24 hours (that is 15 repetitions per minute) whereas a yogi should recite it consciously. This is called *ajapā gāyatrī*. This text explains that by doubling the number of *ajapā*, the *sādhaka* attains the state of *manonmanī* (fixed state of mind). There are no regular *recaka* and *pūraka* in this process. It is only *(kevala) kuṁbhaka*. See *Gheraṇḍa Samhitā*, chapter V, section on *Kaivalī* (84-96).

back. When I explain about stretching, extension or placing the parts of the body in a particular way, I make the pores of the skin as well as each cell to gravitate towards the centre – the self. This way of practice is *rāja yoga*.

No one can demarcate where the *haṭha* ends and the *rāja* begins. You may start with the body, but as you penetrate, you forget the parts of the body but touch the whole – the Soul.

A child playing with clay gives some shape according to its intelligence and says: "This is a mango." We may nod our heads to satisfy the child but we know that it is not the mango. The child has to get enough maturity to know the real mango. Similarly if you just bend the body and say this is the *āsana*, it cannot be an *āsana*. The multi-faceted intelligence flowing in muscles, joints, bones, spine, vertebrae, tissues and nerves as well as in the intelligence must touch the self. This is *rāja yoga*.

In *prāṇāyāma* also, when one inhales, the breath begins from the unknown spot within. We know that air comes from outside but when it touches the space within, it means it touches the Soul *(kṣetrajña)*. That Soul gives room for the in-breath to enter in. At the end of inhalation, the Soul reaches its abode, the body and causes one at once to forget the body. Actually in *kuṁbhaka* we do not hold the breath but we grip the Soul.

In retention after inhalation *(antara kuṁbhaka)*, one connects the Soul to the body. Here the unknown Soul unites with the known body. In the process of exhalation, the breath is made to move out for the self to enter in. In retention after exhalation, the known body is made to unite with the unknown Soul. In this process of *prāṇāyāma* the consciousness as well as the intelligence is transformed equal to the Soul in purity. *Sattva puruṣayoḥ śuddhi sāmye kaivalyam iti* (*Y.S.*, III.56) – when the purity of intelligence equals the purity of the Soul, the yogi has reached *kaivalya*, perfection in yoga.

Do not forget what Patañjali's yoga is, though it is termed by modern commentators as *Rāja yoga; yama, niyama, āsana, prāṇāyāma, pratyāhāra, dhāraṇā, dhyāna* and *samādhi* – all put together is *Pātañjala Yoga* (see II.29).

III.3.19. – *Yama* and *niyama* in *āsana*

Generally the precepts of the ethical practices are thought of objectively, through the books, lectures, and so forth. True ethical practice is a subjective matter. Its practice constitutes a whole way of life. We have to adopt and adapt the ethics in our actions and thoughts. We have to live moment to moment in them and absorb them. Adoption is an objective process, whereas adaptation, absorption and assimilation are a subjective process. Therefore, the principles of *yama* and *niyama* automatically have to flow in the system. This means one has to observe and adopt them while doing *āsana*.

In the *sādhanā* each act has to be disciplined with the principles of *yama* and *niyama*. Do not treat *yama* and *niyama* as separate entities, they need to be crystallised within.

Suppose one is doing *Utthita Trikoṇāsana*, he has to observe his arms. When he stretches the arm he is quick to stretch the front of the arm and not the back of it. On account of this, the front side is overstretched and the back side is understretched. Is this overstretching not violence on the front arm, and a non-deliberate non-violence on the back arm? One over extends the biceps and under stretches the triceps, but does one notice that one is aggressive on the front arm and non-aggressive on the back arm? This practice dominates on one part and does not heed but neglects the other side of the arm. It may be the same with the legs or the flanks of the chest. Is it not that that one side follows *hiṁsā* and the other side follows *ahiṁsā* unknowingly?

Is it not a non-deliberate violence of neglect on the part that is less attended? This way, many do not observe these violent and non-violent movements that take place unknowingly in the practises. So each practitioner has to judge by giving equal opportunity, like walking on a cliff for the front and back of the arms and legs to balance evenly. This way of practice is non-violent practice in a real sense.

This balance leads towards truthfulness *(satya)*. Non-violence is a disciplined freedom, which gives an eye to look at the truth. The mind that is without deviation or diversion lives in truth.

When one does *āsana*, the attention is not the same everywhere. He extends one hand or leg by depriving the other hand or the leg. Therefore, one hand or leg remains lifeless and the other hand and leg gets enriched with energy. This is *steya*. The hand and leg which are enriched with lifeful energy have stolen the energy from the other end. Distribution of energy equally everywhere is *asteya*. The same with the back and front of the chest or its sides.

If one stretches his hand strongly, his intelligence remains strong on that hand. The non-attended hand is neither strong nor intelligent. The hand which is stretched invites attention and becomes a greedy hand. The non-greedy hand remains neglected. Therefore, one has to bring balance between these two states – greed and non-greed. Both the hands and legs have every right to receive the energy evenly in the *āsana*. This is *aparigraha*, in the real sense.

What is *brahmacarya*? Is it mere celibacy? When one balances energy everywhere in the *āsana*, the conscious principle moves within, filling each pore, each cell and each part of the body. The mind does not waver. At that time, the presence of the Soul *(kṣetrajña)* is felt everywhere. *Brahma* is the greatest conscious principle. When he feels this in the *āsana*, his conscious principle spreads graciously and evenly in the body making him experience the pure state of himself. This is *brahmacarya*.

Śauca or cleanliness is from within and without. What is cleanliness within *(antaraśauca)*? One may be attempting the *āsana* physically, without feeling or understanding. This is unclean *āsana*. If one is doing the *āsana* with pride, it is not cleanliness. Pride is a smear of dirt on the mind. If that is there, there is no inner cleanliness. He should attend to *āsana* for the blood to travel 60,000 miles within the body. He has to bathe each cell in blood, supplying pure blood. This is an inner bath *(antaraśauca)*.

Śauca is external as well as internal. In *āsana* both should have a thorough clean bath. Then contentment *(santoṣa)* or the feel of satisfaction is felt. When each cell is provided with energy, the mind is enhanced and feels elated bringing satisfaction to the mind. In the beginning one may do with pride. Then the pride fades and the feel of satisfaction comes. Then restlessness turns into restfulness. It is better to watch these states in the same *āsana* at different times and catch the moment of contentment, satisfaction, exhilaration and elation.

Śauca and *santoṣa* depends upon *tapas*. There has to be a burning zeal in practice with non-stop attention, devotion and dedication.

In *svādhyāya*, the body is the object and the soul is the subject. Interweaving these two with *āsana* connects the body with the soul and soul with the body. Then that practice is spiritual and divine. In each *āsana*, one has to penetrate from the skin to the soul and from the soul to the skin to experience the state of auspiciousness. This is *svādhyāya*. *Sva* is that which belongs to the Soul, and study of all that belongs to the Soul is *adhyāya*.

By studying *sva*, one reaches the *svāmi*, the soul. *Svādhyāya* leads towards *Īśvarapraṇidhāna*. When the Soul is reached, it gravitates towards the Lord within and surrenders to him *(Īśvarapraṇidhāna)*. The realisation of the Supreme brings humility and purity in the *sādhaka*. This is how the principles of *yama, niyama, prāṇāyāma, pratyāhāra, dhāraṇā* and *dhyāna* remain inhibitive in the presentation of an *āsana*. I reiterate that all the eight aspects of yoga inter-link, inter-weave, inter-relate and inter-penetrate during *asana* and *prāṇāyāma* practice.

III.3.20. – The role of *guṇa* in *āsana*

The roots of *prakṛti (mūla-prakṛti)* are constituted of twenty-four principles *(tattva)* with three *guṇa*. The *guṇa* are essentially strong potentials that mould us. The *guṇa* remain in a steady balanced state in root-nature as well as in the causal body. Beyond these twenty-four *tattva* of *prakṛti* there is the twenty-fifth *tattva*, that is *puruṣa*. When *puruṣa* comes in 'contact' with *prakṛti*, it results in vibration. This vibration causes the cosmic intelligence *(mahat)*, the first evolute, to come into action. This cosmic intelligence potentially holds predominantly *sattva guṇa* with a little of the *rajas* and *tamas*. The individual intelligence *(buddhi)*, which is a product of the predominantly *sāttvic* cosmic intelligence *(mahat)*, shines with that same *sāttvic guṇa*. *Ahaṁkāra* sprouts too from here. The *guṇa* of *sattva*, *rajas* and *tamas* begin to express their qualities alternating with one another, which reacts upon the mind, organs of action, senses of perception, elements *(bhūta)* and subtle elements *(tanmātrā)*.

Buddhi, *manas* and *ahaṁkāra* together form *citta*. The *jñānendriya* and *karmendriya* have their origin in gross and subtle elements. The mind works as a middleman, does its job and disappears. It acts as a messenger between the senses of perception, organs of action, intelligence and consciousness. *Guṇa* are a bridge between *puruṣa* and *prakṛti* and they interplay with mind, intelligence and ego. When the intelligence is cultured to an exalted state of purity, it shines in the consciousness as cosmic intelligence and comes closer to the *puruṣa*. This is perfection in yoga.

Guṇa diffuse and flow in the evolutes of *prakṛti (buddhi, ahaṁkāra, manas, jñānendriya, karmendriya* and *bhūta)*. Basically, the body is *tāmasic*, mind is *rājasic* and the intelligence is *sāttvic*. *Ahaṁkāra* is a mixture of all *guṇa* predominating one over the other as occasion arises. We need to make all these evolutes *sāttvic* through yogic discipline. Patañjali has his own terminology. For him *sattva* is inherently illuminative *(prakāśa-śīla)*, *rajas* is inherently active *(kriyā-śīla)*, and *tamas* is inherently inert *(sthiti-śīla)*. *Śīla* means virtue. *Prakāśa-śīlatā* is the virtue of *sattva guṇa*, *kriyā-śīlatā* is the virtue of *rajoguṇa* and *sthiti-śīlatā* is the virtue of *tamoguṇa*. They exist, that is why we exist. Without *triguṇa* our life will be hopeless, tasteless and colourless. These *triguṇa* are inherent in us, but we must work for their disposition, arrangement and utilisation. These are meant to lead us to experience both pleasure *(bhoga)* and emancipation *(apavarga)* – see *Y.S.*, II.18.

Sleep is as essential as food. Sleep is *tāmasic*. It is a natural relaxation or a natural anaesthesia, which makes us forget our pains, sorrows and pleasures. Sleep is absence of memory. Sleep keeps aside our self-awareness. But the moment we are awake, the pains and sorrows surface immediately. In sleep there is no *rājasic* or *sāttvic* quality; only *tāmasic* quality which is virtuous. In sleep you do not feel your existence and this is its blessing. You say you had a sound sleep. Simulating the quality of sleep in watchful state is *dhyāna.* Unfortunately, when you sit for *dhyāna* the mind plays tricks and makes you either go to sleep or invent thoughts and draws you towards the thoughts.

An innocent stupid man has a hidden virtuous nature. He admits his innocence. His ignorance may be *tāmasic* but his innocence is *sāttvic.* The moment he begins to calculate, he loses his virtue because his ego surfaces and pride begins to play upon him to pretend that he knows.

In our *sādhanā,* the *guṇa* play their tricks. As the subject here is particularly on *āsana,* let me express what I understand. When we first begin *āsana,* we act mostly on the body, though it belongs to *tamoguṇa.* We just make the body do without really knowing the head or the tail of the body, nor the *āsana.* Then we begin to connect the mind to the anatomical and physiological bodies. From here, the vibration begins and practice becomes *rājasic* as the mind evolves to reach the subtle parts or the subtle sheaths of the body. The *sāttvic* practice in the *āsana* begins when we change our attention from the anatomical and physiological sheaths towards the intellectual and conscious sheaths of the body. Then we hold the *āsana* anatomically and physiologically in their position throughout the body for the mind to stretch and cover the entire body with conscious alertness and attentiveness. This is *rajas.* From this alert attentiveness, we create an awareness in the intelligence to spread its net throughout the body to get equilibrium and equanimity *(samatvam).* Here the *āsana* is held by *sattva guṇa.* This is how we have to understand the function of the *guṇa.*

In *sādhanā* one may overstretch somewhere and understretch somewhere else as if caught in between the two blades of the scissors. He may remain active somewhere and dull elsewhere. Both the blades need to be sharp to move evenly in cutting the cloth. *Rājasic* nature is like the two sharp blades of the scissors that have to be used accurately to pierce the sheaths of the body with equal alertness and attentiveness. The moment the two blades of the scissors (alertness and attentiveness) enter and pierce the body, they immediately transform one towards the knowledge of illumination. This is the *sāttvic* quality of the *sādhanā.*

This is how we have to study and understand the functions of *tamas, rajas* and *sattva* and hold *sattvaguṇa* to uplift and sustain us in *āsana.* From this comes *āsana-siddhi. Tamoguṇa* supports *sattva* and *rajas. Rajoguṇa* uplifts the body, mind and intelligence to be in *sāttvic* state without wavering.

When one experiences this state, then the *pañcakośa* fade out and only *ānanda,* like the flame in a windless place, blazes. This blazing flame is the Soul.

This is the virtuosity of *guṇa* in *āsana sādhanā.* This is *āsana siddhi.*

III.4 - *Prāṇāyāma*

III.4.1. – Why *prāṇāyāma*

As we breathe day in and day out without a break, we take and carry from each breath the ingredients from the cosmic breath of life-force and we survive.

In order to derive full benefit of these breaths, yogis scientifically studied and experienced the benefit of conserving the value of this life-force, as well as their effects in controlling and minimising the thought waves. In this way *prāṇāyāma* as a science, became an important part of yoga.

One has to practise first *asana* in order to obtain the feeling of getting soaked in the in-breath and the out-breath. Vyāsa, says: *sati āsana jaye....* His insistence on first mastering *āsana* was meant to gain sensitivity of the touch of air soaking the walls of the alveoli. The feel of gradual soaking does not come to those who have not done *āsana*.

Patañjali does not speak of the prolongation of life in *prāṇāyāma*. Rather he says: *tataḥ kṣīyate prakāśa āvaraṇam* (II.52) – the veil covering the light of knowledge gets removed because the brain remains free from clouds or veils. No thoughts pollute the brain or mind, and they gravitate towards spiritual knowledge. This is why *prāṇāyāma* is considered as the hub of life.

III.4.2. – Breath and life

Breath is life and life is breath. "As long as there is breath in the body, there is life; when the breath departs, life departs". Therefore the *Haṭhayoga Pradīpikā* says, restrain the breath.

It is also said that, "When the breath is irregular, the mind wavers; and when the breath is steady, the mind remains steady".

The live body is the dwelling place of the breath, mind, self and Soul. The soul keeps the body, mind and breath alive and the moment the soul leaves all these disintegrate.

Breath and mind are like twins connected by the strong diaphragmatic muscle. Very often fear sets in when the diaphragm hardens. Fear affects the diaphragm first and then the brain. A release in the brain cells takes place the moment the diaphragm starts releasing.

This indicates that the diaphragm is the medium between the physical, physiological and mental bodies, and its importance in *prāṇāyāma* is established when one learns *dīrgha-sūkṣma* method of *prāṇāyāma*.

Because of this value of the diaphragm, *prāṇāyāma* brings mobility and elasticity and its practice builds up confidence in the place of fear. As one builds up confidence, the breath automatically takes his mind to a state of BEING.

Breath is *prāṇa*, commonly known as energy. Wherever energy or *prāṇa* is focussed, there the mind stays and where the mind stays, intelligence and consciousness remain in attention with *prāṇa*.

The importance of *prāṇa* is like the importance of a bridge over a river to cross from one bank to the other. The diaphragm acts like a bridge to cross over from the physical body towards the spiritual body. The carpet of the nostrils filter the drawn-in gross atmospheric air, this filtering is even further in digital *prāṇāyāma* where the passage of air is made to be very fine and subtle, thus more of the gross elements are removed and only the potential nucleaic elements enter into the body. This stimulates the mind for higher thinking with simple living.

Hence *prāṇa* plays a major role in opening the gates of the mind to extend and expend for it to connect the body to the soul.

III.4.3. – Need of *āsana* before *prāṇāyāma* practice

Medical science says that millions and trillions of cells germinate in a split second and die in a split second. But do they all get completely activated before they germinate and die? Do we have that elasticity in our torso to make breathing long and subtle? Suppose one does inhalation by sniffing the air with a strong, rough and harsh sound; does that breath reach the air cells? Do the air cells absorb the energy through this type of breathing? When one inhales soft and long, he allows time for the *prāṇa* to reach the cells for them to absorb the energy. For this the lungs situated on the sides of the chest require elasticity, mobility and pliability. Hence, practice of *āsana* are said to be very important to derive the full benefit of *prāṇāyāma*.

One needs firmness and elasticity in the spine to sit. The body has to co-operate and the nerves should be able to sustain this soft slow deep inhalation and exhalation. One has to learn to quieten the brain. Practice of *āsana* aligns body, mind and intelligence and enables one to withstand or withhold *prāṇāyāma* practice with ease.

III.4.4. – Is *āsana* practice essential for *prāṇāyāma*

All the eight petals of yoga are interlinked and interwoven. If one petal of yoga is explicit, the others are implicit and that is how yoga works. *Āsana* and *prāṇāyāma* bring *saṁyama* in the external *(bahiraṅga)* level. The first five aspects *(yama, niyama, āsana, prāṇāyāma* and *pratyāhāra)* are meant to integrate the *bahiraṅga* (external) body *(annamaya, prāṇamaya, manomaya). Dhāraṇā, dhyāna* and *samādhi* integrate the internal *(vijñānamaya* and *ānandamaya)* bodies. As the five sheaths are interwoven, practice of *āsana* plays a role in co-ordinating by inter-relating the *bahiraṅga* levels with the *antaraṅga* to get rid of diseases. This brings health and mental poise and makes the soul to get established in every cell. The last three aspects *(dhāraṇā, dhyāna* and *samādhi)* bring integration *(saṁyama),* in internal *(antaraṅga)* and inner most *(antarātma)* levels.

Each *āsana* has its own character and value. Therefore it is good to attempt *āsana* to make the blood circulate which soaks each and every cell with life so that they become electrically dynamic.

Amongst so many *āsana,* a few chosen ones can be practised to improve the torso in developing extension and expansion to practise *prāṇāyāma.*

Āsana like *Supta Vīrāsana, Supta Baddhakoṇāsana, Sālamba Śīrṣāsana, Viparīta Daṇḍāsana, Setu Bandha Sarvāṅgāsana, Halāsana, Sālamba Sarvāṅgāsana, Viparīta Karaṇi,* and *Paśchimottānāsana* are necessary to be mastered.

While practising each *āsana,* one has to study the flow of the in-breath and out-breath with keen and clear observation. The breath touches different areas in different *āsana* and aerates. One has to gather the feelings in those areas and with understanding make use of all the areas of the chest in *prāṇāyāma* practice. Then one can begin to experience how the essence of the breath gets absorbed and stored for the psycho-spiritual path.

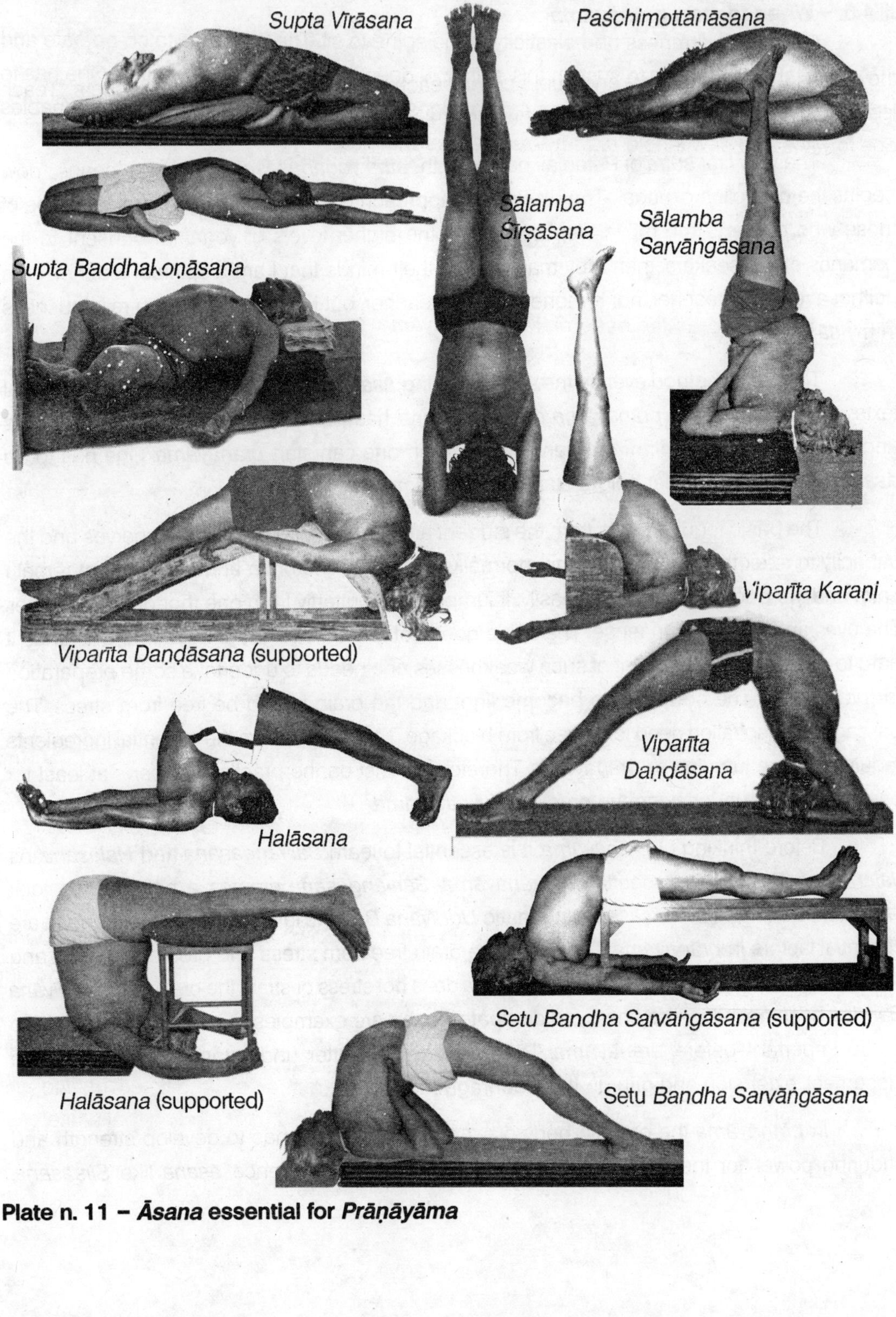

Plate n. 11 – *Āsana* essential for *Prāṇāyāma*

III.4.5. – When to start *prāṇāyāma*

Nowadays, both the teachers and pupils corrupt each other. The pupils ask the teachers, "Teach me *prāṇāyāma*, and meditation," and they do.

The very first *sūtra* of Patañjali begins with; *atha yogānuśāsanam* (I.1) – it means, "now begins the discipline of yoga". The discipline I approach is from the body. I make each one of those who come to me move step by step to the higher levels of yoga. If I consent to the demands of the seekers, then they may think in their minds that I am a spiritual teacher. I am neither a religious teacher, nor a money making teacher, but I am a teacher with religiousness in my *sādhanā*.

There is a method even in the art of teaching *āsana* and *prāṇāyāma*. As per the original texts, one snould begin *prāṇāyāma* only when one has perfected *āsana*. Once the body is under control, the spine firm and nerves calm, then one can start *prāṇāyāma*. One has to do *āsana* for at least one year before starting *prāṇāyāma*.

The basic requirements from the student are the enduring power in the nerves and the capacity to relax the brain. A beginner normally is intense. The brain and mind do not remain calm and the body does not relax easily. It jumps like a butterfly from one thought to the other. The eyes and ears remain tense. The spine does not remain straight or hold firm. One finds it hard to sit straight. On account of such weaknesses one needs to undertake some preparation for *prāṇāyāma*. The body has to become light and the brain has to be free from stress. The passages of respiration need to be free from blockage. These factors are the essential ingredients required before jumping to *prāṇāyāma*. Therefore, I insist on the practice of *āsana* at least for one year before undertaking the practice of *prāṇāyāma*.

Before thinking of *prāṇāyāma*, it is essential to learn *Sarvāṅgāsana* and *Halāsana*. As *Jālandhara Bandha* is essential in *prāṇāyāma*, *Sarvāṅgāsana* creates a natural chin lock (*Jālandhara Bandha*). In *Śīrṣāsana* automatic *Uḍḍīyāna Bandha* takes place. These *bandha* are essential factors in *prāṇāyāma*. They keep the brain free from stress and protect the heart and blood vessels in *kuṁbhaka*. *Jālandhara Bandha* does not stress or strain the brain cells. *Uḍḍīyāna Bandha* does not allow the energy to dissipate. These are examples of why *āsana* are said to be so important before *prāṇāyāma*. They give one a better understanding regarding the placement, extension and grip on the diaphragm.

In *prāṇāyāma* the organic body plays a great role. One has to develop strength and enduring power for the intercostal muscles to gain elasticity. Hence *āsana* like *Śīrṣāsana*,

Sarvāṅgāsana, *Halāsana*, *Setu Bandha Sarvāṅgāsana* and *Supta Vīrāsana* are to be done to gain elasticity in the lungs. Then one is able to do the slow, soft, deep inhalation and exhalation.

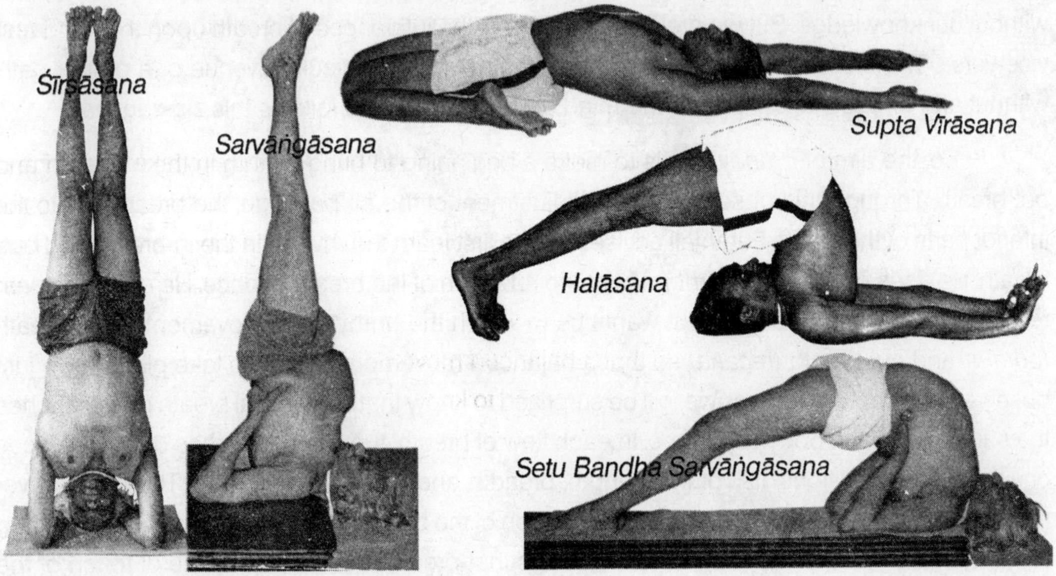

Plate n. 12 – *Āsana* that bring elasticity to the lungs

Need or greed is not easy to define. One's liking or demanding to begin *prāṇāyāma* and *dhyāna* may not be from need, but for greed. If a student asks for heaven, can a teacher take him to heaven without clean body, clear mind and untainted heart? Are they not belonging to *tapas?* My advice is to learn *āsana* properly and then do *prāṇāyāma* and enjoy its subtlety.

III.4.6. – Difference between deep breathing and *prāṇāyāma*

As breathing takes place from birth to death it becomes the link between body, mind and self to survive. Realising the value of breathing that takes place in life, the saints and yogis discovered these techniques to trace the difference between normal breathing, deep breaths and *prāṇāyāmic* breathing.

All of us breathe but unconsciously. We are aware of food while eating, but we are unaware of the breathing that goes on constantly except at the time of illness. The moment we become conscious of our breath, the pattern of the breath changes, and that is its beauty.

Breath has three movements, *pūraka, kuṁbhaka* and *recaka.* Patañjali calls it *śvāsa (pūraka)* for inhalation and *praśvāsa (recaka)* for exhalation. These two movements happen without our knowledge. But we are often ignorant of the influences of breath upon the mind and vice-versa. The breath moves in a zigzag way, without any particular avenue or a proper path, without aim or destination. So too the mind also functions and follows this zig-zag way.

So, the aim of *prāṇāyāma* is to make a beginning to bring rhythm in the in-breath and out-breath. Through this observation and adjustment of the air passage, the breath soaks the interior parts of the lungs. Patañjali advises one to first learn the rhythm in the in-breath and out-breath. He does not jump to *kuṁbhaka* or the retention of the breath at once. He does not even recommend any specific type, but wants us to watch the unrhythmic movements of in-breath *(pūraka)* and out-breath *(recaka),* so that a balanced movement begins to take place. If we just observe its normal movement, we will be surprised to know that the normal breath never touches the same part of the body each time. In each flow of breath, the breath touches different places changing their positions. Its volume, length, breadth and dimension all differ. The lungs never respond to a single breath at once. The absorption of the breath by the lungs changes according to the touch of the breath. The part of the lungs that breathes, feels that sense of touch of the breath. If the lungs need energy, they take the initiative. If the abdomen needs energy, the abdomen takes the initiative. At times if some other part feels the need, they take the initiative. This way the path of the breath moves and changes its avenue according to the need of the place in the body.

Though one breathes constantly, he realises that each in-breath and out-breath has its own avenue and its own chosen place. In a *prāṇāyāmic* way, attention is brought on the mind to do controlled breathing. It is through this process of breathing that one realises the empty parts of the lungs according to the contact or touch. Attentive awareness brings the mind to feel those parts that were unattended in the natural breaths. From this understanding, one begins to learn how far inhalation and exhalation move and where these end.

Medical science says that we take about fifteen breaths a minute. Even if one observes these fifteen breaths, one can notice that each one breath is quite different to the other. By these observations and study, Patañjali begins the science of breath. He wants us to adjust and re-adjust the flow of the breath by study and observation. This means that it must be a controlled and sustained flow from the beginning to the end in each breath. This is *gati viccheda,* or controlling the interruptions of the unrhythmic flow of each in-breath and out-breath. This is the beginning stage of learning the art of breathing in yogic *prāṇāyāma.*

As one enjoys watching sunrise or sunset and listening to the sounds of birds and animals, the practitioner has to listen and watch his own breath for a few minutes; so that he begins to understand its flow and at the same time enjoy the flavour of each breath. Watching the breath from the starting point of inhalation to its end point, and exhalation from its starting point to end point, is *gati viccheda*. Watching carefully the termination of in-breath and out-breath, gives a sense of understanding to feel whether it is a false end or a real end.

This way each one has to develop the art of observation to watch the in-flow and out-flow of breaths, and learn to control and adjust the breath to touch all parts of the lungs. This way one single breath does the job of fifteen; spacing and touching the lungs from one end to the other longitudinally as well as laterally. This not only minimises the cycles of breath per minute, but makes the breath to fill the lung cavity with ease, comfort and a feel of plentifulness. This is the first step of *prāṇāyāma*.

After the mastery of *āsana* Patañjali introduces one to begin *prāṇāyāma; tasmin sati śvāsa praśvāsayoḥ gativicchedaḥ prāṇāyāmaḥ* (*Y.S.*, II.49). It conveys the idea that *prāṇāyāma* is the regulation of the in-breath and the out-breath.

After defining the quality of the in-breath and the out-breath, he explains various facets of *prāṇāyāma: bāhya ābhyantara stambha vṛttiḥ deśa kāla saṁkhyābhiḥ paridṛṣṭaḥ dīrgha sūkṣmaḥ*. It means that the breath has three movements – inhalation, exhalation and retention, mentioning the control of them quality-wise and quantity-wise. This has to be followed with precision according to the space in the torso. Quality-wise means refinement and quantity-wise means prolongation.

The *dīrgha-pūraka* and *dīrgha-recaka* are known as deep inhalation and deep exhalation. Deep inhalation and deep exhalation means to prolong the process of breathing-in and breathing-out more than what one normally does.

Prāṇāyāma has two functions; *dīrgha* and *sūkṣma*. *Dīrgha* means prolonged. Deep breath does not mean puffing the chest. It is not just the expansion of the chest wall but the smooth touch of the breath from the interior most part of the trunk to the skin of the torso. This touch of the inhaled air by the lungs and the seepage of air by the alveoli have to be felt by the practitioner. It is through *āsana* practice that such elasticity of the lungs has to be developed.

What is *sūkṣma?* Take a bucket of water and spread a thin and fine cloth and dip it in the bucket without pressing the cloth. Observe how the thin and fine cloth slowly and gradually gets soaked into the water. As the weight of the wet part increases, it draws the rest of the cloth to get soaked. In this manner, the inner chest – the wall of alveoli – like the texture of a cloth with fine pores, has to get completely soaked and impregnated with each breath. This is *sūkṣma pūraka* and *sūkṣma recaka*. This shows that our normal breathing is shallow and deep breathing is rough. A yogi, knowing about the compact lungs, develops the art of *prāṇāyāma* to make full use of them. He not only prolongs the breath but makes it finer. This prolonged, refined breath makes him realise that the vital energy is made to circulate and be stored inside without allowing it to dissipate. The normal breath does not penetrate deep into the lungs. Hence Patañjali advises to learn the art of slow soft deep inhalation and exhalation; so that the breath that is soaked by the lungs is not only deep *(dīrgha)* but also subtle *(sūkṣma)*. The breath has to be penetrative and tangible. It has to embrace all the parts of the alveoli for storing the energy.

Inhalation or *pūraka* is the generator of energy. If one doesn't inhale, life ends. It is not that one takes the air inside, but the atmospheric air is drawn in by the *jīvātman* – the indweller. Some who do not understand the core of life force, may call this as consciousness or mind. The one that is the source of our existence within, known as *jīvātman*, draws the breath.

The moment *jīvātman* witnesses the breath; there is a long pause – a long gap of pure moment. This does not happen when witnessing the normal in-breath or out-breath. During normal breathing one does not witness. The moment one witnesses, there is no more normal breathing. If inhalation is done consciously from the beginning, one observes along-side the breath and feels the inner torso. This is how *prāṇāyāma* takes one to feel the core of life.

Retention or *kuṁbhaka* is the organised distribution of that generated energy that is drawn. *Kuṁbhaka* is not holding the breath. Holding the breath for one minute is pride and not *prāṇāyāma*. According to yogic science, *kuṁbhaka* is to make use of the generated energy for organised distribution for absorption and sustenance. During and after the distribution of energy, the unwanted toxins created by the used energy are allowed to leave slowly. This is the art of exhalation. The air that is destructive is expelled.

When one exhales, it is not expulsion but the release of the breath. Correct releasing of the breath is an art. Patañjali uses the word *sūkṣma*. It should move like the water that evaporates from the sea to form the clouds. The art of exhalation is the way in which it evaporates and comes into contact with the external atmospheric air. Here it gets cleansed for us to take a deep inhalation again.

Patañjali first introduces *prāṇāyāma* at a peripheral level. Without going into its depth, he just says to arrest the movement of inhalation and exhalation.

During the *prāṇāyāmic* breathing there has to be a clear understanding between the physiological body and the mental body. The mental body is dependent on the physiological body and vice-versa. In normal breathing, the physiological body acts on its own and the mental body does not. As it acts on its own, understanding between the mental and physiological bodies is not there. Patañjali ties the mind to the flow of breath in *prāṇāyāma* to understand the connection between mind and breath. It also does not mean counting of breath or saving of breath or prolonging the span of life. These kinds of explanations are given just to attract people.

The difference between normal breathing, deep breathing and *prāṇāyāmic* breathing is that normal breathing is zigzag. Deep breathing is a rough and forceful physiological movement with no understanding of the depth of the flow of energy inside. *Prāṇāyāmic* breathing is that in which the energy seeps and touches from the core of the being to the periphery and from the periphery towards the core.

I hope through this understanding one captures the transformation that occurs in *prāṇāyāmic* method. When the normal breath is converted into *prāṇāyāmic* breath, it gets filled with vitality, charging life's nectar into divine energy.

III.4.7. – Why some inhale with ease and some exhale with ease

A person should not inhale or exhale from the brain, but from the lungs. If a person inhales longer than his capacity, it means he uses the potency of the lungs more than the lungs can take. Secondly, one should not allow the brain to take the lead in doing deep breaths. The lead should be from the intercostal muscles of the chest. Practise inhalation and exhalation by watching the ability and the elasticity of the intercostal muscles. Listen to the lungs and do not use force on them for inhalation. Then it is bound to affect the exhalation.

Basically have a good understanding of the interaction between the chest, the lungs and intercostal muscles. Prolonged deep inhalation makes the exhalation go unrhythmic or fast; similarly, if the exhalation is deep and prolonged, inhalation goes zigzag. For this, one has to learn to judge and balance the power of the lungs while inhaling and exhaling deeply. It should be like a shopkeeper weighing the produce on a scale. If the pressures are used on the intercostal muscles in deep exhalation, then one cannot do a deep rhythmic inhalation.

Therefore, avoid using chest muscles; rather use the intercostal muscles during deep inhalation or exhalation. Learn to create softness in the inner and outer intercostal muscles in deep inhalation movements and to gain control on deep exhalations, though a certain amount of grip on them is needed.

Factually if the length of inhalation disturbs the rhythmic flow of exhalation, one has to adjust the intercostal muscles to lessen the length of in-breath, so that the zigzag movement of exhalation is minimised. Similarly, if the prolonged exhalation disturbs the smooth flow of inhalation, then shorten its length, so that the inhalation moves in rhythm.

This is how one has to learn by adjustment, to get a good grip on *prāṇāyāmic* practice.

III.4.8. – Caution for the unprepared *sādhaka*

If one reads *Light on Prāṇāyāma,* he will know how I struggled to learn *prāṇāyāma*. In my youth I was suffering from tuberculosis. If I took one deep inhalation I could not exhale or take a second deep breath. Please read about my efforts in this book which I am sure with not only encourages but inspires you all for practice.

Today I can inhale at a stretch for forty seconds and exhale forty seconds with uninterrupted flow. I do an hour each day. When I started I had to wait for normalcy to return to my lungs with each slow breath before I tried the next one. I used to perspire and feel the load in the brain. From that state I am now at this level. Even now my lungs are tender even though my chest is broad. In my early days I used to get up each morning with a religious thought to do *prāṇāyāma*, but in a few moments I was preferring to sleep in *Śavāsana*. My mind was prepared but not my lungs. Hence I know how difficult it is to learn *prāṇāyāma*.

First watch how the breath moves in its natural way and then build working on it gradually. As one learns the letters of the alphabet to read and write, learn to be patient and cajole. Do at least two deep breaths, rest for a while and repeat. Then in the course of time lessen the interval and practice. In the beginning learn to do in pauses. If one feels uncomfortable, wait for some time and proceed. When freshness in the lungs is felt, then try again. This way try to master *prāṇāyāma*. If one sows the seed today, does he expect the fruit tomorrow? Sow the seed of deep breaths before going to enjoy the fruits of *prāṇāyāma*. Here *Haṭhayoga Pradīpikā* says, *Yuktam yuktam tyajet vāyuṁ yuktam yuktam ca pūrayet* (*H.Y.P.*, II.18) – slowly and cautiously exhale and inhale. Only when this is mastered does the text advise *kuṁbhaka* and not to start with retention. Patañjali too guides *prāṇāyāma* the same way by using the word *gati vicchedaḥ*.

Patañjali concisely uses the word *gati vicchedaḥ*. It means to regulate the flow of *pūraka* and *recaka* and to stop the zigzag flow. The movement of inhalation or exhalation should be in the regular order *(yukta)*. *Haṭhayoga Pradīpikā* compares the taming of the breath to the taming of lions or tigers.[1] Can you tame them in a day? You have to wait for an appropriate time to make the breath to move with rhythm. This comes with patience and perseverance. Then toning and tuning takes place.

III.4.9. – Can *prāṇāyāma* be done in the lying or sitting position

One needs a stable spine, and firm spinal muscles to sit in *prāṇāyāma*. All the thirty-three vertebrae of the spine have to be balanced one over the other carefully, maintaining the space between each vertebra. At the same time one has to keep the muscles of the body passive and receptive.

If a person is weak, as I was, then I certainly advise him to begin soft deep breathing lying in *Śavāsana*.

Only one has to remember that in *Śavāsana*, the head has to be placed on a folded blanket on a pillow, so that the strain is not felt on the brain, but on the chest and lungs. If the head is not kept a little above the level of the chest, one feels the load and strain on the brain. In the sitting position, the strain is not felt on the brain because one follows *Jālandhara bandha*. In sitting position, the brain is kept passive through *Jālandhara bandha* but the firmness of the spine has to be maintained. In *Śavāsana* the brain and the spine remain receptive. Never forget to use a pillow or a folded blanket for the head to make the brain to rest slightly above the chest. In *Śavāsana,* besides resting the brain one learns to extend the spine with the support of mother Earth to expand the rib-cage with ease.

In case of fear, a beginner may keep his eyes slightly open to observe the movement of the chest during soft slow deep breaths. It is my experience that many people are afraid to close their eyes in *Śavāsana* due to the feel of emptiness. Hence, it is better to keep the eyes slightly open, looking at the sternum in practice.

---

1 *Yathā simhō gajōvyāghrō bhavedvaṣyaḥ śanaianaiḥ* I
tathaiva sevito vāyuranyathā hanti sādhakam II *(H.Y.S.,* II.15)

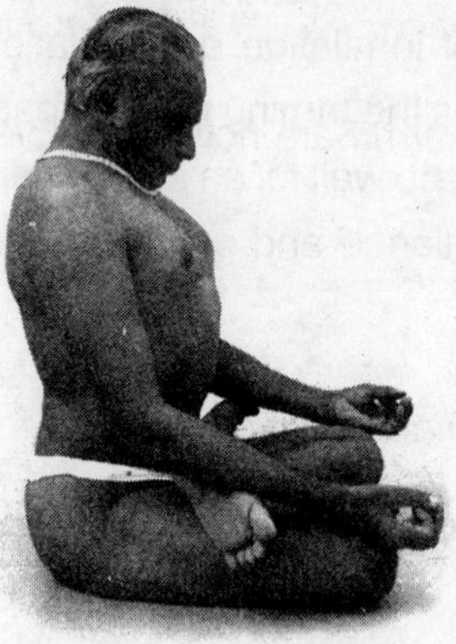

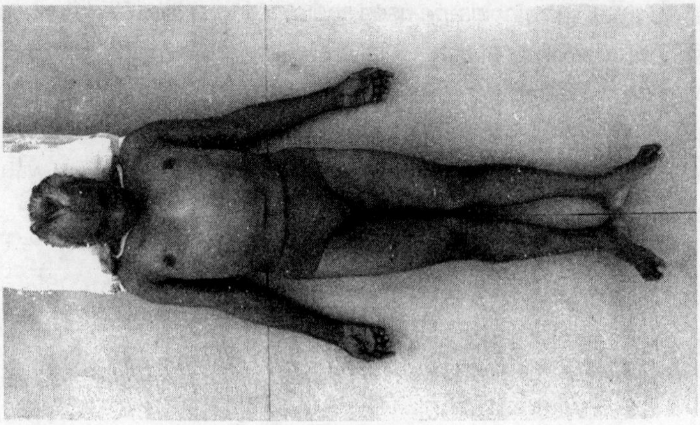

Plate n. 13 – *Prāṇāyāma*

At the beginning of *prāṇāyāma* in a sitting position, one is unaware of shifts and disturbances that take place in the body. The stronger side of the spine, functions more and takes the lead disturbing the position of the body as well as the channels in the flow of the breath. Whereas in *Śavāsana* one will be able to judge the correct or incorrect movements of the chest by positioning the back evenly by measuring the back from the centre of the spinal column.

In *Śavāsana* study the even movements of the spine and the ribs on either side and learn to maintain those in sitting position without stooping the spine. In the sitting position, develop intelligence to keep the spine firm and erect but mobile, and the brain as passive as in *Śavāsana*. If it is possible, then I say do the *prāṇāyāma* in the sitting position, maintaining serenity in the brain and mind and dynamic action of the body during the practice.

III.4.10. – Is *ṣaṭkarma* essential for *prāṇāyāma*

There are two methods of treatment in medicine: one treatment is from conventional means and the other is by drastic means. Yoga has both conventional and drastic methods. *Neti, dhauti, basti, trāṭaka, kapālabhāti* are drastic methods, whereas *āsana, prāṇāyāma* and *dhyāna* are conventional methods. *Ṣaṭkarma* are neither conventional nor classical yogic methods.

Classical texts prefer *prāṇa-neti* i.e., *prāṇāyāma.* Here the breath *(prāṇa)* is used as a thread to pass through the nostrils.

Haṭhayoga Pradīpikā mentions in clear terms that the *ṣaṭkarma* are not for all. Even great yogis like Vāsiṣṭha were not for *ṣaṭkarma:*

Medahśleṣmādhikaḥ pūrvam ṣat karmāṇi samācaret I
anyastunācaret tāni doṣāṇām samabhāvataḥ II *(H.Y.P.,* II.21*).*

The six acts *(ṣaṭkarma), dhauti, basti, neti, trāṭaka, nauli* and *kapālabhāti* are advised to be done only by those who are obese and phlegmatic, but they are not advised to be done by those who have no such defects and whose humours are almost balanced.

Further the author says:

Prāṇāyāmaireva sarve praśuṣyanti malā iti I
acāryāṇām tu keṣāncidanyat karma na sammatam II *(H.Y.P.,* II.37)

Some of the *ācārya* (teachers) emphasise that all the impurities are removed by *prāṇāyāma* alone and *ṣaṭkarma* are not accepted by them.

Prāṇāyāma practice is *bahiraṅga* as well as *antaraṅga sādhanā. Ujjāyī, Viloma, Bhastrikā, Kapālabhāti* are *bahiraṅga prāṇāyāma. Anuloma, Pratiloma, Sūrya bhedana, Chandra bhedana* and *Nāḍī Śodhana* are *antaraṅga prāṇāyāma.* Today many do *Ujjāyī* and actually call it *Nāḍī Śodhana* not knowing the placement of the fingers on the nostrils.

In the *Haṭhayoga Pradīpikā*, it is said that the *sādhaka* has to use the tip or the head of the thumb, the ring finger and the little finger, but the method of placing them is not described. This has created confusion in many. See *Light on Prāṇāyāma* for details. The way people practice pseudo *Nāḍī Śodhana* may disturb the electrical nerves of the brain, so too with *Bhastrikā* or *Kapālabhāti.* This way of practise pressurises the brain, bloats the eyes, sucks the flesh of the nose and the in-breath is drawn forcefully. If proper placement of the fingers on the nostrils is learnt, then the refined process of breathing process takes place. Today the way *prāṇāyāma* is taught is to sniff the air and blow out in exhalation. I have seen people who did wrong *prāṇāyāma* and came to me with problems.

Many doctors are against yoga as they had to treat people who had practised *sūtra neti, jala neti* and *dhauti* where threads of the cloth were removed and they were treated for puss formation in the passages. These methods were used by yogis to treat *rogi* (diseased), they are not classical practices as per the texts.

The yogic texts say that in *prāṇāyāma* one has to keep the ears alert and receptive to hear the sound *(nāda)* of *pūraka* and *recaka.* It means *nāda anusandhāna. Bhastrikā* is done for blocked nostrils to bring out the mucous. Except a little bit of exhilaration in the brain, it does not take the *sādhaka* close to the core.

One has to differentiate one *prāṇāyāma* from the other as one compares one *āsana* with the other. Quality-wise comparison is important for each one to trace better quality through refining the breath. If some say that *Kapālabhāti* and *Bhastrikā* are the major *prāṇāyāma*, and if one takes it for granted, then it is his decision.

It is better to study the yogic texts where cautions are given for the practice of *prāṇāyāma*.

III.4.11. – Is *Bhastrikā* a panacea

Bhastrikā is a good type of *prāṇāyāma*. It is a part of yogic discipline. *Kapālabhāti* is a milder form of *Bhastrikā*. In *Bhastrikā*, the blasts are strong and forceful, while in *Kapālabhāti*, the blasts are mild. Some call *Kapālabhāti prāṇāyāma* while some others classify it with *kriyā*. Both can be introduced for a short time before starting subtle *prāṇāyāma* to keep the nostrils and brain fresh.

For instance, while doing digital *prāṇāyāma*, if one finds that the nostrils are not responding or the head is heavy, a few blasts of *Bhastrikā* or *Kapālabhāti* is good. It opens the blocked nostrils and one feels light in the head. Then it is comfortable to proceed with digital *prāṇāyāma*. One should not do *Bhastrikā* and *Kapālābhāti* without knowing one's inner strength and capabilities. When the nostrils are blocked, sinus passages get choked; a short practice of *Bhastrikā* or *Kapālabhāti* will clear the passages. Similarly, if the brain is dull, a few blasts of *Bhastrikā* bring mental vigour and clarity. *Bhrāmari prāṇāyāma* is also good for lungs and brain, as the long exhalation with the humming sound quietens the brain.

One has to be cautious in these two *prāṇāyāma* practices. They may inflict something like micro haemorrhages in the brain cells or in the capillaries of the eyes; nostrils may bleed; or they may block the ears inviting deafness. Hence, my advice would be to practise these when necessary and not to be included in daily practices.

a) – How about *Bhastrikā* for women

It can be done with limited dosages. Anything over done is harmful.

Women did talk to me about *Bhastrikā* in private. Through them, I learnt the other side affect of *Bhastrikā* and am careful about it and tell my female pupils that their lungs are not as strong as those of men and in this *prāṇāyāma or Kapālabhāti,* they lose the shape of their breasts due to the force of these *prāṇāyāma* which may affect their family relationships.

My advice is that women do *Bhastrikā* or *Kapālabhāti* only to clear the nasal passages and devote their practice to more subtle types of *prāṇāyāma.*

III.4.12. – Aerobics and *prāṇāyāma*

Regarding aerobics and *prāṇāyāma* I confess that I have not done aerobics and therefore I cannot speak about that method of breathing techniques or what it follows.

Secondly, comparisons are always odious. As a dedicated yoga practitioner I worked on for health and went on giving demonstrations after demonstrations to ignite people into yoga.

I confess that I started *prāṇāyāma* late as I had no lungpower. We breathe from birth to death, but this cannot be called *prāṇāyāma.* Aerobics is an exercise. *Prāṇāyāma* is not. The *prāṇāyāmic* inhalation, exhalation and retention are not the same as in aerobics. The variance between these two is like the distance between earth and sky.

Āsana and *prāṇāyāma* give a feel of energy circulating and energising the body all over. The nerves and the brain experience placidity. Aerobics are exhaustive and irritative and yogic practices are stimulative and exhilarative.

III.4.13. – Tremor in *prāṇāyāma*

When one becomes tremulous it means he is unconsciously tightening his chest and brain. As one breathes in, the duty of the intelligence is to watch, observe and work to remove tautness and strain in the lungs, chest and head. Make the lungs listen and be subordinate to the intelligence. Tautness and hardness lead to tremor. The breath has to move like a needle that injects the fluid carefully into the tissue, to accept the fluid without creating bubbles. Start with two or three slow and soft deep breaths and do normal breathing for sometime to stop the tremors. Then repeat two or three slow and soft deep breaths and wait. By this way the cells of the lungs are rested to become fresh soon so that one does it with ease and wins over tremors. Passivity in the head is a must, both in inhalation and exhalation!

One should not force the breath into the lungs beyond one's capacity. The walls of alveoli are tender. The breath should not rape the lungs. Do not prolong the exhalation when the lungs cannot tolerate the prolonged exhalation. As over-nourishing and under-nourishing are both harmful, forced inhalation over-nourishes, and then exhalation goes out fast and by this undernourishing takes place. First understand and attend to the needs before forcing the breath. Forcefulness is a form of greed.

III.4.14. – Does practice of *prāṇāyāma* make teenagers pre-mature in age

Generally *prāṇāyāma* does not lead to fast aging. It is a life-giver and not a life-taker. Right practice of *prāṇāyāma* does not bring any adverse effect on the practitioners. It keeps one young, provided one does it according to one's age and condition. As we do a right thing at the wrong time and a wrong thing at the right time, my advice would be to do the right thing at the right time. Having said this much, I say that *prāṇāyāma* is not good for children or teenagers.

I was invited sometime ago to visit Bangalore to attend a conference where experts would meet to discuss introduction of yoga in schools, from the third standard to the tenth standard.

Many were officials who had no knowledge of yoga.

When I asked them what was the feedback they got from teaching yoga in schools so far, none knew or had any experiences. Their concept on yoga was just imaginary ideas, whereas my teaching experience in schools for girls and boys goes back to 1936. Even now many of my students teach yoga in schools on a voluntary basis. When others were discussing on the level of experiment, we had experiences. Unfortunately, their heads could not accept experiential knowledge.

During discussions I realised that these people wanted school-children to do *ṣaṭkarma* such as *dhauti, basti, neti, trāṭaka, nauli* and *kapālabhāti.* They wanted *prāṇāyāma* also to be taught. They had a fixed idea that if *prāṇāyāma* had to be introduced then *ṣaṭkarma* too are a must. A lot of discussion and argument took place.

I wanted the curriculum to be suitable to everyone in all schools, whether urban or rural according to their age-level and capacity.

Now, the *ṣaṭkarma* practices require clean cloth, clean vessels and pure water. One of the schools of yoga was keen to introduce *śankha prakṣālana kriyā* also, in which one needs plenty of water to drink as well as a lavatory because the practice of this *kriyā* requires one. Suppose, the *kriyā* has to be introduced, can the school authorities provide water and toilets? In villages one does not get water to drink, how can they provide water or clean thread for *neti* and cloth for *dhauti?* In case the thread or the cloth gets stuck in the nose or throat, it may create medical problems. If the thread or cloth is unclean, it may introduce unnecessary infections. But the committee was least bothered about these practical problems.

Then the discussion on *prāṇāyāma* was taken up. There, I said that children look prematurely aged, if they are taught to hold the breath in *prāṇāyāma*. Retention makes the tender faces prematurely aged. I suggested deep breathing only. They could not conceive *prāṇāyāma* without *kuṁbhaka!*

I still emphasise more on the practice of *āsana* than *prāṇāyāma* in schools, since *āsana* are effective and helpful for the proper growth of children. If the *āsana* were well taught at that age, then *prāṇāyāma* would be easy to learn when they enter that age where the right thing can be taught at the right time.

Children's lungs are tender and delicate. The intercostal muscles are soft and tiny. I think forcing children to do *prāṇāyāma* on such tender bodies and soft muscles is not safe.

I was against the introduction of *prāṇāyāma* for children at a wrong time and I stand for it even now I am in touch with children and guide them in yoga though I am ninety years young.

Childhood is the right time to nurture the body. The moment one asks children to draw in the breath, they use force. They jerk and inflate the eyeballs, choke the ears and strain the brain-cells. These kinds of harsh breaths injure the brain-cells and delicate lungs and make them look more aged than their actual age.

The format should be with caution, harmonious and smooth in introducing *prāṇāyāma*. Otherwise children get parochial and develop lonely, sad and dispirited.

Practice of *prāṇāyāma* needs physical stability, mental maturity and intellectual sensitivity, which children do not have. *Āsana* develop their active physical stability, emotional strength and intellectual sensitivity and enthusiasm. There need to be gradual stages or phases, which have to be attended to in educating children in yoga. If you ask children to sit quietly with eyes closed, they either blink or wink. They burst into laughter without any reason, indicating their restlessness. Children should not be forced to concentrate. If one teaches skilfully, children automatically concentrate. Let interest be kindled in the subject rather than involving them seriously.

Children's thoughts are basically out-going. They are predominantly concerned with external things or objective considerations. Practice of *āsana* develops their mind to be positive in their thinking angle. If one forces their extrovert mind towards introversion, it may possibly take then to become lonely and depressed and damage their nerves, brain and mind.

Before introducing them to the deeper practice and spiritual quest *(antaraṅga sādhanā* and *antarātma sādhanā)*, they have to be trained in an active external phase of endeavours *(bahiraṅga sädhanā)*.

Children want to know everything. They grasp fast. They have both one-channelled and all-pointed attention, and they should be encouraged to develop this faculty.

There might be a few cases of child prodigies but they are rare. Dhruva, Prahlāda are the cases of *bālayogi* (child yogi). According to the *Vishnu Purāṇa*, Dhruva, as a child, performed severe penance and attained self-realisation at a tender age. Prahlāda, the son of a demon king, Hiraṇyakaśipu, was devoted to Lord Vishnu. In their cases the previous birth's impressions *(saṁskāra)* carried them to reach that highest level at that early age. So what we can do is to create good imprints *(saṁskāra)*, in the pure heart of children.

Some yoga teachers teach retention with *Uḍḍīyāna Bandha*. Once I saw on T.V., children doing *Nauli* and *Uḍḍīyāna*. Children who suck their abdomen along with their chest are bound to damage their growth. Therefore, one has to be careful and constructive. Teachers must sit together, discuss the pros and cons and introduce those techniques, which are harmless and encouraging to that age.

Children have prolific energy. Their enthusiasm, courage, flexibility and endurance keep them dynamically active. The varieties of *āsana* appear natural for them. First, let us channel their energy in *āsana*, so that when they reach adult age they do *prāṇāyāma* healthily. *Prāṇāyāma* as a separate subject can be taught when they grow, let us say after sixteen years of age.

Therefore, the best way to start and keep them in touch is with the *āsana*. One may not accept my factual suggestion, but time alone will prove that what I say is right.

So, my suggestion is to avoid retentions of breath and forceful sucking of the breath, contracting the facial muscles and brain.

a) – Can breath control postpone old age

If one wants a good garden, he needs to tend it each day. The moment he stops taking care of it, it dries up. If one does not use a blade, it rusts. If one needs to play a violin each day, he needs to tune it as well. It is the same with the body, breath and mind. They need to be tuned each day. Otherwise they become insensitive. Body is like a garden. So one has to take care of it through discipline each day and tend it carefully, in a right way.

Practice of *prāṇāyāma* keeps the respiratory system healthy. Each alveolus gets nourished with the in-breath, otherwise it gets dry. *Prāṇāyāma* practice brings indirect control on the mind. The energy produced by *prāṇāyāma* with favourable mental disposition keeps one young even in old age and one may postpone old age as he lives in the present watching the movements of his own breaths.

Death is certain. Why worry about it? But have a deliberation on this moving life that is dynamic.

III.4.15. – On *bandha*

Regarding *bandha*, my advice to all is to read *Light on Prāṇāyāma* and to learn first the principles of *prāṇāyāma* but forget about *bandha* for the time being, as there are many things to learn before jumping to *bandha*.

One should first learn the art of inhalation and the art of exhalation. The basic *prāṇāyāma* begins in *Śavāsana*, as there is a lot of scope for learning through observing the flow of the movement of energy in inhalation and exhalation. The awakening of breath consciousness comes in the movement of chest, intercostal muscles without stress through the firmness of the spine and non-obstruction of the flow of energy in the nerves. In sitting *prāṇāyāma, Jālandhara Banaha* is advocated to keep the brain free from tension and strain. On this bandha I have cautioned not to force the head or neck down. Then the *Antara Kuṁbhaka* is introduced to get a better grip on *Jālandhara Bandha*. When one is stable in *Antara Kuṁbhaka*, then he is introduced to suck the abdomen from the pubis for the diaphragm to move closer towards the back-bone after exhalation *(Uḍḍiyāna)*. It is not to be done in each exhalation, but to rest the organs before one sucks again. Here, the most important thing to keep in mind is NOT TO CONTRACT THE CHEST BOX.

Mūla Bandha comes later.

In order to do *Mūla Bandha* in *prāṇāyāma* one has to practise *Aśvini Mudrā* in *āsana*. *Aśvini Mudrā* happens spontaneously in *Tāḍāsana, Paścimottānāsana, Śīrṣāsana, Ūrdhva Dhanurāsana* and in all other backbends. Later the *Mūla Bandha* is done with attention as a separate practice in *prāṇāyāma*. Read the cautions that are in *Light on Prāṇāyāma* on *Mūla Bandha* and then think of its practice when you are sure of doing correctly. Remember not to attempt *Mūla Bandha* without perfecting *Uḍḍiyāna Bandha*.

III.4.16. – What is *kāla* (time), *saṁkhyā* (precision), *dīrgha* (long) and *sūkṣma* (fine and soft) in *prāṇāyāma*

Let me explain these terms in brief. *Kāla* indicates chronological time. *Saṁkhyā* means counts, which indirectly conveys time. It also stands for calculation, deliberation, reasoning, reflection and precise understanding. *Dīrgha* suggests a chronological time or the length, or duration of the breaths, whereas *sūkṣma* means intellectual attention where subtle and refined adjustments of the breaths are to be made.

Dīrghatā indicates expressiveness whereas *sūkṣmatā* indicates non-expressiveness. The former indicates effort and the later effortlessness. *Dīrgha prāṇāyāma* suggests intentional manifestation, while *sūkṣma prāṇāyāma* is non-manifest and unintentional. *Dīrgha* indicates the phenomenal aspect and *sūkṣma* indicates noumenal aspect in *prāṇāyāma*.

Dīrgha prāṇāyāma expresses pronounced sound and vibration, whereas *sūkṣma prāṇāyāma* expresses feeble sound with least vibration.

Dīrgha breath is fathomable. *Sūkṣma* breath is sacred because it is unfathomable. *Dīrgha prāṇāyāma* is like a crown, while *sūkṣma prāṇāyāma* consecrates.

Dīrghatā is a process for cultivation and *sūkṣmatā* is for culturing. *Dīrghatā* brings dignity to *prāṇa* while *sūkṣmatā* brings divinity involving both evolution and involution. Hence, *kāla, dīrgha, sūkṣma, saṁkhyā*, convey different facets of *prāṇāyāma* and cannot convey the same meaning.

Though Patañjali speaks of *kāla, sāṁkhyā, dīrgha, sūkṣma* these apply to all the eight petals of yoga: *bāhya abhyantara staṁbha vṛttiḥ deśa kāla sāṁkhyābhiḥ paridṛstaḥ dīrgha sūkṣmaḥ* (*Y.S.*, II.50). It conveys that *prāṇāyāma* has three movements, inhalation, exhalation and retention. These three movements have place *(deśa)*, time *(kāla)* and precision *(saṁkhyā)*. Tracing the source root of the breath in the torso and measuring the length of the breath is *kāla*. Prolongation of the in-breath, out-breath and retention is *dīrgha*, and to adjust the gates of the breath for minute flow of inhalation and exhalation is *sūkṣma*.

The regulated inhalation, exhalation and retention are the three components of *prāṇāyāma*. They are to be observed place-wise, province-wise, length-wise, breadth-wise, depth-wise, duration-wise, subtlety-wise and precision-wise.

Now, take *deśa*. *Deśa* means place, province or region. It could be in the body such as abdomen, chest and back. It could be a geographical place, which could be on different altitudes. A yogi not only conquers his body but also conquers the place. For me, it does not make a difference whether I am in India or Switzerland or South Africa. I do maintain the same length, depth and subtle quality of *prāṇāyāma* as I practise in my hometown.

About *kāla*, it is time, or duration or season. *Prāṇāyāma* should not change quality-wise or quantity-wise whether it is morning, noon, evening, night or midnight or winter, summer, spring or fall. It should not change under any conditions.

Saṁkhyā often means number or number of cycles of inhalation, exhalation and retention as fixed duration as well as fixed number of cycles. For many these two factors appear to be the same.

I have already mentioned at the beginning of this topic that *saṁkhyā* conveys several meanings besides knowing the soul through *buddhi*.

The *Sāṁkhya Darśana* – one of the six systems of philosophy, codified by Kapila Muni indicates the quality and the counts. It means number, intellect or intellection. It conveys the method of logic and the root-cause of creation and motion of cosmogony. He is the first one to put the cosmogony of *prakṛti* with twenty-four evolutes that are categorically explained. It also means arranging, doing precisely and decisively.

Patañjali Muni accepts the evolutes of *prakṛti*.

In the *sūtra* II.50 he arranges the words like *deśa, kāla, sāṁkhya, dīrgha* and *sūkṣma* thoughtfully and sequentially. The exhalation, inhalation and retention (*bāhya, abhyantara* and *stambha*) have a sequence. He wants us to do *prāṇāyāma* thoughtfully with long, deep and fine movements studying the length, breadth and depth of the torso.

Between each exhalation and inhalation, or inhalation and exhalation, there is an unknown pause *(stambha* or *kumbhaka)*.

Vṛtti means movement or modification. This word indicates movements and varieties of *prāṇāyāma*. Breathing differs from person to person on account of physical structure and mental conditions. *Prāṇāyāma* arrests these zigzag movements of the breath. In order to make the foundation of *prāṇāyāma* firm, one needs to know the origin of the in-breath *(pūraka)*, with its termination as well as in the out-breaths *(recaka)*. To experience this, several types of *prāṇāyāma* were introduced in various yoga texts to improve and gain mastery over inhalation, exhalation and retention, place-wise, time-wise and precision-wise.

Patañjali's *dīrgha* and *sūkṣma* indicate circumferential expansion, extension, length, width and breadth whereas *sūkṣma* indicates subtlety, softness and fineness. *Dīrgha* indicates quantity, density and volume, while *sūkṣma* indicates quality of flow which should be thin, transparent, clear and precise.

See what *Haṭhayoga Pradīpikā* says on *kāla* and *saṁkhyā*.

Svātmārāma says that *prāṇāyāma* has to be done four times a day, i.e. dawn, noon, twilight and midnight. This is time-wise, with a quantitative approach. He says that one perspires in a lowest type of *prāṇāyāma (kaniṣṭha prāṇāyāma)*. In the middle type of *prāṇāyāma (madhyama prāṇāyāma)*, the body vibrates, tremors and shakes. In the finest *prāṇāyāma (uttama prāṇāyāma)*, one advances towards the spiritual path. This last one seems to indicate the *sāṁkhya* factor as it is said to be qualitatively the finest. He indicates this difference in II.12: In the first stage, there is perspiration; in the second, tremor is felt throughout the body; and in the highest stage, the *prāṇa* goes to the [chief] place [*Brahmarandhra*]. So he says that one should control the breath.

If one observes carefully, *prāṇāyāma* done place-wise brings health to physical and physiological bodies covering the lungs, chest, respiratory, circulatory and glandular systems.

Time-wise, it works effectively on nerves, brain and mind bringing calmness and quietness.

Saṁkhyā-wise, it ushers change at the intellectual level and the *citta* undergoes transformation leading the aspirant on to the spiritual path.

Though the adjunctions of *prāṇāyāma* undoubtedly seem to make it a complicated practice, it takes one to the depth of spiritual endeavour. A beginner cannot practise with all these details. Hence, he is taught to do at gross level and gradually initiated to the subtleties.

In some of the *purāṇa*, the method of calculating the *prāṇāyāma* time-wise is given in various types of *prāṇāyāma*, namely; *Ujjāyī, Nāḍī Śodhana, Sūrya Bhedana* and so forth. But whatever the *prāṇāyāma*, the base of *deśa, kāla, saṁkhyā* and *sūkṣma* is advocated.

The crux of the matter is that whatever *prāṇāyāma* one does, it should be done quality-wise.

The efforts involved in *prāṇāyāma* cannot be minimised. These texts expound that one has to observe where the breath is manifesting. In the age-old method, a piece of grass straw or a stalk is held in front of the torso and a long exhalation is attempted to test the subtleness of flow of exhalation by bringing the stalk close to the nose and seeing that it does not move.

If the stalk is near the throat and shakes, then this short-distance of exhalation is considered to be of *kaniṣṭha* or inferior *prāṇāyāma*. If it shakes somewhere near the chest-region, it was said to be *madhyama* or medium *prāṇāyāma* and if it moves somewhere near the navel or below the navel it is superior or *uttama prāṇāyāma*. Our ancestors were using this type of gauge to measure. Have I not often stressed that one has to master the chronological time (not clock-time).

Bhagavad Gītā says:

Apāne juhvati prāṇam prāṇe apānam tathapare I
prāṇāpānagati ruddhva prāṇāyāma parāyaṇāḥ II (*B.G.*, IV.29)

Here, Lord Krishna explains *prāṇāyāma* as *prāṇa yajña* (a sacrifice). Inhalation is *apāna kriyā* and exhalation is *prāṇa kriyā*. The act of sacrificing the inhalation into exhalation is *pūraka yajña* and the act of sacrificing the exhalation into inhalation is *recaka yajña*. The inhalation begins from the *apāna-sthāna*, which is below the navel. The exhalation begins from the *prāṇa-sthāna*, which is the top chest. The retention is done after the inhalation as well as after the exhalation. These retentions are *kuṁbhaka yajña*. Here it is explained place-wise, with *dīrghatā* and *sūkṣmatā*. Between *prāṇa* and *apāna* there are the provinces of *udāna*, *vyāna* and *samāna*. The *deśa* is quite an extensive territory. It is said that if our lungs, alveoli are spread out, they are as huge as a tennis court. In this spacious place, if the breath has to spread all over, how subtle it should be?

These things cannot happen unless there is precision and perfection. At one place Svātmārāma, speaking about retention, says: *ā keśāda nakhāgrācca nirodhāvadhi kuṁbhayet* – retain it in such a manner that the energy is stabilised even in the hair-end and nail-end. In other words the *prāṇa* has to pervade the whole of the body from the head to the toe. A complete quietness in *kuṁbhaka* alone can bring this effect. This is *saṁkhyā* – precision. For example, one might have seen how the water is drawn from the well. A pulley is fixed in the middle; a coir-rope is moved on the track of pulley. The pot is fixed to the hook or noose of the rope. The pot is released in the well. And when it is filled with water, it is drawn up from pulley.

Consider the body as a well, and the area behind the nose and above the palate, i.e. the sinus passage, as a pulley. The awareness of *citta* is a coir-rope. The exhalation is like the pot released into the well and inhalation is like pulling the pot from the well. While releasing the pot into the well it is empty and while pulling it up it is filled with water.

When the empty pot is allowed to move into the well, it will move fast since the movement is towards gravity; while pulling it up, it is against the gravity. Often one finds the exhalation going faster than inhalation.

If the coir-rope is released faster into the well, it cuts the palms and the palms burn with heat. To avoid this injury, one releases the coir slowly and carefully. So also while exhaling one has to release the breath slowly and carefully, until one reaches the end part of the torso – *apāna sthāna*.

Here the *prāṇa* meets *apāna*. During inhalation the energy is drawn from the bottom of the pulley, i.e. from abdominal walls to the nose. The filled pot cannot be pulled up fast. One has to pull it slowly so that water is not spilled into the well and again with the light touch the pot is released into the well. Similarly, during the inhalation the breath has to follow the consciousness as the coir pulls the pot up.

During exhalation, the coir follows the pot. In the same way, the consciousness *(citta)* has to follow the exhalation-breath.

When the empty pot is released in the well-water, the coir also touches the water. One does not feel the heaviness of the pot and need not grip the coir either. The coir is kept loose to allow the pot to get filled. After exhalation and during *Bāhya Kuṁbhaka* (exhalation-retention) neither the chest nor the consciousness should remain heavy. Svātmārāma says: *kuryāt cittam nirāśrayam,* meaning make *citta* supportless. It becomes so light during the *Bāhya Kuṁbhaka* that it does not need the support. *Citta* is light and empty along with firmness.

In *Antara Kuṁbhaka* (inhalation-retention), it is just the opposite. The pot filled with water is lifted up from the well and care is taken that water does not spill back into the well. In *Antara Kuṁbhaka*, the *citta* is full, dense and firm along with the energy. This is the precise adjustment during the *kuṁbhaka*. The inhalation and exhalation should not be in a flux. Stability in mobility should be balanced evenly. Neither the inhalation nor exhalation should move as a tide.

In case we like to take the fragrance of the flower, we inhale very slowly and softly to retain the pleasant feeling of fragrance in our memory so that the flavour may not fade out.

Similarly, while exhaling, the consciousness retains the fragrance of air though the breath is allowed to go out.

Do *prāṇāyāma* this way so that the awareness does not fade. Maintaining the cool sensation in the brain is precision in *prāṇāyāma*. Often we see people doing retention with a taut brain and head. To keep the brain-cells in a quiet state during inhalation is an art. Basically, inhalation is a *bruḥmaṇa-kriyā*. *Bruḥmaṇa* means to nourish, to make oneself strong. Inhalation nourishes and energises the cells of the body. If one makes the brain-cells taut and inflates them, then one ends up in *prāṇāyāma* with dissipation of energy.

Exhalation is a *laṅghana kriyā*. *Laṅghana* means fasting or starving. In exhalation the brain-cells deflate bringing lightness. If one does forceful movements in exhalation, it leads towards dissipation of energy. The precision in *prāṇāyāma* should come without dissipation of energy retaining silence in its mental movements. This is *saṁkhyā*.

The original or *mūla citta* is basically quiet. The flow of quietness in its very nature is *svarasa-vāhini* or flow of the self's fragrance. The *praśānta vāhini* or flow of peace has to flow in *prāṇāyāma*. These two rivers, the *svarasa vāhini* and *praśānta vāhini*, have to have confluence with the *gupta vāhini*, i.e. *ātmā vāhini*, which is hidden and concealed. This is real *prāṇāyāma*. In order to bring this ultimate effect of freedom, it is essential to know the *saṁkhyā* as precision.

Therefore, don't take the meaning of *kāla* and *saṁkhyā* as time and cycles or duration but take it as precision. By following the time and number of cycles mechanically one neither feels the precision nor the Soul – the very source which is felt in *prāṇāyāma*.

III.4.17. – The interaction of five *vāyū* (energy) with *bhūta* (elements)

Prāṇa is *viśva prāṇa* or *viśva caitanya śakti*. When this universal energy *(viśva caitanya śakti)* is individualised through *prāṇāyāma*, it becomes *vaiyaktika śakti*. Each one of us is born with universal energy. The energy *(prāṇa)* hidden in the sperm and the ovum of our parents, yields us some potential energy which we absorb genetically. This *prāṇa* functions in our body according to its province *(deśa)*, quality *(guṇa)* and action *(karma)*. This universal energy power *(śakti)* is divided into five as *prāṇa*, *udāna*, *vyāna*, *samāna* and *apāna*. Provinces are allotted to each one in our body according to its characteristics and functions. The area below the navel is *apāna kṣetra;* the chest and the brain is *prāṇa kṣetra* and the abdomen is *samāna kṣetra*. The region of the chest and the throat is *udāna kṣetra* and the whole body which has its own net of circulatory and nervous systems covered by the skin is *vyāna kṣetra.* In the same way, the elements of the body have their own provinces. *Apāna kṣetra* has earth element; *prāṇa,* water element; *samāna,* fire; *udāna,* air and *vyāna,* ether. These elements and *prāṇa* exist in us to produce the vital energy.

Table n. 1 – *Viśva prāṇa* or *viśva caitanya śakti*

	Prāṇa		Element		*Kṣetra* / Province
i.	*Apāna*	–	earth	–	below navel
ii.	*Prāṇa*	–	water	–	chest and brain
iii.	*Samāna*	–	fire	–	abdomen
iv.	*Udāna*	–	air	–	chest and throat
v.	*Vyāna*	–	ether	–	all over

Let us now consider the impact of the five elements and the five *prāṇa* on the senses of perception. We will see how they intermingle, interact and collaborate with each other in order to keep our senses functioning.

Chāndogya Upaniṣad says the eyes belong to *prāṇa.* The brain and eyes have a close connection. I often say that eyes are the windows of the brain. If the brain is tense, the eyes are tense and vice-versa. If the brain relaxes eyes relax and if the eyes relax the brain relaxes. All this happens because of *prāṇa.* The eyes also have fire element *(darśanāgni).*

Samāna kṣetra is the province of fire which yields digestion. When the stomach is full one feels drowsy. The place of fire element being the *samāna kṣetra,* it invites bile *(pitta)* to come to its help to digest the food. If one is hungry and thirsty for a long time, the eyes close automatically. When light food is taken the eyes and brain gain back their sharpness. This is the relationship between the fire element and digestion. Intelligence is again a fire element *(jñānāgni)* and it also belongs to air element.

The ears belong to *vyāna vāyu* and ether element. *Vyāna kṣetra* is in the heart as well as in the whole body. This indicates the circulatory system as the blood supply takes all over the body through *vyāna.* Here, I also say that as ears belong to air element, they act as the windows of the mind.

Prāṇa controls the five senses, which are situated in the head. *Prāṇa* plays a great role in sensory perception. The ears hear because of ether. Blocked ears, perforation in the eardrums or the bone growth indicate derangement due to the earth and air element.

The tongue belongs to *apāna* though its province is water element. *Udāna* and *prāṇa* govern it. Salivary glands are watery but they are provoked when one is hungry. Hunger is fire. With fear the throat and the tongue get dry and become speechless. When the *udāna* flow is low, the saliva fails to function and one needs water. The tongue is to feel the taste, yield speech and sing. The action of speaking and singing is by *udāna*, which operates the larynx. The tongue is also related to the *apāna* though its province is below the navel. The taste buds are basically of the earth element, though the sensation of taste is from the water element (saliva), which is stimulated by *prāṇa*. See the paradox. Saliva is watery but hunger is fire. When you are hungry the saliva oozes. When one has fever, or constipated, or stomach upsets, there is loss of taste. If one has facial paralysis, the tongue gets affected with or without loss of speech. This is the effect of *apāna,* though the speech is the function of *udāna*.

Because of *prāṇa* one's intelligence remains in a wakeful state. In old age or disease a person loses his speech on account of *apāna*. The tongue, larynx and mouth express the words but the origin of speech is in the area of the navel, the province of *apāna*. When *apāna* fails, the voice fails. The nerve supply controlling the tongue gets affected.

Basically *apāna* gives the physical and physiological strength and *prāṇa* the intellectual and spiritual strength.

Again according to *Chāndogya*, the nose is *samāna* and as per *yogaśāstra* and *āyurveda* the seat of *samāna* is the abdomen. Again the nose is the province of the earth element, which gives sensitivity of smell, yet comes under the province of air. Nostrils too yield breathing. So the question arises in the mind, how to associate nose, *samāna vāyu* and earth element with its function of smelling and breathing?

Respiration and digestion are related to each other. If the digestion is poor, respiration is poor. If one has overeaten, the nostrils get blocked. Breathing becomes hard as *samāna* gets congested and the fire blocks the nostrils. If both the nostrils have to remain open, *samāna* has to maintain its balance. The province of fire in *samāna* is to keep one healthy. *Samāna* means evenness or balance. If one has to do *Uḍḍīyāna* in *prāṇāyāma, samāna* has to function healthily. Normally the breathing is done alternately by the nostrils, yet they do not remain open evenly. The flow of the breath changes every one to one and half hours in the nostrils in turn. When *samāna* is controlled, both the nostrils keep open. This shows that the respiratory system is dependent upon the rhythmic function of *samāna*.

The skin belongs to *udāna*. Yoga as well as *āyurveda* relates it to the air element and touch as its sensitivity, though it has the quality of the earth element – the smell. *Vyāna* controls the blood circulation and energy flow in the nerves. The space, the element of ether, makes blood to flow in their channels by sensitising the system to carry messages through the nerves. The province of the air element is in the throat and upper chest, though this area belongs to *udāna*. Its job is to respond and reflect to the senses of perception like a mosquito bite, touch of a fly or skin burns.

While doing *āsana* or *prāṇāyāma*, the *udāna* plays a great role of giving sensitivity and lightness to the skin, though *vyāna* maintains the sensitivity of touch. Thus *vyāna* introduces sensitivity as well as contraction or expansion and *udāna* brings action on the skin.

In *Vibhūti Pāda* Patañjali says that *udānajayājjalapaṅka kaṇṭakādiṣvasaṅga utkrāntiśca* (*Y.S.*, III.40) – By mastery of *udāna vāyu*, the yogi can walk over water, swamps and thorns without touching them and he can also levitate. As *udāna* gives sensitivity, it can also withdraw the touch perception and bring lightness in a person to levitate. *Vyāna* brings the lightness as well as the mobility.

Matsyendranātha and Gorakṣanātha could go from place to place by levitating through *udāna jaya* and speed up through *vyāna*. The space travelling (*ākāśa gamanam*) is possible thanks to *vyāna*. And the lightness by eliminating the weight factor making one as light as the cotton fibre is of the *udāna*.

Kāya ākāśayoḥ saṁbandha saṁyamāt laghutūlasamāpatteḥ ca ākāśagamanam (*Y.S.*, III.43) – by knowing the relationship between the body and ether, the yogi transforms his body and mind to become as light as the cotton fibre. He can levitate in space. This is the conquest of ether. *Udāna* and *vyāna* work co-ordinating with each other.

Though *Upaniṣad* differ from yoga and *āyurveda* regarding the positions of *vāyu*, one needs to know the depth of the *prāṇa śakti* through experienced knowledge as they function differently when brought under control.

The eyes can see through the power of *prāṇa*. Ears hear through the power of *vyāna*. By the power of *apāna* tongue tastes food without consuming it and develops divine speech. Through the power of *samāna* the nose smells and controls digestion. This is how the cosmic energy engulfs the entire body as *Vaiśvānara agni*.

The brain is the main province of *prāṇa* and functions as controller and activator of the senses of perception and makes the skin to feel the whole body. The *prāṇa* from the brain, and *apāna* from the bottom of the body have to reach the core for the life force to be active. If *apāna* is the base, *prāṇa* is the roof. Between *prāṇa* and *apāna*, the *samāna*, *vyāna* and *udāna* function.

The organs of excretion and reproduction as *karmendriya* are under the regime of *apāna*. The excretion indicates the health of digestion, absorption and assimilation. The reproduction announces the health of the next generation. The seven ingredients *(saptadhātu)*, which hold and support the body, point out the whole metabolism of the body, which begins from *rasa* and terminates in semen.[1] These ingredients need to be healthy and proportionate. *Apāna* generates the energy and *samāna, udāna* and *vyāna* organize and distribute the energy. *Prāṇa* throws and destroys the unwanted, polluted energy. Inhalation is *apāna kriyā*, which starts from the navel. Exhalation is *prāṇa kriyā*, which starts from the chest. The retentions in both ways organize and distribute the energy. *Samāna, vyāna* and *udāna* help to sustain the energy.

Thus, we learn that the five elements (earth, water, fire, air and ether), their fine infrastructures (odour, taste, shape, touch and sound), five *vāyu (prāṇa, apāna, samāna, udāna* and *vyāna)* are all interwoven, inter-relate and inter-function with the five principles of the body *(annamaya, prāṇamaya, manomaya, vijñānamaya* and *ānandamaya)*, uniformly balancing the body for the Soul to travel freely.

If disturbances take place in these interwoven elements, diseases take place creating chaotic *(astāvyasta)* state in health of body, mind and Soul.

In order to observe and understand these interwoven functions in these various facets of life and to develop balance, harmony, concord and at the same time bringing sensitivity and clarity, long uninterrupted practice of all the aspects yoga alone are the means to live dynamically with an electrifying life.

III.4.18. – *Kevala Kuṁbhaka*

Patañjali explains yoga as *yogaḥ citta vṛtti nirodhaḥ* – yoga is to restrain the fluctuations of the consciousness. Though the meaning is simple, how many of us know the depth of this statement?

Citta is simply an instrument, but the constituents that are sheltered by it are many. These are organs of action, senses of perception, mind, I-ness, intelligence and ego. Therefore

[1] **Seven ingredients** – ***Saptadhātu***

chyle	*rasa*
blood	*rakta*
flesh	*māṁsa*
fat	*meda*
bone	*asthi*
bone marrow	*majjā*
semen	*śukra*

a yoga *sādhaka* has to begin to look into the content and understand them. Then *citta* reveals its simplicity.

This gives the idea that, in order to create silence in consciousness, one has to first restrain the senses of perception and mind. From this restraint, one will be able to do *prāṇāyāma* directly from the consciousness.

As *citta* has *vṛtti, prāṇa* too has its *vṛtti,* which are *bāhya vṛtti, abhyantara vṛtti* and *staṁbha vṛtti.*

If inhalation is *abhyantara vṛtti*, exhalation is *bāhya vṛtti* and steadiness of *prāṇa* is *staṁbha vṛtti. Nirodha vṛtti* of *citta* is synonymous to *staṁbha vṛtti* of *prāṇa.*

Patañjali explains *kevala vṛtti* or *kevala staṁbha* or *kevala kuṁbhaka* clearly in *sūtra* II.51 – *bāhya ābhyantara viṣaya ākṣepī caturthaḥ.* It is a state of non-deliberate retention of *prāṇa* where the consciousness fades out on its own (*svarūpa śūnya*).

As the *vṛtti* of *citta* are afflictive and non-afflictive, the *vṛtti* of *prāṇa* also are afflictive and non-afflictive by nature. *Prāṇāyāma* regulates the irregularities of the breath *(prāṇa vṛtti nirodha)* and affects the consciousness to remain still.

When *prāṇāyāma* transcends the known towards the state of aloneness *(kevala)*[1] consciousness also transcends its level to become one with the Soul. This shows the co-relation between *prāṇa* and *citta.* The word *viṣaya ākṣepī* is *akalpitā vṛtti* (inconceivable *vṛtti).* As consciousness has *akalpitā vṛtti* (Y.S., III.44)[2] so does the *prāṇa.* This is the *viṣaya ākṣepi* of *prāṇa vṛtti,* identical to the ultimate state of consciousness. By this *prāṇa viṣaya* the consciousness becomes *prajñā viṣaya.* This way Patañjali brings the union *(saṁyoga)* of *prāṇa* with *prajñā* and *prajñā* with *prāṇa.* This state is nothing but *ātmā bhāva bhāvanā nivṛttiḥ (Y.S.,* IV.25), fading of the sense of separation between consciousness and soul. Others call this state *Kevala Kuṁbhaka.*

---

1 *tasmin sati śvāsa praśvāsayoḥ gativicchedaḥ prāṇāyāmaḥ* (Y.S., II.49) – *prāṇāyāma* is the regulation of the inbreath and the outbreath.

bāhyābhyantara stambha vṛttiḥ deśa kāla saṁkhyābhiḥ paridṛṣṭaḥ dīrgha sūkṣmaḥ (Y.S., II.50) – *prāṇāyāma* has three movements – deep and fine inhalation, retention and exhalation. They are measured according to the space in the trunk, time and precision.

2 *bahiḥ akalpita vṛttiḥ mahāvidehā tataḥ prakāśa āvaraṇakṣyaḥ* (Y.S., III.44) – in the disembodied state, the consciousness acts outside the body, the veil covering the light of illumination is destroyed.

III.4.19. – Effects of *prāṇāyāma*

The different types of *prāṇāyāma* are meant to bring changes at all levels of the body whether they are physical, physiological, psychological, emotional or intellectual or spiritual. Basically the process of *prāṇāyāma* rotates around five major factors, though there are varieties of *prāṇāyāma*.

These are, a) inhalation *(pūraka)*, b) inhalation-retention *(antara kuṁbhaka)*, c) exhalation *(recaka)*, d) exhalation-retention *(recaka kuṁbhaka)*, and e) retention beyond the imaginable thoughts of inhalation or exhalation *(kevala kuṁbhaka)*.

Patañjali covers the science of *prāṇāyāma* and its techniques in three *sūtra* and their effects in three. He explains in I.34 and II.49 to 53.

In the second chapter, he gives a guideline on *prāṇāyāma*, where he initiates the pupils of yoga to regulate the movements of breath (*Y.S.*, II.49) – when the perfection is achieved in *āsana*, he advises one to attempt to regulate inhalation, exhalation and retention. The *sūtra* indicates a format mainly to improve the movements like expansion and extension of physical and physiological bodies through the breath. Here he wants one to observe the movements of breath and learn to adjust for smooth flow.

In *sūtra* II.50, Patañjali fastens disclpline and asks one to acquire control over the breath. By this, Patañjali wants the yoga practitioners to go to the subtle techniques of *prāṇāyāma*, where he shows spacing of the breath in the torso, by making full use of the trunk. Then he wants them to maintain the depth and precise flow of breath. Here he advises not only the precise flow of breath but also its cessation to be prolonged and refined according to one's capacity.

Then *Bāhyābhyāntara viśayākśepi caturthaḥ* (*Y.S.*, II.51). He wants us to transcend the previous stages of *prāṇāyāma*, explaining how to make it natural after efforts are ceased. As the *sūtra* 49 and 50 indicate effortful effort, the 51st *sūtra* indicates an effortless state of *prāṇāyāma*. This *prāṇāyāma* is beyond the regulated inhalation and exhalation recognised as *kevala kuṁbhaka* by other yogic texts. Here the practice of *prāṇāyāma* for the *sādhaka* becomes effortless, non-thoughtful and non-deliberate. These explanations in three *sūtra* show cultivation, culture, crystallisation and reaching the ultimate fruit in *prāṇāyāma*.

Now let us study what *pratipakṣa bhāvanā* means. *Pratipakṣa bhāvanā* literally means, "cultivating of the opposite". Patañjali says, *vitarka bādhane pratipakṣa bhāvanam* (*Y.S.*, II.33). The principles that run contrary to *yama* and *niyama* are to be encountered with knowledge and awareness. In *prāṇāyāma* he wants all opposing forces to be sublimated to develop the smoothness and crystallisation.

Pratipakṣa bhāvanām means to develop the awareness to counteract the wrong feelings and tendencies. *Pratipakṣa bhāvanā* is a counteracting force, or a counter-thought to check wrong acts or wrong thoughts. So we have to bring opposite acts or thoughts to fight with those acts and thoughts that overpower or weaken us. This is known as *pratipakṣa bhāvanā*.

The nose seems to be the entrance for the flow of the breath. But actually the inhalation originates from the navel and not from the nose. When one begins to inhale, he needs to remain alert and silent to find out the exact origin that takes place before the start of inhalation. For this, silence is needed to observe and see that no other thought-sound arises in the mind in order to trace the vibration before the movement of inhalation.

The question here is not about how long one breathes, but how one watches the breath without any other thought or chain of thoughts. For this, he has to see that silence is established in the head and heart before he begins *prāṇāyāma*. He should not oscillate the mind but use it to witness the flow of the breath. These phenomena are opposite by nature. The movement of breath stimulates and creates thoughts in the brain. Here begins *pratipakṣa bhāvanā* where he has to discipline the brain to remain quiet while doing the deep in-breath, out-breath or retention. If the brain is not quietened, then the thoughts interrupt the movement of breath and drive it to be sucked by the brain. Hence, one has to develop deliberation on the line of *pratipakṣa bhāvanā*. He has to learn to develop the sovereignty of intelligence and sobriety of brain, so that the brain remains as a witness and not an actor. This is called *pratipakṣa bhāvanā*. The *vitarka bādhanā* is the stimulation of brain cells, leading to arousal of thoughts. If *pakṣa* is action of the brain, *pratipakṣa bhāvanā* is to make it a witness and to remain silent.

Often prayers, *praṇava japa* or *gāyatri mantra japa,* are introduced to check the thought waves and make the mind to focus on one point. This is also a kind of *pratipakṣa bhāvanā,* as arousal of thoughts is arrested with prayers.

Watching the movement of respiration makes the mind rewind itself to feel the touch and the way the breath percolates and expands along with its vibration. By this method, the mind merges with the breath and the breath with the mind arresting the thought movements. This is also *pratipakṣa bhāvanā*.

Again, one finds that one lung or one nostril or one side of the torso responds to the breath more than the other side. Or one side takes the initiative and the other may remain inactive. The one that acts is *pakṣa,* and making the other side to act along with *pakṣa* is *pratipakṣa bhāvanā.* Weighing the imbalanced side with the balanced side is also a sort of *pratipakṣa bhāvanā.*

It is interesting to observe that in the process of *recaka* there is a non-deliberate *kuṁbhaka.* If the torso is not gripped firmly, exhalation cannot be moved smoothly. *Prāṇāyāmic* exhalation has a utility purpose and it is this. Due to soft, slow and subtle exhalation in *prāṇāyāmic* method, the lungs get a chance to re-absorb the residual *prāṇic* energy that is drawn through subtle inhalation, which remains till the end of exhalation. This is how the energy gets stored whereas in the normal breath, the chances for lungs to re-absorb are remote.

Normally the chest and the diaphragm move faster than the release of the breath. In *prāṇāyāmic* breathing the diaphragm is controlled, the intercostal muscles are gripped for smooth flow of breath. It is interesting to observe that the chest-box and diaphragm are held firm in exhalation whereas they are kept passive and pensive in the movement of the inhalation.

In inhalation, the intelligence remains passive in order to keep the lungs receptive, whereas in exhalation the intelligence controls the movement of the breath.

When *Antara Kuṁbhaka* is done, study how the self engulfs the chest with firm spine and relaxed brain, while in *Bāhya Kuṁbhaka* the intelligence gets subdued and reaches the self.

Due to want of understanding, if the physical grip overpowers the mental grip in *kuṁbhaka,* shift the grip from the body to the mind. This is also another kind of *pratipakṣa bhāvanā.* In *kuṁbhaka.* Learn to bring alignment and grip evenly at the physical, physiological, psychological and intellectual levels.

Then this type of *kuṁbhaka* is restful and peaceful. When one has crossed the deliberate *prāṇāyāma* technique, then arises, *Kevala Pūraka, Kevala Recaka* and *Kevala Kuṁbhaka. Kevala* means natural.

In inhalation see that the energy reaches every nook and corner of the chest. In exhalation see that the effortful state of releasing reaches an effortless state. Do not do *prāṇāyāma* movements unmindfully.

See that no micro-ventilation takes place in *kuṁbhaka.* If so, then that *kuṁbhaka* is not a divine *kuṁbhaka* as *kuṁbhaka* is nothing but to be in contact with the Supreme within.

Patañjali refers to the effects of *prāṇāyāma* in two *sūtra.* He says that the mastery of *prāṇāyāma* removes the veils covering the intelligence, and leads one towards knowledge and understanding. He does not speak of lungs. Here he mentions in simple terms that *prāṇāyāma* brings clarity in the brain and purity in the heart. Then he says that since the mind has acquired the competence to move on towards the gateway of concentration *(dhāraṇā),* it indicates that perfection of intelligence *(buddhi śakti)* takes place in *prāṇāyāma.*

Also in *sūtra* I.34, *pracchardana vidhāraṇābhyāṁ vā prāṇasya,* Patañjali brings to our attention how rising thoughts can be subdued. Is it not *pratipakṣa bhāvanā,* as one can notice how in exhalation *bhāvanā* disappear into thin air which makes the mind quiet and pensive.

Therefore, the effect of *prāṇāyāma* and *citta vṛtti nirodha* are identical as both *prāṇa vṛtti nirodha* and *citta vṛtti nirodha* leave no imprints of *bādhanā, bhāvanā* or *pratipakṣa bhāvanā.* All these three states fade out totally, without disparities for one to experience oneness of the Soul.

III.5. – *Pratyāhāra*

III.5.1. – *Pratyāhāra* in practice

Pratyāhāra actually is a resting time to feel the behavioural pattern of the peripheral mind, the organs of action and senses of perception by keeping them in their places or abodes like the restraint of the consciousness that makes the soul to rest in its abode.

Pratyāhāra can be compared to *virāma pratyaya* state as a threshold between *bahiraṅga sādhanā* and *antaraṅga sādhanā.* Patañjali explains the four states of *samādhi,* namely, self-analysis, synthesis, bliss and the feel of the pure soul in *sūtra* I.17, in the succeeding *sūtra* II.18, he speaks on the pause that happens between the states of *samprajñāta samādhi* and *asamprajñāta samādhi.* It may be possible that in this state of pause (*virāma*), a stalemate may occur in one and he may miss the road towards further progress or it may make him to leap towards the innermost quest *(antarātma sādhanā).*

In *pratyāhāra* state, Patañjali guides us in such a way that the evolutionary methods so far followed may not bring a downfall but may act as a stabilising state from where one proceeds to climb the top-most point of yoga.

In order to grasp the fullness of this *sūtra,* let me elaborate, how it works in the presentation of *āsana.*

Most of us practise *āsana* and *prāṇāyāma* using our senses of perception for perceptibility. This perceptibility creates an organisation of external stimuli, and an ability to process, act and interpret according to the imprints derived from the senses of perception.

Āsana like *Utthita Trikoṇāsana, Utthita Parśvakoṇāsana, Pārśvottānāsana, Prasārita Padottānāsana, Paśchimottānāsana, Bharadvājāsana, Ardha Matsyendrāsana,* can be engaged through the senses of perception for recharging the mind and intelligence. In these *āsana* the senses of perception act as messengers of the mind to bring various forms of attention on one's practice. The external senses take the lead to process, act and interpret the *āsana*. This according to Patañjali is learning through external means *(bahiraṅga sādhanā).*

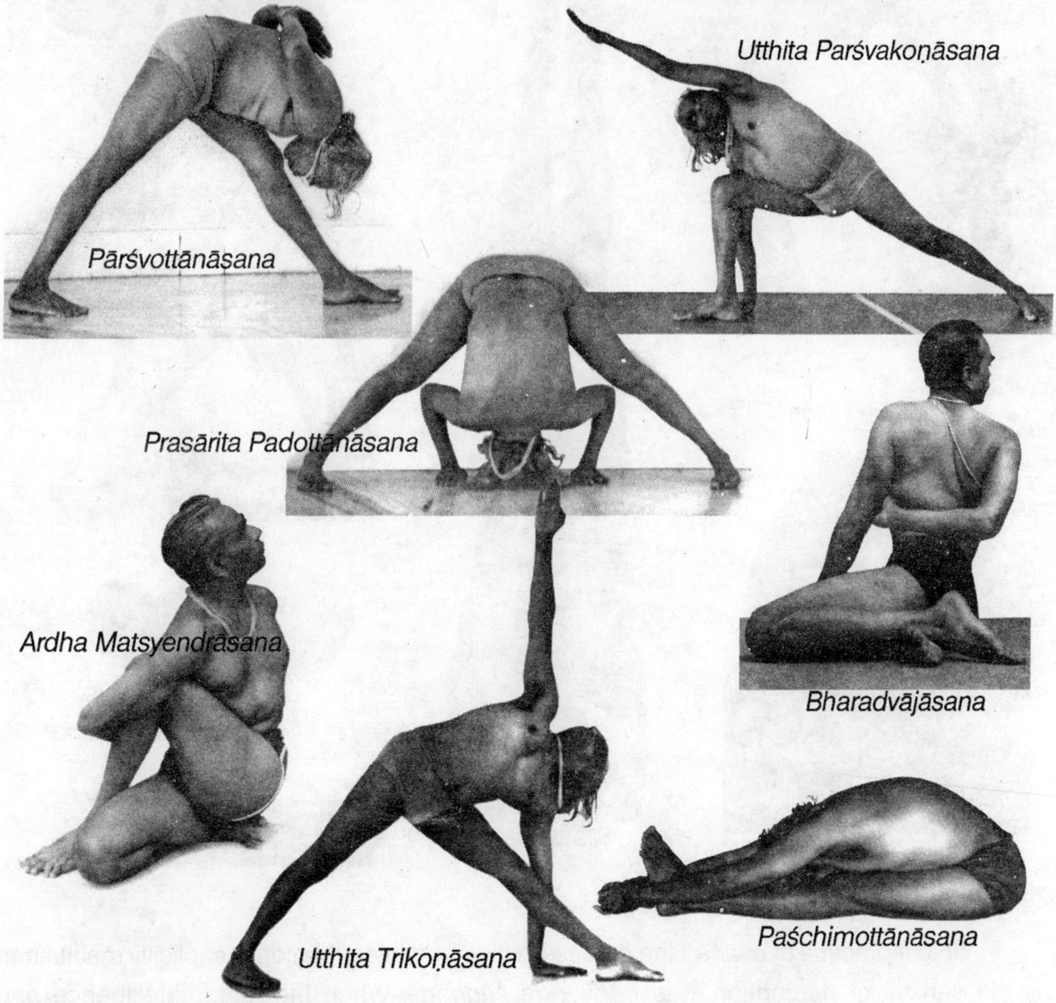

Plate n. 14 – Perceptual *āsana*

Āsana like *Śīrṣāsana, Ūrdhva Dhanurāsana. Kapotāsana, Vṛṣchikāsana, Ūrdhva Kukkuṭāsana, Pārśva Kukkuṭāsana,* are conceptual *āsana.* They are to be processed, acted and interpreted through the conception of the mind. The feeling that is sensed in the body by the mind acts as an internal stimuli to re-act in bringing right-action for stability in the body, awareness in the mind and attention in the intelligence. This conceptual practice of *āsana* and *prāṇāyāma* is done through the internal organs like mind, intelligence and consciousness. This is actually as internal practice (*antaraṅga sādhanā*).

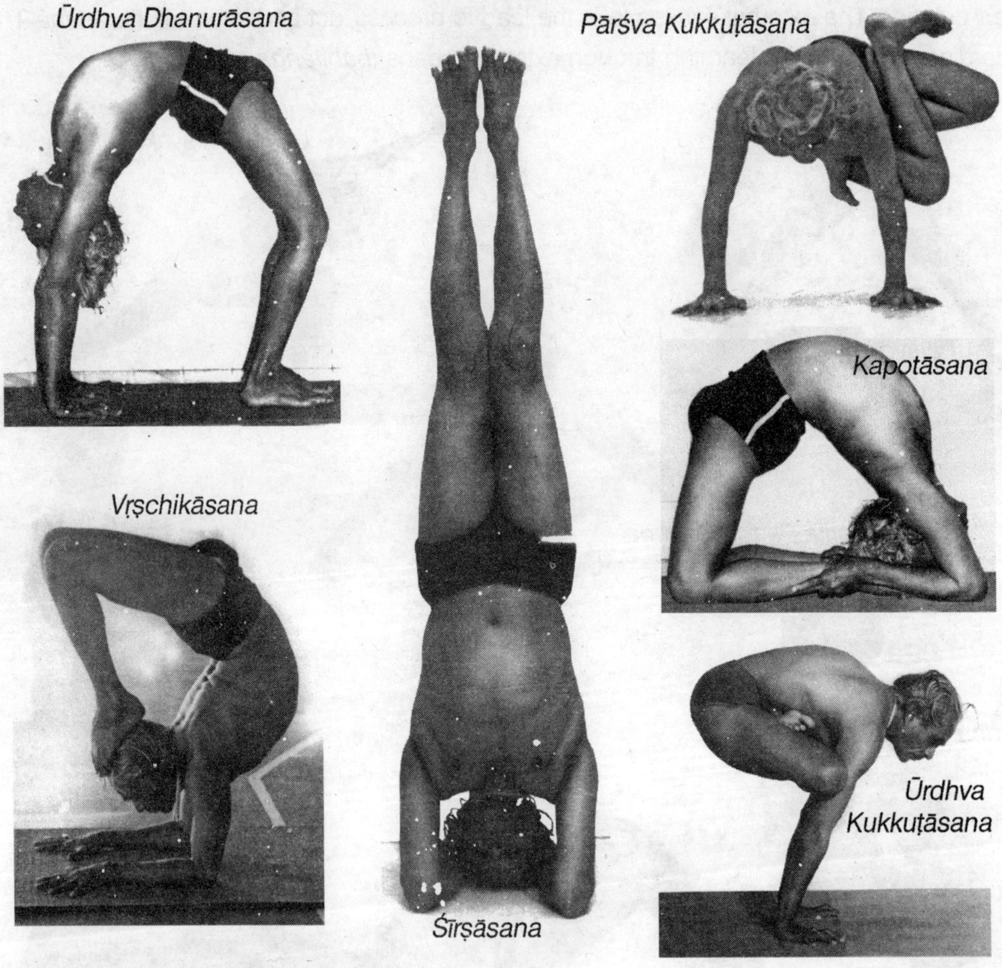

Plate n. 15 – Conceptual *āsana*

In our practice of *āsana* if the process, action and interpretation is explicitly maintained by the senses of perception, it is *bahiraṅga sādhanā.* When the mind, intelligence and consciousness explicitly manifest in process, action and interpretation it is *antaraṅga sādhanā.*

As I have said on several occasions, a bird flies with two wings, here, *āsana, prāṇāyāma* or *dhyāna* have two wings to reach the ultimate goal of achievement. These two wings are the external stimuli, by the senses of perception and internal stimuli by the mind and intelligence.

Patañjali explains that *dhāraṇā, dhyāna* and *samādhi* are internal *sādhanā* compared to the other external aspects of yoga *(yama, niyama, āsana, prāṇāyāma, pratyāhāra): trayam antaraṅgaṁ pūrvebhyaḥ* (*Y.S.*, III.7).

For me *pratyāhāra* conveys that the moment one moves from external stimuli, through the senses of perception, towards earning knowledge to trigger the internal stimuli, for intellectual wisdom and conscious awareness, even the earlier five aspects of yoga, become internal *(antaraṅga)*. So *pratyāhāra* is an adaptation and hence is not a disciplinary methodology.

This is an important stage to cross over, from the perception of the senses towards the conception of the mind.

When the self is not in contact with the thought waves or afflictions, it rests in its own abode. Similarly, in *pratyāhāra* the senses of action and perception are made to rest in their abodes by making them to get non-attached to the external objects of the world.

Tataḥ paramā vaśyatā indriyāṇām (Y.S., II.55) – thus, *pratyāhāra* results in the absolute control of the sense organs. The ways of quietening them have been dealt with by Patañjali in: *viṣayavati vā pravṛttiḥ utpannā manasaḥ sthiti nibandhani (Y.S.,* I.35). Here the senses, mind, intelligence and consciousness are held in an attentive awareness on a pleasing thing or an object congenial to spiritual aspirations. As such, *āsana* is also a part of that contemplation.

For the *sādhaka,* the adolescent period is a crucial time, where one begins to desire the taste of the pleasures of the world. Nature keeps adolescents and youths in the highest peak of physical power with expressions of emotions, desires and physical instinctive wants. Their minds are caught in the web of pleasures and enjoyments. Though the mind is considered as the king of senses of perception and organs of action, it falls prey to the cravings of the senses. This is the time for them to think and channel their energy in the right direction for a disciplined way in the benevolent art of living.

Children are not aware of such pleasures of life of which adolescents are aware. Their heart is pure and hence they need not be deliberately taught to control the senses and mind. They are not aware of the problems of the future. Why create confusion in their minds for unknown things to toss over? The sensual pleasures that remain dormant in childhood grow in the adolescent period. What we need to think of is how to find ways and means of guiding them in their adolescent period so that they are disciplined to grow themselves in positive and constructive ways. As they are educated by the time they reach adolescence, they can use their discriminative knowledge in disciplining their senses and mind for manhood or womanhood. Elders have to live as examples so that children follow their footsteps in order to build right discipline without speaking on *pratyāhāra.*

Children follow by looking at elders. The modern life has changed the concept of life. Parents go astray and children follow and imitate them. If the parents take to smoking and drinking, children follow them and when they grow up they literally become the victims of such habits.

Moral practices of *yama* and *niyama* are common to all religions. It is advisable to follow these universal moral principles as much as possible, which cover all sections of society irrespective of place or class.

These universal disciplines as well as individual disciplines along with *āsana* and *prāṇāyāma* act as a backbone for *pratyāhāra. Āsana* individually guides one to bring his body, brain and nerves under control, whereas *prāṇāyāma* cultures the mind. Then intelligence establishes in building up a state of stability in body, senses, and mind.

Pratyāhāra is not a practice but a will to maintain what has been earned and progressively cultured to establish a permanent imprint in the head and heart.

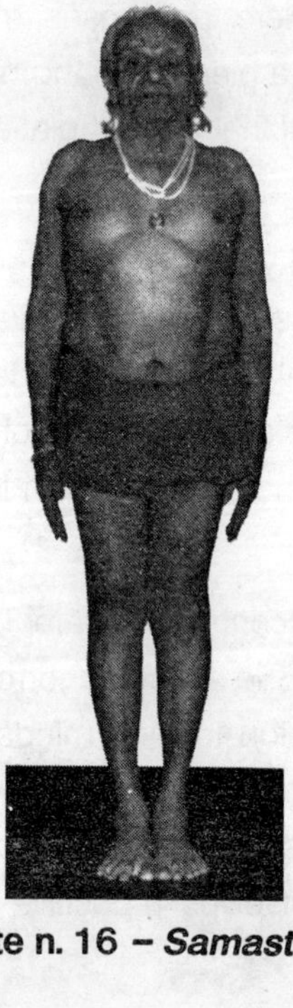

Plate n. 16 – *Samasthiti*

One knows *Samasthiti,* in which he holds the body in an upright position. Does his awareness spread all over the body without disparity? Here the importance of the combined knowledge of perceptivity and conceptivity comes in to play which is the key of *pratyāhāra.* In my teaching, I use these two stimuli to bring awareness to spread from the top of the head to the bottom of the feet, so that the flow of intellectual attention and conscious awareness is felt evenly on the outside and the inside, as well as the front and back of the body in the performances of *āsana* and *prāṇāyāma.* Here I make them to bring right alignment not only in external actions but in the internal ones to move towards the self. This is *pratyāhāra* in action.

In the second chapter of the *Bhagavad Gītā* Lord Krishna speaks about the characteristics of *sthitaprajñan,* the one whose wisdom is firmly established:

Yadā saṁharate cāyaṁ kūrmo'ṅgānīva sarvaśaḥ I
indriyāṇī indriyārthebhyah tasya prajñā pratiṣṭhitā II *(B.G.,* II.58)

One who withdraws his senses from the sensual objects as a tortoise draws its limbs into the shell from all directions, establishes the intelligence firmly in wisdom. As the practitioner learns to withdraw the limbs, senses and mind inwards like a tortoise, he is a *pratyāhārin.*

Practice of *āsana* works on the cells of the body, and *prāṇāyāma* controls the flow of the breath and stills the oscillations of the mind. These two aspects put a brake on the out-going and distorting mind and protect the practitioner from lack of attention, awareness and alertness.

No doubt, stress, strain and fatigue are felt in the beginning, as one has to discipline and culture the body, senses, mind and intelligence. This happens because he does not link these two together. The moment he feels that they are gradually integrating, he is inspired and feels energetic to go ahead.

Patañjali defines *pratyāhāra* as withdrawal of the senses from external objects bringing control over them. He defines *pratyāhāra* without a methodology. While teaching *āsana*, I make all adjust each and every part of the body judiciously and conspicuously using understandable terminologies so that they draw the senses and mind towards the interior body. This is a process where I draw their intelligence towards *pratyāhāra.* For example, *Kṣurikopaniṣad* says, "Bring the *citta* to the feet, toes, ankles, knees, anus and abdomen and establish there". Am I asking anything different? *Triśikhi brāhmaṇōpaniṣad* asks to establish *citta* on thighs, reproductive organs, heart, throat, palate, root of palate, tongue, root of tongue, nose, forehead, eyes, hands, joints of hands, and all the sensitive areas of the body where *prāṇic* energy is stored *(marmasthāna).* In each *āsana* I take the attention wholistically to all these areas in the body and show ways to adjust so that the energy is enthused and not wasted. Is it not *pratyāhāra* according to the *Upaniṣad?*

Years ago, I had compared the four corners of the bottom of the feet to the four tyres of a vehicle, where air pressures are measured and the tyres filled accordingly. This explanation was meant to position the body in *Tāḍāsana* in such a way that energy flows without interruption from the feet to the head. It is the restraint of energy or *prāṇabandhana. Darśanopaniṣad* defines *pratyāhāra* as retaining and maintaining energy in its place; *prāṇabandhanam vāyudhāraṇātmakam pratyāhārah* (7, 10, 11-12).

In my early days of practice, my sincere approach was to reach perfection in *āsana.* Later this approach revealed to me the process of travelling inwards, which I then read about in the *Upaniṣad.* This confirmed that I was in the right direction as per the valid knowledge of the scriptures *(āgama)*. If I were devoid of faith *(śraddhā)*, I would not have reached this level. Unfortunately, our doubting minds differentiate *āsana* and *pratyāhāra* as separate entities.

The question is how to bring our attention to focus within. Stop differentiating between doing, doer and done or the knower, the instrument of knowing and the known, and see all these three flow as a single unit. Whether it is *āsana* or *prāṇāyāma*, make the attention to go centripetally and centrifugally to spread all over the body. This state becomes the state of *pratyāhāra*.

In our spinal column, we have six *cakra* where the physical, mental and spiritual energies are stored and intersect. Through *āsana* and *prāṇāyāma*, the energy is stored and stimulated as self-enlivening energy *(svarasavāhini)* to penetrate the source, and this is the stabilised point of *pratyāhāra*. So do not conclude that practice of *āsana* or *prāṇāyāma* is done to gain mere physical health.

In *prāṇāyāma* the inhalation is a journey from the soul to the skin and in exhalation it is a journey from the skin to the soul. In *kuṁbhaka*, the soul is lifted along with its dwelling place, the chest. These expressions are not easily understood. The soul has freedom to move all along its frontier. The Soul is the King. The *pañca prāṇa*, *pañca karmendriya* and *pañca jñānendriya* as well as the *manas, buddhi* and *ahaṁkāra* are like attendants who move with the king. When indiscipline besets the attendants, it is the King who becomes the victim. If the King (Soul) disciplines his subordinates it means he is teaching them *pratyāhāra*.

Placed as the fifth limb, Patañjali has rightly sown the seed in the form of *yama* and *niyama* along with *āsana* and *prāṇāyāma* to grow as fruit in *pratyāhāra*. When *pratyāhāra* is fully ripened *(paripakvata)*, it transforms to savour the essence of experienced wisdom *(rasātmaka jñāna)*.

III.5.2. – Should the eyes be kept open or closed in our practices

The eyes are meant to see. We can see and experience the world through the eyes. Eyes play a double role. They may lead one to live in the pits of pleasure or they may guide one to rest on the bed of the soul.

The eyes are the windows of the brain and the ears are the windows of the mind. Both the eyes and ears follow the outgoing thoughts or the incoming thoughts. Hence it is essential for the mind and intelligence to train the eyes and ears. The brain helps in controlling the eyes, and the mind helps in controlling the ears, or the eyes may discipline the brain and ears the mind.

While doing *āsana*, the eyes are kept open so that the brain remains alert and gets charged to connect itself to all parts of the body to perfect the *āsana*. If the body is left unseen then the *āsana* takes a wrong shape. Eyes are there to perceive and the mind is there to conceive. As one can peep out from windows, one can also peep in. *Āsana* makes the intelligence peep into the body, asking for measured guidance. Practice of *āsana* with closed eyes disconnects the body from the mind and intelligence. Hence, it is better to keep the eyes open for the conscious brain to get connected to the action as well as to the body.

In *prāṇāyāma*, the eyes play a different role. Here they are made to close while the ears are made to listen to the resonance of the sound of in-breath and out-breath. This way *prāṇāyāma* acts on the mind and makes it to extend at the threshold, for spiritual awareness. If the eyes are kept open in *prāṇāyāma*, restlessness sets in, whereas closed eyes quieten and pacify the brain. This is how eyes and ears are trained to bring stability in the mind for it to enter the gates of the Soul.

III.5.3. – Effect of *pratyāhāra*

Patañjali makes an authoritative statement in *sūtra* II.17; *draṣṭṛdṛśyayoḥ saṁyogaḥ heyahetuḥ* – association of the seer with the seen is the cause of distress. Avoidance of union between them is the remedy for distress. The contact of nature with *puruṣa* is the cause of all unhappiness in the world. It is a guide to all of us to learn to detach from the world to find liberation. No doubt, it appears as a sweeping statement. But later he realises: *prakāśa kriyā sthiti śīlaṁ bhūtendriyātmakaṁ bhogāpavargārthaṁ dṛśyam* (*Y. S.*, II.18) – nature, with its three *guṇa (sattva, rajas* and *tamas)*, exists for the enjoyment of pleasures, or for the emancipation of man.

Nature has certain qualities and virtues like *sattva, rajas* and *tamas*, which have their own importance in life. The *guṇa* are so powerful that they pull us either towards *bhoga* or yoga. So he instructs us to understand the good qualities of *tamas, rajas* and *sattva* to learn about the world without being a part of it. *Kṛtārthaṁ prati naṣṭam api anaṣṭaṁ tadanya sādhāraṇatvāt* (*Y. S.*, II.22) – the relationship with nature ceases for the emancipated beings as its purpose having been fulfilled, but its process continues to affect others.

Normally, we surrender to the flow of these qualities and move with them as they take us, and we use them mostly for *bhogārtham,* as pleasures are our basic instincts. We need to recognise the *śīlatā* or the virtuosity of senses because the senses can also be used for *apavargārtham.* In *Yoga Sūtra* II.23, Patañjali clearly says that the senses are for the evolution of the soul. Understand their purpose: as soon as they have fulfilled one's purpose they withdraw and he realises his position.

He wants us to use them as the instruments for progress to achieve spiritual realisation. "They are there only to serve us, not to rule over us". Yoga is that method which teaches us to draw the senses towards the soul. For example, when we do *Paśchimottānāsana,* we cannot look at the world: we have to look within ourselves. When we do *Adho Mukha Śvānāsana* (dog pose), the moment we stretch the spine, we look through our mind and feel the back. By this we learn to turn the mind inwards. This way we discipline the senses of perception and organs of action and draw them towards the seer. Let the seer benefit from these agents. If we use the agents of the seer for the sake of enjoyment, then we are caught in the web of worldly pleasures.

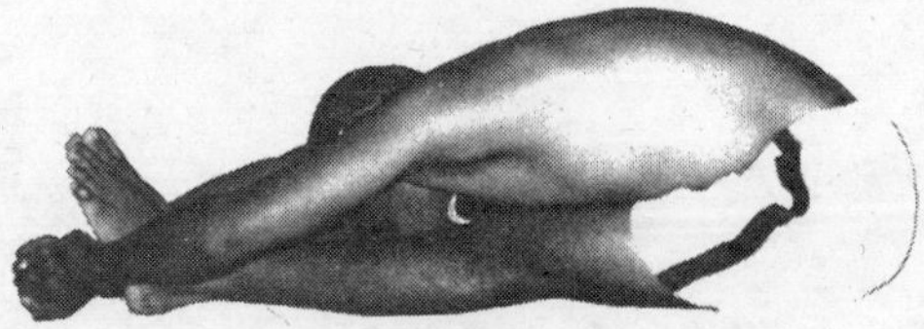

Paśchimottānāsana

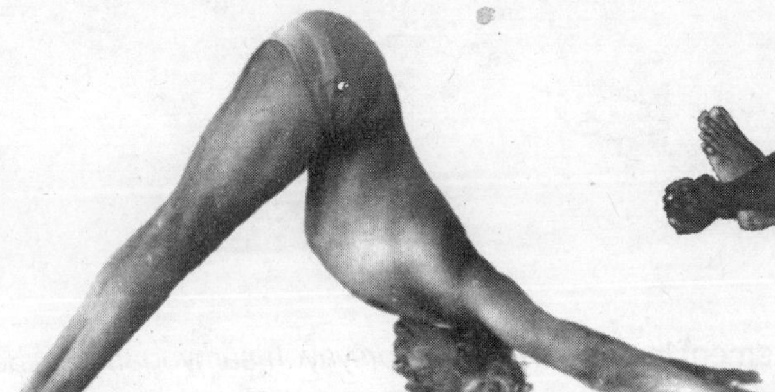

Adho Mukha Śvānāsana

Plate n. 17 – *Paśchimottānāsana* and *Adho Mukha Śvānāsana*

So distinguish between tainted pleasures *(bhoga)* and the unalloyed bliss *(apavarga)* and get disciplined in yoga.

Memory influences the mind. It does not allow the intelligence to interfere with the mind. Because it knows that if the mind listens to the intelligence, it loses its identity. So memory tries to grip the mind and see that it does not listen to the intelligence though the intelligence reminds the mind not to get caught in the net of memory. When the mind loses its balance, it talks to itself, "I should not have listened to the memory." When this dawns, it is too late for the mind. If the intelligence transforms the mind and wins it, then it is *pratyāhāra.* In this *pratyāhāra,* the memory is superseded and sublimated by the intelligence and takes the mind towards the Soul. Here the true *sādhanā* begins for the *sādhaka,* as he is made to proceed towards the domain of the Soul.

III.6. – *Dhāraṇā*

III.6.1. – What is *dhāraṇā*

Dhāraṇā is a process in which our consciousness *(citta)* is channelled and disciplined to focus on or associate with a chosen object. *Citta* is the composite of three components – mind, intelligence and "I" *(ahaṁkāra). Dhāraṇā* is a process to unite the above three components on a desired object or thought centripetally.

We may have the will *(icchā)* to achieve our wishes or our desired objects, and the power to act *(krlyā),* but lack of understanding *(jñāna)* may cause frustrations and failures. Want of knowledge and lack in dynamic action become hurdles in our aims. Sometimes we are blessed with will-power *(icchā),* knowledge *(jñāna),* but lack on the driving force to act *(kriyā śakti).*

In *dhāraṇā* we need the powers of *icchā, jñāna* and *kriyā* to reach the desired goal. If any of these fade, pursuit becomes casual. Hence, Patañjali advises the *sādhaka* to practise first *yama* to *pratyāhāra* so that the *citta* gets firmly moulded for *dhāraṇā.*

Patañjali defines *dhāraṇā* in the first *sūtra* in *Vibhūti Pāda*: *deśa bandhaḥ cittasya dhāraṇā* (*Y.S.,* III.1) – fixing the consciousness on one point or region is concentration. But he speaks on *dhāraṇā* also in *Samādhi Pāda* without the term *dhāraṇā:*

In *viṣayavati vā pravṛttiḥ utpannā manasaḥ sthiti nibandhani* (*Y.S.,* I.35) – he says that, by concentrating on an object that helps to maintain steadiness of mind and consciousness, is *dhāraṇā.* Or, *viśokā vā jyotiṣmatī* (*Y.S.,* I.36) – by contemplating on a luminous, sorrowless, effulgent light in order to gain stability. Or, *vītarāga viṣayaṁ vā cittam* (*Y.S.,* I.37) – by contemplating on divine objects, or attentively thinking on those enlightened sages who are free from desires and attachments, calm and tranquil. Or on *svapna nidrā jñāna ālambanaṁ vā* (*Y.S.,* I.38) – by recollecting and studying the experiences of dream-filled and dreamless sleep during a watchful, waking state. Or through *yathābhimata dhyānāt vā* (*Y.S.*, I.39) – meditating on any desired object conducive for stilling the consciousness.

In *dhāraṇā* the *citta* with its three components *(manas, buddhi, ahaṁkāra)* are brought to focus on a point or on an idea. One attentively focuses while reading, writing or solving the riddles.

Often we fail to co-ordinate and co-operate when we are in want of stability and will-power. Sometimes haziness makes the mind to jump from one thought to the other. *Dhāraṇā* is to tone and tune the mental faculty in such a way that the mind, intelligence and I remain in a non-wavering state with attentive awareness.

Āsana, prāṇāyāma and *pratyāhāra* practices, trains and moulds the body, mind and intelligence to be friendly and conducive towards steadiness. This steadiness *(sthiratā)* is nothing but auspicious moments *(sukhatā)* in *āsana* practice. *Prayatna śaithilya ananta samāpattibhyām* (*Y.S.*, II.47) – when the effort to perform becomes effortless, perfection in an *āsana* is achieved; *dhāraṇāsu ca yogyatā manasaḥ* (*Y.S.*, II.53) – the mind too becomes fit for concentration. *Svaviṣaya asaṁprayoge cittasya svarūpānukāraḥ iva indriyāṇāṁ pratyāhāraḥ* (*Y.S.*, II.54) – by this dawn of wisdom, the mind controls the organs of action and the senses of perception, and takes an inward journey towards the seer. *Tataḥ paramā vaśyatā indriyāṇām* (*Y.S.*, II.55) – with this control, the mind turns ripe and avid to reach its maker – the seer. It is from this state of the *citta* that the *sādhaka* moves towards *dhāraṇā*. He chooses a place *(deśa)* or a spot so that he is not distracted, but remains steady for the ripe knowledge to be revealed. This in turn purifies the mind and intellect.

The beauty of *āsana* and *prāṇāyāma* is that one extends the rays of consciousness to reach from the disk of *citta* to the extreme frontiers of the body to make the abiding *citta* to be lively in its existence as one with the body. This is *dhāraṇā* in *āsana*.

For example, when one does *Viparīta Daṇḍāsana* the consciousness has to be in that *āsana* with its rays spreading evenly from the head to the feet as a single consciousness. One cannot look here or there or make the mind shift from place to place. One has to feel in that *āsana*, not only the contact with the spine, feet, abdominal and chest region, neck and throat, but make oneself to be totally engrossed with the rays of consciousness engulfing without division the end points of the body. This way one experiences *dhāraṇā* in *āsana* where *citta* gets confined to the *āsana* and *āsana* to the *citta*.

Dhāraṇā demands only sharp *icchā śakti, jñāna śakti* and *kriyā śakti* so that the physical, mental and intellectual energies do not deviate from position to position.

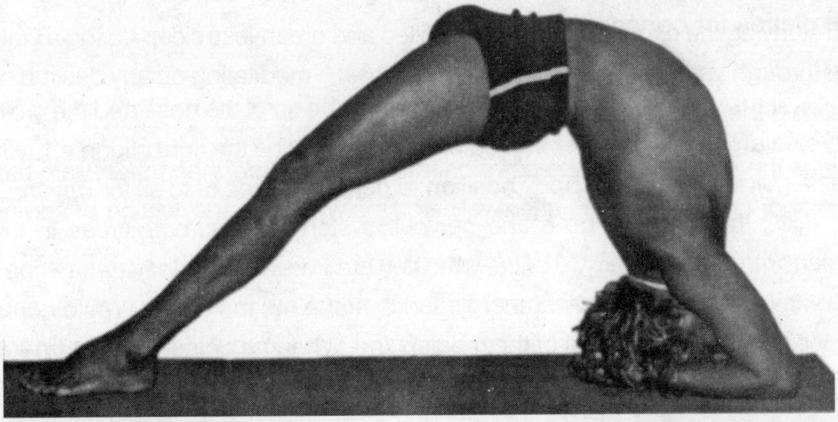

Plate n. 18 - *Viparīta Daṇḍāsana*

III.6.2. - Is effort needed in *dhāraṇā*

Yoga cannot be achieved effortlessly. All the aspects of yoga have to be done effortfully in unison. Intellectual attention and expansion of consciousness are the golden keys involved in the effective effort.

If tension is felt on the navel, the quietness on the *citta* is interrupted. If the breath changes its channel, *citta* gets disturbed. One needs *dhāraṇā* to eliminate the fluctuations in *citta,* which requires sustained effort to start with. When *citta* remains without movement and without any connection of the objects as the sun without its rays, then it is effortlessness *(samāpatti).*

In *dhāraṇā* efforts are centripetal while in *dhyāna* efforts are centrifugal. *Dhāraṇā* is like a strong coffee decoction, while in *dhyāna* the *citta* is spread all over without any dilution. In *dhāraṇā,* the *citta* is bound *(bandha)* and in *dhyāna,* its flow is like oil that flows evenly *(ekatānatā)* from one vessel to the other. This way, *dhāraṇā* and *dhyāna* silence the *citta* for the *puruṣa* to establish as Soul *(svarūpa pratiṣṭhā).*

III.6.3. – The places for concentration

The navel, the spiritual heart, throat, the tip of the tongue, the tip of the nose and the crown of the head are the median line of the inner and outer body. It explains the right alignment, which one has to use as a guide to study the body position to perform *āsana* or to sit for *dhyāna*. According to *yogic* texts, the median line of the nervous system is *suṣumṇā*. Areas in the spinal column are rich with *prāṇic* energy. That is why they are known as *prāṇāyatana* – the abodes of *prāṇa*, the vital areas. *Prāṇa* means energy and *āyatana* means abode. While commenting on dhāraṇā, Vyāsa speaks in places of the median line. When he points to *nāsāgra* – the tip of the nose, it indicates the entrance of *prāṇa*.

Similarly, *jihvāgra* or the tip of the tongue, which controls speech, indicates the connection with the mouth cavity, throat and larynx. The *jihvāgra* also indicates *mauna*. *Mauna* is to keep silence. One can keep silent outwardly, but the vibration of speech continues internally. This *antar-mauna* is important for *dhāraṇā* and is possible only with the silence of the tongue *(jihvā)*. One may stop talking externally, but to stop talking internally he needs to still vibration and create quietness at the navel. The stillness and quietness at the navel brings silence in the mind. That is why when we sit for *dhyāna*, the position *(āsana)* should be correct; breathing *(prāṇāyāma)* should be accurate and non-disturbing, the senses and mind should be at peace *(pratyāhāra)*. The *citta* should concentrate on the centre or median line of the body, that is, the spiritual heart.

It is very interesting to see these points in a different perspective. Though the tongue, mouth cavity and larynx are involved in talking or speech activity, the area below the navel is the origin of sound vibration where *apāna vāyū* rules. From this vibration, expression or pronunciation of speech takes place.

Though language is learnt by the brain, the vibration of speech first takes place at the navel. Even the mental thoughts vibrate in the navel region; therefore, stilling and silencing the navel region is essential for creating quietness in the brain and calmness in the mind. As wars take place between the head *(kurukṣetra)* and the heart *(dharmakṣetra)* the *ṛṣi* of yore therefore insisted on serenity and composure *(śanti)*, for establishing freedom to think and for maintaining peace within oneself.

Emotional disturbances create tremors in the navel and affect the heart *(hṛdaya)*. When these two get disturbed, the digestive system gets disturbed showing signs of indigestion, diarrhoea, irritable bowel syndrome, high blood pressure, palpitation, diabetes and so forth. Even the respiration or rhythm of the breath becomes laboured. Hence, the practice of *āsana* helps to co-ordinate the various functions of body to maintain both physical and mental peace.

All these suggest that the practitioner has to maintain the elements and energies (five *bhūta* and five *vāyu)* of the body in a balanced state for *dhāraṇā*.

The external objects chosen for *dhāraṇā* lead towards external knowledge, which has been explained in the *Vibhūti Pāda,* but when *dhāraṇā* is held on the inner parts, they lead towards *prakṛti-jñāna* and from *prakṛti-jñāna* towards *puruṣa-jñāna.*

Patañjali says that one acquires the knowledge of the body and its interconnected components through *saṁyama* on the navel. *Nābhicakre kāyavyūhajñānam* (*Y.S.,* III.30) – he has perfect knowledge of the human system. By *saṁyama* on the heart one acquires a thorough understanding of the consciousness *(citta),* its contents and tendencies. *Hṛdaye cittasaṁvit* (*Y.S.,* III.35) – by *saṁyama* on the core one has thorough knowledge of the functions of the consciousness. By *saṁyama* on the crown of head one gets vision of those who have reached perfection. *Mūrdhajyotiṣi siddha darśanam* (*Y.S.,* III.33) – by *saṁyama* on the crown of the head, the yogi has visions of perfected beings. Through *saṁyama* the intelligence reaches the state of *sattva* leading towards *puruṣa jñāna. Sattvapuruṣayoratyantāsaṁkīrṇayoḥ pratyayāviśeṣo bhogaḥ parārthatvāt svārthasaṁyamāt puruṣajñānam* (*Y.S.,* III.36) – by *saṁyama,* the *yogi* easily differentiates between the intelligence and the soul which is real and true. Thus, the integration *(saṁyama),* done on the internal parts of the body is meant to unite *prakṛti-śakti* or *prakṛti-jñāna* with *puruṣa-śakti* or *puruṣa-jñāna.* The choice is given to us by Vyāsa whether we want to reach self-realisation or accomplishments *(siddhi),* which are explained in *Vibhūti Pāda* from *sūtra* 15 onwards. It is a challenge thrown to us by Vyāsa – whether we want *siddhi* or *ātma-jñāna.*

Please note that *dhāraṇā* and *dhyāna* are not for peace; but peace of mind is required for *dhāraṇā* and *dhyāna. Dhāraṇā* is the focus of attention, *dhyāna* is the union of attention with intelligence and awareness of consciousness.

III.6.4. – Difference between *dhāraṇā* and *dhyāna*

Though Patañjali does not give specific techniques, he touches the subject indirectly. Yet the word *deśa* is enough for us to grasp that there is a technique for *dhāraṇā. Deśa* means region, area, place or spot. For example if I say that I stay at Shivajinagar in Pune, it indicates location but not the exact place. When I give the name of the road as Hare Krishna Mandir road, and door number of the residence, then the spot is located. Similarly, I adopt the same procedure in guiding you to perform *āsana*, concentrating on the specific areas to reach *dhāraṇā*.

Patañjali does not specify *deśa* but Vyāsa does. He says that it could be either an internal place or an external place. He enlists regions of the navel, the heart, light in the head, the tip of the nose and tongue and ends with the word so on and so forth. He also explains that *dhāraṇā* could be on an external object in space or place.

It will be interesting for one to note that Patañjali uses the word *citta* and not *citta vṛtti*. From this, it appears that *dhāraṇā* is done not only with modifications *(citta vṛtti)* but with *citta* and its rays *(citta kiraṇa)*. *Dhāraṇā* indicates *bandha* or control on these rays of consciousness. As clouds interrupt the rays of the sun, the mind interrupts the focal point. The intelligence penetrates these obscurations of the mind. This is *bandha*. Hence, the word *bandha* is used in the sense of removing the veil that blocks the rays of consciousness and obstructs it to be in connection with the Soul.

Many mistake *dhāraṇā* as *dhyāna*. *Dhāraṇā* is like the rays of the sun at its zenith holding no shadow; blazing, illuminating and penetrating where nothing remains unseen. Whereas *dhyāna* is like the rising and setting sun, low on the horizon; as if its rays were fully absorbed into one bright luminous disk. It is brimming, resplendent and complete. No excess, no lack, no waver.

Often, I am criticised that I practise and teach *āsana* and not *dhāraṇā* or *dhyāna*. If one examines my method of practice and teaching, one realises how close I am with the *sūtra* on *dhāraṇā*. My insistence on the correct posture of the body in *āsana* without any contortion, distortion and refraction is a movement in the direction of *dhāraṇā*. It makes the rays of consciousness to move uninterruptedly with full interpenetration and attention of intelligence to experience what *dhāraṇā* is. It may appear as though I am demanding the correction in the external parts of the body, but I make one to use the external body as the foundation to place the *citta* precisely to get established everywhere as one with the body. I go part by part while teaching *āsana* so that one day one reaches the whole body as *citta* expands.

Again, I would like to draw your attention to 6.13 of the Bhagavad Gītā where Lord Krishna explains the position of sitting for dhyāna. I have taken his words: *samaṁ kāya śiro grīvaṁ dhārayan acalaṁ sthiraḥ,* literally. For me it is a transformation and enlightenment. I started re-practising all *āsana* measuring the circumference of the body and balancing the right and the left sides, legs and arms to be exactly equidistance in line with the crown of the head, the centre of the neck, the sternum, the navel and the middle of the pubis and lastly the core or the centre of the self. Deciphering the message of the *Bhagavad Gītā* cleared my doubts in understanding *sthira sukhamāsana* of Patañjali.

If one jumps to *dhāraṇā* without going through the preliminary aspects of yoga, then it is like those who search for a black object in a pitch-dark place. While performing the *āsana* one has to feel each particle of the muscle and each part of the organ of the body pulsating. Body being *tāmasic,* practice of *āsana* transforms into *rājasic* nature for it to get enlightened. Hence, *āsana* are a stepping-stone for *dhāraṇā.* By *prāṇāyāma* the mind sharpens the intelligence to go towards *dhāraṇā.*

Often beginners ask where they should be seeing in the *āsana.* In fact, there is a lot of difference in seeing and looking. Looking requires attention, while seeing may remain casual. It is not bringing the eyes to see, but to look from the intellectual eye to the centre of the Soul in order to align each and every part of the body in line with the Soul.

While doing *āsana* one needs to keep the eyes open. With open eyes one maintains the brain to remain alert to look within and explore; while in *prāṇāyāma* one needs to keep the eyes closed to the feel of touch, and the ears receptive to listen to the smooth sound of the flow of each breath.

Dhāraṇā needs the internalisation of the eyes and ears to increase the attention of intelligence *(prajñā)* and flow of energy *(prāṇa),* establishing oneness in both. I ask all to penetrate through the outer body to reach the inner body and to find the source of energy mentioned by Vyāsa. To feel the inner body or cause body, the outer body has to act as a gate and therefore in *āsana, dhāraṇā* progresses from the periphery towards the core.

Vyāsa wants the *āsana* to be done by using the internal apparatus of the *citta* as *deśa,* which covers the mind, intelligence and I. All these have to work in total unison to reach the inner 'abode' or 'place'. If it is an external object *(bāhya viṣaya)* then the externalisation of attention is needed with the integration of the senses of perception and mind for *citta* to function. Here, the *citta vṛtti* become the instrument along with *citta.* As I said before, Vyāsa comments that *dhāraṇā* is fixing the mind through its modifications on different places.

As per Vacaspati, the *vṛtti* need to be disciplined for the *citta* to project on the external objects in *dhāraṇā.*

In external *dhāraṇā* the knowledge gained through *pramāṇa vṛtti* and *smṛti vṛtti* has to be very accurate. Regarding internal *dhāraṇā,* if one has to concentrate on Lord Vishnu or Jesus Christ, he needs to know the image or idol of Lord Vishnu, the significance of all the symbols, his incarnations and on Jesus Christ, he needs to know Jesus Christ, his work, historical background, his teachings, the significance of the cross and so forth. One has to concentrate and embrace wholly the personified image. While doing the *āsana* it is the same. One connects the consciousness *(citta)* directly to the chosen spot in the body for *vṛtti* to fade. Then he is wholly within himself.

Vyāsa mentions two alternatives; the first one for beginners to mould and direct the *vṛtti* to draw the attention, while the second method is meant for those who have toned their bodies and minds to focus and concentrate. According to Vacaspati, only discipline is needed. By disciplined practice one intensifies the *sādhanā* and make *dhāraṇā* easy.

As far as my way of approach is concerned I transform the rays of thoughts *(vṛtti-kiraṇa)*, and use the *citta* without the rays for attention and awareness, drawing back the rays *(vṛtti-kiraṇa)* towards the *citta*, confining within the disk of *citta* only.

III.7. – *Dhyāna*

III.7.1. – What is meditation

Meditation is to bring the complex state of mind to a state of simplicity and serenity. When one gets completely involved and integrated in the subject, it is meditation. Sitting in a corner and closing the eyes and remaining empty in body and mind does not mean meditation.

Japa, repetition of a *mantra*, is not meditation but a way towards it. Patañjali gives not only *praṇava japa* but also other methods to train the consciousness to move towards meditation. Relaxation is not meditation, but it is a state to experience the glimpse of its quality. Meditation is an experiential state and not a subject of study. It has no expression. Vanquishing the sense of ego (*ahaṁkāra*) is *dhyāna*. It is possible only to experience *dhyāna* when one is ripe both in action *(karma)* and knowledge *(jñāna)*.

III.7.2. – Preparation for meditation

Patañjali in his eight-petalled yoga has given six preparatory backgrounds before the seventh aspect – meditation. The logic behind this is to show that each aspect of yogic discipline has its own depth which makes the disciples to climb the rungs of the yogic ladder. We are composed of body, mind and soul. Therefore the mode and direction of endeavour in *sādhanā* basically starts from the periphery to the sublime, i.e., the external body towards the innermost Soul.

If the soul is the seed, mind is the tree and the skin of the body is its fruit. All the three layers that is, the seed, the tree and the skin of the body need a right treatment for the life to be tasty. As the care and treatment begin from the planting of the seed, so too the body, mind and soul require treatment with three tiered practice called *bahiraṅga*, *antaraṅga* and *antarātma sādhanā*. As the journey from the seed to the fruit cannot be demarcated, so it is in yoga *sādhanā*. Do not demarcate the physical endeavour or mental training and spiritual bliss as different to each other. All these endeavours co-exist and co-ordinate with each other. For the sake of convenience and for want of knowledge, endeavours are graphed to begin from the external *(bahiraṅga)*, terminating in the inner most *(antarātma)*. We have a *śloka* which is recited from the *Sandhyāvandanam* and is very well known to us:

Ākāśāt patitam toyam yathā gacchati sāgaram I
sarva deva namaskārah keśavam pratigacchati II

As the rains from the sky flow to the ocean, similarly the salutations done to any Deity or any God ultimately reach Keśava alone, i.e., Lord Krishna. It is the same with sādhanā, which ultimately reaches them. Hence, the *sādhanā* begins from the outer quest by moulding and culturing body and mind terminating at the innermost quest of the Self.

Guṇa are influential in the Universe and also in man. In order to have the predomination of illumination *(sattva guṇa)* one has to decrease the domination of vibrancy *(rajas)*, and inertia *(tamas)*.

In order to counterbalance the pull of the *guṇa*, Patañjali gives us the clue in *pratipakṣa bhāvanam*. When one's action is tainted, he asks us to deliberate on it thoughtfully before attempting to act. Here the light of right judgement begins. This is the beginning of churning *sattva guṇa*. When one is confused, perturbed or angry, actions and thoughts are also inevitably perturbed and unclear. We often say remain calm when disturbed, or do a few cycles of soft smooth breathing. Obviously, this changes the thought-process and clears such minds to endeavour in a right way.

Lord Krishna says in Bhagavad Gītā that all actions *(karma)* done in the past or going to be done now or in future, may be with the admixture of effects of *sattva, rajas* and *tamas:*

Na hi kaścit kṣaṇam api jātu tiṣṭhaty akarma kṛt I
kāryate hyavaśaḥ karma sarvaḥ prakṛtijair guṇaiḥ II (*B.G.*, III.5)

Everyone is impelled and incited to act according to the qualities he has acquired from the modes of material nature; therefore no one can refrain from doing something, not even for a moment.

He says that faith *(śraddhā)*, food *(āhāra)*, sacrifice *(yajña)*, austerity *(tapas)* and giving gifts or alms *(dāna)* are done with three types of intentions dependent upon the predominance of *sattva*, *rajas* and *tamas*. Our *sādhanā*, *tapas*, *abhyāsa*, *vairāgya*, *Īśvara praṇidhāna* are also categorised upon *sattva*, *rajas* and *tamas*.

In order to reach emancipation, Patañjali says that a practitioner has to pursue the practice of yoga with trust, confidence, vigour, keen memory and the power of absorption. These potentialities may be varying in each *sādhaka* according to his *guṇa-dharma* as soft or mild *(mṛdu)*, moderate *(madhya)*, keen *(adhimātra)* and intense *(tīvra)*. Knowing the interplay of the *guṇa* and the practitioner's capacity in *sādhanā*, Patañjali opens out the eight petals of yoga from *bahiraṅga sādhanā* to *antarātma sādhanā*.

If he wanted everyone to initiate their journey with meditation, he need not have taken trouble to explain the earlier six aspects. In order to travel one needs a passport, visa, ticket, endorsement, boarding pass and so forth. Similarly, the foundation for meditation is required to be established to build up that state of absorption through the earlier six petals of yoga.

One must undergo self-education and self-training following the yogic discipline from *yama* to *dhāraṇā* in order to embark on *dhyāna*. The first six aspects of yogic approaches are to be attended to train and discipline the body, organs of action, senses of perception, mind and intelligence.

The food that comes on the dining table has undergone lots of preparation and processing. The cooking process, taste-wise quality control, required spices or dressing of salads are behind a tasty food processing. Similarly, each aspect of yoga has to undergo the process in order to reach the next stage. When there is a lack in preparation, meditation ends up in *tāmasika* state or a dull state of quietness.

The *aṣṭāṅga yoga*, from *yama* to *pratyāhāra*, is known as *pūrvāṅga* and is meant to eradicate faulty erroneous state of *cittavṛtti*. Such a solid background given by Patañjali has been callously forgotten.

I am for *dhyāna* through purification of *jñāna* and *karma*. So I ask my students to follow each aspect of *aṣṭāṅga yoga* in order to reach finally the state of absorption *(samādhi)* with illumination and light of wisdom.

I advise the practitioners to read the story of Rāvaṇa, Vibhīṣana and Kumbhakarṇa in *Uttara Rāmāyaṇa.*

Kumbhakarṇa's meditation ended in sleep, Rāvaṇa could not control lust of love whereas Vibhīṣaṇa was completely non-attached and detached to everything in life except *Īśvara.*

III.7.3. – A guideline for meditation

First of all one should know what meditation is. Meditation is to bring the complex mind to an innocent state of humility where the intelligence of the head and the heart unite as one.

Take the water of the ocean. The water in the ocean, over all, appears to be on a level, but at the bottom, it has dents. The non-changing Self from birth to death is the same. But consciousness and intelligence act like the dents of the ocean. These dents make the waves of the ocean to move in different directions, like currents in the ocean. If this intelligence is levelled in the body through *yogic sādhanā*, it transforms itself into meditation. Witnessing or reflecting is meditation; acting is concentration. Making an effort to get for what one attempts is concentration. When that effortful effort becomes effortless or natural, it turns into meditation.

I always guide how to focus while practising *āsana* or *prāṇāyāma,* indicating the expansion of the consciousness and extension of the intelligence spreading on each area in the body.

In order to get the knowledge of the world *(laukika jñāna)* one uses the senses of perception *(jñānendriya)* and draws the intelligence to go with them. In order to get spiritual knowledge *(adhyātmika jñāna)* the intelligence takes the initiative and directs the senses to function accordingly. While teaching or doing *āsana* I reverse my intelligence from the senses of perception and mind to move towards the Self. This practice and teaching is meditation for me.

If one advances in the practice of *āsana* and *prāṇāyāma* he will soon not only learn meditation, but live in meditation. First involve the wealth of yoga to bring calmness in the mind and consciousness. From this calm state of consciousness move towards the light of all lights - the *ātman.* Here culminates *dhyāna.*

III.7.4. – Stress management and *dhyāna*

The root cause of stress today is the competitive living standards that bring symptomatic effects on body, mind and nerves. But it is also true that stress is a natural phenomenon. No one in this world is free from stress. Men of wisdom framed and presented yoga to be free from stress. Meditation is not going to remove stress as mind is not the goal of meditation. Mind is just a threshold between body and intelligence as well as ego or 'I'-ness. Meditation is to subjugate the pronoun "I", hence I do not like to lower the quality of meditation to the mind. Before meditation, one needs to culture the brain and mind and learn how to relax and quieten them.

Brain is the instigator of action in the art of living. *Āsana* and *prāṇāyāma* keep the brain cells passive and receptive. It is better to practise them to relieve stress and to keep the nerves free from turbulence.

Āsana and *prāṇāyāma* certainly help to de-stress the nerves and lead one to experience the real unchangeable *(kūṭastha)* Self, which perpetually remains the same from birth to death. Instead of advising to relax the brain, I take stressed people and put them in certain *āsana* where the brain goes automatically silent. *Āsana* like *Uttānāsana, Śīrṣāsana, Viparīta Daṇḍāsana, Nirālamba Sarvāṅgāsana, Halāsana, Setu Bandha Sarvāṅgāsana, Viparīta Karaṇi* in *Śīrṣāsana* and *Sarvāṅgāsana* and *Śavāsana* not only quieten the brain and mind but cool the nerves. They refresh one far more than sleep because these *āsana* allow the energy of the brain to be passive and rejuvenate the nerves soon. The chemical changes that take place on the mind in *āsana* are a hidden secret and beauty.

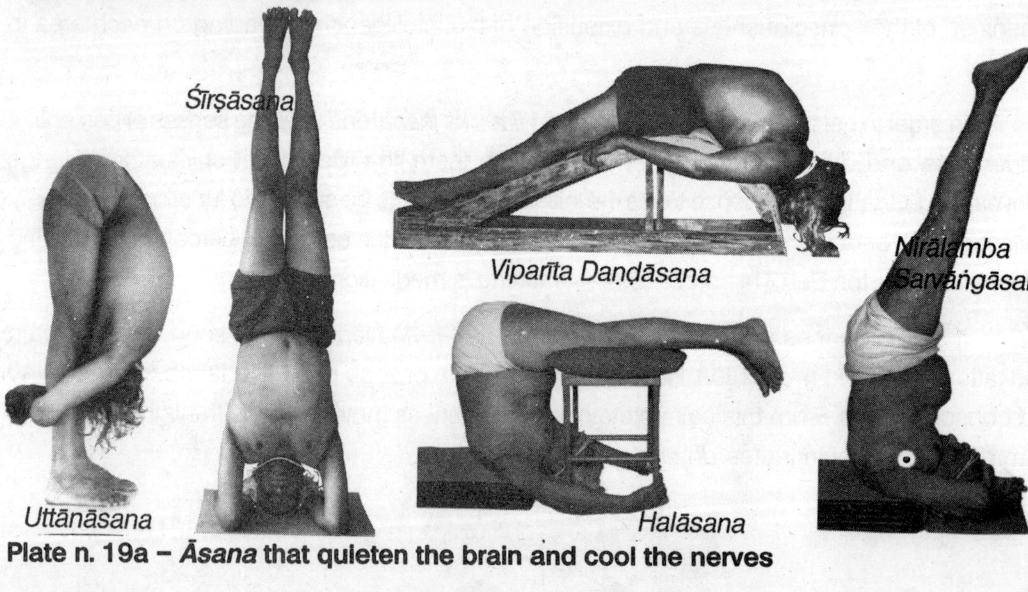

Plate n. 19a – *Āsana* that quieten the brain and cool the nerves

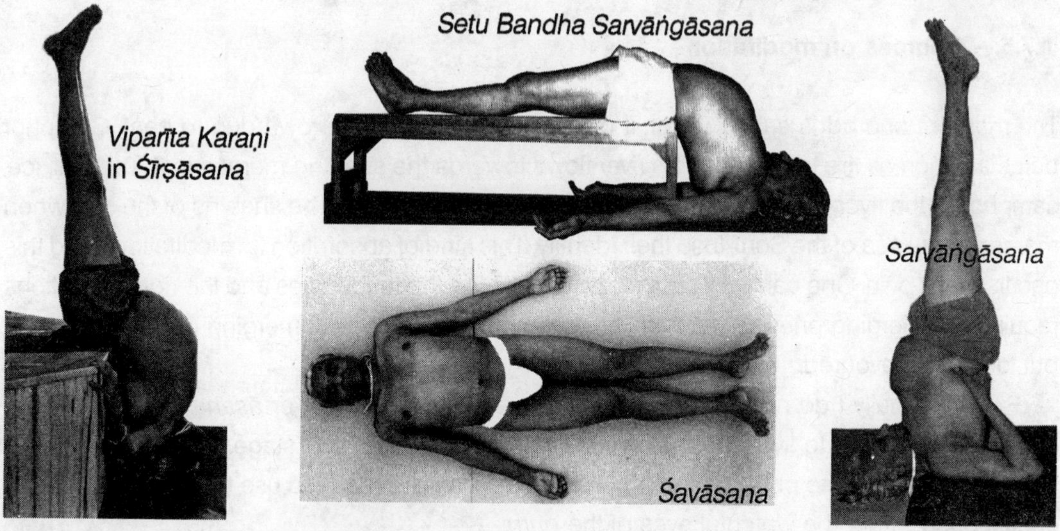

Plate n. 19b – *Āsana* that quieten the brain and cool the nerves

It has been beautifully said in the *Haṭhayoga Pradīpikā,* "Mind is the king of the senses; breath is the king of the mind; and the nerves are the king of the breath". If one knows how to keep the nervous system for the energy to move uninterruptedly, then it takes away the load without the feel of stress. Even *Śavāsana* is a stress, but thinking and thought processes are minimised and one feels happy. Even in sleep there is a stress factor as one changes the position often. In meditation also there is a stress factor because one has to keep the spine erect and struggle to disconnect the senses of perception from the brain and mind. Walking, eating, reading are also stresses. Everything is stress in this world including the fear of death, except actual death. So consider voluntarily how to culture the cells and receptivity in the brain.

If it rains torrentially, the water does not seep into the earth; if it showers continuously, then the water seeps deep into the earth, which brings us good harvest. In the same way one has to think and act to change the stress factor. This change happens in the presentation of various *āsana* where extension and expansion reach the interior parts of the body triggering and invigorating the nerves, brain and mind to a new life. *Āsana* and *prāṇāyāma* practices diffuse the strain and stress and bring rhythm between the nerves and mind, and lead one to know the higher state of life,[19] the Self.

Once one gets refreshed, then he is fit for meditation. Actually *dhyāna* needs a quiet and fresh mind. *Dhyāna* is the penultimate state of *yoga sādhanā.* Meditation certainly is not meant for relieving the stress factors. Meditation is a state where one experiences the untainted, unalloyed eternal bliss and make the consciousness to rest on the lap of the Soul.

III.7.5. - Courses on meditation

The moment one adds salt to water, it dissolves. Ice melts on its own due to heat. Camphor burns as soon as fire touches it. The river flows towards the sea and merges in it. The salt, ice, camphor or the river, all lose their marks on one way or the other. The sheaths of the self, when merged in the sea of the Soul, lose their identity. This kind of absorption is "meditation"; and this occurs on its own. One can only show ways to develop the tendencies and the right conditions required for merging oneself into that Supreme. But the process of merging cannot be taught but to be endeavoured.

Personally I do not believe in short courses on meditation or *āsana*. In the *Gurukula* system, pupils used to live with their *guru* throughout the learning stage. A constant contact was there between the pupils and the *guru*. The pupils were made to use their time in learning continuously under the watchful eyes of the *guru*.

All arts like music, yoga and dance were taught in such a manner that one was really drawn and soaked into it. Now the days have changed. This approach is lost and not only arts but also camps on *dhyāna* (meditation) are treated on superficial levels.

An emerging consciousness *(vyutthāna citta)* cannot be converted at once into a cultured, balanced, harmonious state *(samāhita citta)*. At our Institute we build up yogic attitudes with a definite aim. Here, *aṣṭāṅga yoga* is taught progressively, building up physical power, mental stability and intellectual clarity. In meditation camps no qualitative considerations of the *sādhaka* are attended to before taking the subject of *dhyāna*. It is like a blind man leading the blind or like sheep leading the sheep.

Many are of the opinion and declare that we do not teach *dhyāna*. *Dhyāna* is not idle sitting. While teaching *āsana* and *prāṇāyāma*, we guide how to move towards *pratyāhāra*, *dhāraṇā* and *dhyāna*. As *dhyāna* is a dynamic flow of intelligence and consciousness, we make these two to flow concurrently in all the sheaths of the fort of the soul, without actually using word "meditation" but by making the students to experience meditation in action. Only we don't call it *dhyāna* or meditation classes. We teach all aspects of yoga and dhyāna being a part of yoga, special mention of it is unnecessary.

Here we teach how to watch the movements, moment to moment. How to know and change, while doing *āsana* and *prāṇāyāma*, the thoughtless moments turn into thoughtful moments, which turn into auspiciousness. Is this not an auspicious state, a state of meditation? If I define and declare this as meditation, you may accept it. But I don't because meditation can never be taught, but one can only guide towards it.

In *aṣṭāṅga yoga*, the first two aspects–*yama* and *niyama*– are the foundation or receptacle for the other six aspects of yoga to develop and strengthen *samāhita citta* or *citta prasādana*.

Āsana acts as *jñāna mārga*. Its practice generates knowledge to reach perfection and maturity. For example, in an *āsana*, if one reaches a state wherein the dualities fade,[1] the breathing pattern begins to change. It runs soft, smooth, rhythmic, subtle and often quiet in between breaths. Even his mind along with organs of perception and action reach a subdued stable state in the *sādhanā* as if one is in *pratyāhāra* and *dhāraṇā*.

Through the practice of *āsana*, one recognises the various parts of the body. As mind has no place, one has to provide a space for it to remain, as if it has a place. Mind will be there, but also it will be hard to locate as it moves in the body like a bird in space. *Āsana* practice stabilises the mind to remain steady. If *āsana sādhanā* helps us to gain knowledge, practice of *prāṇāyāma* guides and takes us towards *bhakti* or the path of love. As *sādhaka*, one has to trace this state of *jñāna* and *bhakti* that arise for himself.

First a *sādhaka* has to begin to control the organs of action and senses of perception as he can find and locate their places. But mind is mercurial and slips like mercury subject to sudden changes and moods. *Pratyāhāra*, one of the petals of yoga, helps the inner planet of man to remain steady as the stem of banana plant, which is straight. When this steady attention *(dhāraṇā)* is maintained and made to expand without losing the focal point, it turns into *dhyāna*. The special feature of *dhyāna* is the uninterrupted maintenance of focal attention, expanding uniformly, evenly and totally covering the space within the body as well as outside the body on all points without a fixed point.

Dhāraṇā has a double duty. Not only does it bring the focus of attention on one point, or on the symbol *āuṁ*, or the image of the desired deity, but it arrests and eradicates the fluctuating thought-waves. In *dhyāna* the emphasis is to maintain throughout a constant and continuous attention. So much is the difference between *dhāraṇā* and *dhyāna*.

This process cannot be taught by force. One has to be established in training in the first six petals of yoga from *yama* to *dhāraṇā* to understand *dhyāna*.

Dhyāna humbles the 'I' and makes it to dissolve in the Soul like camphor in fire. I can go on pointing to the ego and hit the ego to ensure that it does not raise its hood. But each one alone has to work to extinguish it. The use of prayers and *praṇava japa* are meant for cultivating

---

[1] *Tataḥ dvandvāḥ anabhighātaḥ* (*Y.S.*, II.48) – from then on the *sādhaka* is undisturbed by dualities.

bhakti. Bhakti helps in dissolving the ego a great deal. Ego cannot be conquered without *bhakti. Bhakti* is impossible without *jñāna* and *jñāna* cannot be acquired without right *karma.*

Through profound meditation the knower, knowledge and the known become one. The seer, the sight and the seeing have no separate existence. When a musician becomes one with his instrument, music emanates from it. Similarly, meditation is not created, it just happens. It is entered into.

Therefore, courses on *dhyāna* are brain-washing and an eye-wash. When the tree has grown from the best of seeds, nurtured and nourished, it bears healthy fruit. One has to wait until the tree grows for it to give those fruit. But people have become immature and impatient, they want everything ready-made. They want the fruits before the tree grows. Without proper nurturing and maturing of all aspects of *sādhanā* and *anusṭhāna*, people want to jump to meditation, which takes them nowhere. Momentary sensual peace is neither real peace nor to be considered as meditation.

III.7.6. – Is meditation isolating

Isolation means to cut off from everything and to live a dejected lonely life. It is a self-abnegating and nihilistic approach. Isolation is not meditation.

Isolation *(kevala)* means isolating the agents or the tributaries of the sea of the Self and to experience the state of self-aloneness. This aloneness stands for the establishment of the Self, or explicitness of the Self *(swami svarūpa)*, this is what commentators mean.

Look at myself and my life.

Am I isolated from society? Am I morose and lonely or am I full of energy? Do I not practise and do I not teach? Do I not look after all those who come to this Institute, for their well-being? I am doing all this as an offering to that Unlimited Force and that is my meditation. I am not sitting in a lonely place, but see all the faces of life! I am enjoying the joy that comes from my *sādhanā* and at once share with all what I experience for them to feel that auspicious joy. Is it not for me total involvment and absorption in what I do that I share the good with all?

Transforming the objective knowledge into subjective experience and then make others share that subjective experience is meditation for me. Meditation is meant to reach the source seat of energy and help others from that state so that all experience the electrical way of living sharp and bright.

III.7.7. – On Transcendental Meditation

Meditation is only one (*Y.S.*, III.2) and always transcendental (*Y.S.*, III.3). In meditation the *citta* transcends from its usual object of experience. As far as I am concerned, there is no such thing as Transcendental Meditation. Going beyond the present state of consciousness and moving towards further states is transcendental. When all conditioning ceases to operate for the meditator (the subject), then there is no meditator separate from the object (of meditation).

The essence of meditation is to draw the eyes and ears towards the seat of the soul by keeping the spine erect and the brain quiet, so that the energies from the senses, mind, intelligence, I-ness and I-consciousness are reversed towards the soul. The outgoing energy is made ingoing. The outlets are closed and inlets are opened. For this reason the nature of all these has to be changed and transformed. This transformation from one to the other is called 'transcendental' because one transcends *(pariṇāma)* from one state to the other state. This does not come under normal experience as our senses, mind, intelligence are accustomed to outgoing thoughts and objects. We are all accustomed to the disturbances in one way or the other. Hence, we hunt and search for peace. Peacefulness is a rare experience while disturbance is a normal experience. Therefore, for *citta* (consciousness) it becomes a rare experience to transcend from the usual experience. This experience becomes a state of transcendence to the consciousness. Transcendence towards the Self is meditation.

III.7.8. – Different types of meditation

Some attribute various names and titles, saying that there are various types of meditation. As truth is one, meditation is one and the effect of experience also is one. Concentration *(dhāraṇā)* may have different avenues to focus attention, but not so in meditation *(dhyāna)*. **Meditation** is only one (*Y.S.*, III.2). It makes the objective Self, subjective. Meditation is meant to experience what Self is. The Self, is concealed by the mind, the intelligence and the consciousness, and it has to be uncovered through meditation. To experience this state, one begins with concentration, which is a process of maintaining an uninterrupted flow of attention on a fixed point, a fixed region or a fixed object. In concentration, the thoughts flowing towards an object may change. In meditation no change in thoughts takes place, but the agents of the self get overwhelmed.

One has to understand that there is a vast difference between the mediator – the consciousness, and the meditator himself.

Consciousness *(citta)* is a mediator between the outgoing and incoming thoughts. The job of the mediator is to intervene and establish peace through agreement or reconciliation. At the beginning consciousness acts as a mediator, as it has to convince the outgoing thoughts of the mind, which hunts for pleasure, to move inwards. When the mind begins to move inwards then the door of the consciousness gets turned towards meditation. The moment this happens the consciousness functions as a meditator.

Meditation is a steady and continuous flow with single-pointed attention towards the chosen object or the self.[1] The object of meditation depends upon the aim. One may concentrate by fusing the attention on a chosen point or object either within or outside the body. One may focus on the navel, heart, root of the tongue, tip of the nose, centre of the forehead or the crown of the head. These places are such that they should be conducive to the practitioners to go towards meditation. Or it could be on the idol of God, symbols like *āuṁ* or *swastika*, but the technical process is the same.

Plate n. 20 – *Āuṁ* and *swastika*

As far as the *praṇava japa* is concerned, I said that doing the *japa āuṁ* does not make any sense when you have no discipline. Muttering and repeating vocally or verbally does not make any sense. Having the moral, physical and mental discipline, aiming constantly and reverentially at the omnipresent, omnipotent and omniscient God who is symbolised by the

---

1 *Tatra pratyaya ekatānatā dhyānam* (*Y.S.*, III.2) – a steady continuous flow of attention directed towards the same point or region is meditation.

syllable *āuṁ,* with attention, contemplation, understanding the meaning and feeling of its auspiciousness is meditation.

The *praṇava japa* is given by Patañjali to remove not only the diseases of the body but of the consciousness. The disease belongs not only to the body but also to the consciousness. Patañjali includes the physical and mental diseases in the list of impediments. He does not say that *praṇava japa* is meditation but advises the *praṇava japa* for meditation's sake.

III.7.9. – Is meditation active or passive

Meditation is one. Some sit and keep themselves quiet and call it meditation. I am active and keep myself totally attentive, forgetting myself. For me it is total attention in activity.

Suppose a child is made to go to university as soon as it has learnt the ABC, what will be his fate? Shockingly, as well as surprisingly, this is what happens to many in meditation courses. If meditation is so simple, then Patañjali could have brought it at the place of *yama,* and not as the penultimate aspect in *aṣṭāṅga yoga.* When one is physically, morally, mentally and intellectually unsteady, and is forced to create intense attention, one either goes to sleep or damages one's brain and nerves. Recently I saw some people "meditating", with sunken chests, collapsed spine, hard eyeballs and shallow breathing.

Meditation is not a sedative or a drug. It is an alert dynamic state of intelligence demanding total integration of body, mind and intellect. It is not an empty state of consciousness *(śūnyāvasthā)* but an absolute state of consciousness *(aśūnyāvasthā).* It is not a restful state *(manolaya),* but an alert state of dynamic fullness of the self *(amanaskatā).* It is not a mindless state but a state where mind dissolves and self shines.

Let us take the example of an artist. He gets completely absorbed in his art and forgets himself. As an artist, he has an object to meditate upon, whereas a yogi has consciousness itself as his object, and it becomes hard for him to have a total involvement. Therefore, some introduce passive thoughts for meditation, which calm the mind, but this should not be considered as meditation.

There is a story from the *Purāṇa.* There was a farmer who used to pray to God regularly and religiously in the early mornings and the rest of the time remained engaged in his farming work.

Once Nārada Muni asked Lord Vishnu: "Who is the best among the *bhakta?*" Lord Vishnu replied that he had seen a farmer on the earth as the best of *bhakta*. Nārada could not believe this. So he came down from the heaven to the earth to see this farmer, the best among the *bhakta*. He found him praying early in the morning for a while and then working in his farm. Nārada asked him how many times he prays. He said: "Where is time to think of the Lord when there is plenty of work left to do on the field?" He said that he prays and thinks of the Lord only once in the morning. Nārada went back to the Lord and asked Him why He considered the farmer as the best among the *bhakta*. The Lord replied, instructing him to take a vessel filled with water to the brim and perform three circumambulations around the temple without spilling water, taking the name of the Lord. Nārada took the vessel with brimful of water, went for circumambulation and returned to Lord Vishnu. The Lord asked him whether he spilled any water. Nārada replied: "No." Then the Lord asked him: "How many times did you remember me"? Nārada, in a bashful state replied: "Not even once." The Lord said that He appreciated and ranked the farmer as the best because when he prayed and worked in the field, he was fully engrossed and had the power to surrender to God as well as to his work in the field with total attention.

If one remains in that non-oscillating state, he is in meditation. Here, the consciousness remains alert and totally engrossed in the object that is meditated upon, whereas in forced meditation he remains with an identity mark on his body or mind and intellect.

The story of Nārada illustrates *dhyāna* for anyone.

III.7.10. – *Trāṭaka* and *dhyāna*

Yoga and meditation are not separate from each other. Meditation is a part of *aṣṭāṅga yoga*. Therefore do not treat meditation as separate from yoga. *Trāṭaka* is a part of *ṣaṭkarma*. It does not come in *Yoga Sūtra*.

If yoga is for silencing the *citta*, *dhyāna* is for subjugation of *ahaṁkāra*, which is the other side of the *citta*. *Dhyāna* is an experiencing state of consciousness merging in the seer. As the moon draws the energy from the sun, consciousness draws its energy from the seer. Consciousness waxes and wanes like the moon. Meditation is a leaf in yogic *sādhanā* where the *sādhaka* succeeds in maintaining the consciousness in a steady state of awareness and attention without waxing and waning, for a long time, and makes the consciousness lose its identity and realise its master with a non-oscillating awareness and to become one with the seer.

Although one may say that he sits for meditation, he actually does concentration *(dhāraṇā)* and not *dhyāna*. In order to bring the mind to a state of one-pointedness, certain objects are given to focus on. Gazing *(trāṭaka)* is one of those. This is not *dhyāna* but a gaze of the eyes. During the practice of *trāṭaka* there are certain pressures in the eyes and those pressures bring out colours of light, except a dark spot at their centre. As practice increases, these various colours of light disappear. These colours should not be misinterpreted as spiritual success. *Trāṭaka* cleanses the eyes as they water and helps for physical concentration. *Trāṭaka* also has a bad effect. Its prolonged practice leads one to day-time blindness. But mental and intellectual concentration is different from *trāṭaka*.

The important thing for a *sādhaka* is to become ripe in *jñāna* so that the light of wisdom dawns. This happens when the *sādhaka* becomes one with the practices and loses the sense of both. This is meditation.

Do not conclude that *trāṭaka* is meditation. It is one of the ways for meditation.

III.7.11. – *Āsana* and *dhyāna*

Āsana is a part of *aṣṭāṅga*, hence I do conclude that there is an effect of *āsana* on *dhyāna*. Most of us relate yoga only to the *sūtra; yogaḥ cittavṛtti nirodhaḥ* (*Y.S.*, I.2) – stilling the fluctuations of consciousness as yoga. But Patañjali continues and explains to understand the other 195 *sūtra* for us to ponder over. This makes one ponder. Meditation is not closing the eyes and remaining silent. We all go to sleep eight or ten hours a day and remain silent. But do we call this a meditation? In sleep, stilling of the mind does not take place. Hence, we cannot call sleep as meditation. But meditation is not only stilling the mind, but also silencing it. In sleep there is no *jñāna*. In *dhyāna* or meditation *jñāna* plays a major role.

Yoga is a journey from *jñāna* to *dhyāna*. Hence, meditation is not a separate aspect of yoga. As humans we have mind, intelligence, ego, consciousness, awareness, memory, emotions and so forth, which we cannot deny. Can we stress on one of these and neglect the other sheaths? Each and every part of yoga is as important as another. *Dhyāna* is not an expressive subject, but experiencing the integrated state of living.

If one says that the body is different, mind is different, brain is different, it means he is a disintegrated person. Meditation is possible only if one integrates the body, brain, mind, and intelligence with the Soul. Meditation being very subtle; Patañjali has placed it as the penultimate aspect.

Vyāsa, equates yoga with *samādhi*. He says, "Yoga is *samādhi*." He does not mean that one tries to jump at once directly to *samādhi*. He only emphasises the meaning of yoga. Yoga being joining or yoking, this is possible only in *dhyāna* and *samādhi*. All the components of yoga are meant for man to get integrated to the soul. Though this integration happens in *dhyāna* and *samādhi*, one has to follow *yama, niyama, āsana, prāṇāyāma, pratyāhāra* and *dhāraṇā* as preparations for *dhyāna* and *samādhi*.

Some think that sitting silently or chanting the name of God or making a prayer is meditation. This is not meditation but a *japa*. You must differentiate the meditation from the preparations for it. In meditation the river of *citta* is made to flow with its single content and with a single thought. There cannot be any taint on the consciousness. The consciousness must be stainless *(vimala)*. The mind has to flow continuously with a single thought. Mind naturally gets crowded with several thoughts and the true goal of life remains far off. Hence, one needs to channel them, as a preparation towards meditation.

At the moment of stilling the mind, opposing forces actively dominate. There is a tug-of-war between restraint and opposing thoughts. But we do not witness the silent gap that takes place between restraint and rising thoughts (III.9). In that silent moment there is a sign of tranquillity (III.10). If we increase the period of that pause, the state of *ekāgratā* sets in (III.11). Probably many have not heard of Patañjali speaking of *nirodha pariṇāma, samādhi pariṇāma* and *ekāgratā pariṇāma*. The transformations from a state of restraint to a state of tranquillity, and from the state of tranquillity to a state of single uninterrupted point of awareness have to be achieved. These transformations happen only through the practice of *dhāraṇā, dhyāna* and *samādhi*.

We know that *ekāgratā* means one-pointed attention. The exact meaning of *ekāgratā* is to bring the wandering mind to a state of focus – *eka* means one, *agra* means tip, apex or end, and *agratā* means priority. Here the priority is given to reach the soul. The body, mind and energy are completely focussed towards that *eka*, the single one, the one without second – the soul. The foundation is the soul or the core of the being because our existence depends upon it. But in reality it is the apex. To keep our energy and attention pointed at the apex, the soul, is *ekāgratā*. As the magnet draws the iron filings towards it by its force pull or attraction; we need to develop that attraction towards the soul. The pensive state between the rising and restraining thoughts draws the consciousness and intelligence like a magnet towards the core of the being. To live totally as a single unit knotted together with one's energy, intelligence and consciousness to the core, is meditation.

Sometime ago, I saw in France many handbills, advertisements of *kuṇḍalinī, cakra* and colours as if it is so easy to awaken the divine force. As there is *iḍā* and *piṅgaḷā* in the body, so there is *suṣumṇā.* The starting point of *iḍā* and *piṅgaḷā* is in the spine, which supplies energy to engulf the body, making it possible for *suṣumṇā* to flow everywhere. But besides physical energy and vital energy, *suṣumṇā* supplies, the spiritual energy to flow in every cell of our body. This can be felt only if one is a true *sādhaka.* One sublimates his senses of perception, mind, brain, intelligence, consciousness and the conscience through *tapas,* and turns his vision towards the core or the Self.

One may be doing meditation in sitting at one corner, creating emptiness within. I do meditation in every action I perform. *Āsana,* for me is a meditation. I make my intelligence and consciousness to run parallel in my entire body without disturbing the body. For me meditation is not emptying the mind but spreading it fully from the Self throughout the entire body. I want my mind, intelligence and consciousness to shine like a full moon *(purṇimā),* and today's meditation is taught like the fading moon as new moon *(amāvāsya).* I am alert and allow my mind to diffuse and cover the whole body to be one with my mind, my brain, my consciousness, my intelligence and my soul, without creating divisions. That is how I practise and hence I see no difference between *āsana* and *dhyāna.* For me, where *dhyāna* is, *āsana* is. Where *āsana* is, there is *dhyāna.* I bring all the principal aspects of yoga in my practice of *āsana* and *prāṇāyāma* and hence, they merge in *dhyāna.*

Bhagavad Gītā says:

Samaṁ kāya śiro grīvaṁ dhārayan acalaṁ sthiraḥ I
Samprekṣya nāsikāgraṁ svaṁ diśascānavalokayan II (*B.G.,* VI.13)

Holding the body, head and neck erect and steady without motion, he should fix his gaze on the tip of his nose, without looking around.

By keeping the right and the left, front and back of the body, in a rhythmic harmonious state, without any variation, measuring it from the middle of the perineum to the middle of the throat, which is the central part of the inner body, I adjust the various parts of my body, mind and intelligence to run parallel to that central line. Think of this *śloka* of the *Bhagavad Gītā* and question yourself – "Can I sit like that?"

Many advise repeating *auṁ* in meditation to still the mind. I use each *āsana* as *praṇava*. There is a beginning to *āsana* **(ā)**, then there is stable maintenance of the *āsana* **(u)**, and lastly I bring advertence in ending the *āsana* **(ṁ)**.

The type of *dhyāna* I learnt through my practice of *āsana* and *prāṇāyāma* is like the midday sun. As the sun's rays at midday are in its zenith, in my practice of *āsana* and *prāṇāyāma* I extend the rays from the disk of my consciousness to penetrate and pierce each and every cell of my body. This made me to bring the consciousness to touch and reach all areas of its frontier evenly, everywhere without division. I learned to remove any inattention in the dark spots of the body that were obstructing and interrupting the rays of my consciousness. This way I learnt *dhyāna* by bringing equivalence between the Soul and its dwelling place – the body. This is how I bring *dhyāna* in *āsana*.

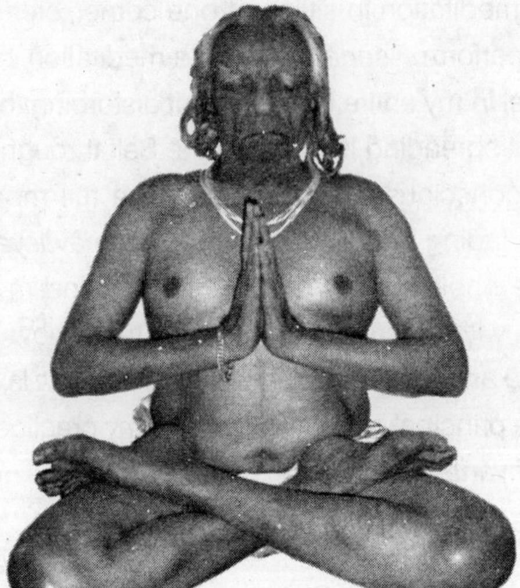

Plate n. 21 – *Dhyāna*

III.8. - *Samādhi*

III.8.1. – *Saṁprajñāta samādhi* and *asaṁprajñāta samādhi*

In yoga, *samādhi* is considered as the ultimate fruit. When one gets accomplished in the first seven aspects of yoga, the eighth one expresses on its own. Though *samādhi* is mentioned as a last, singular aspect, it has been described in two phases, namely *saṁprajñāta* and *asaṁprajñāta*.

Patañjali speaks of *saṁprajñāta samādhi*. These are: *savitarka, nirvitarka, savicāra, nirvicāra, sānanda* and *sāsmitā*. He connotes them as *sabīja*. However, he does not mention the name of *asaṁprajñāta samādhi*. His commentators have used the word *asaṁprajñāta*, but he has not. Though he doesn't, Patañjali uses *sabīja* which he says leads one later towards *nirbīja samādhi*.

If *sabīja samādhi* stands for *saṁprajñānāta samādhi, nirbīja samādhi* may stand for *asaṁprajñānata samādhi*.

Between *sabīja* and *nirbīja* there is a transitory state or a phase. Patañjali defines this intervening phase as *virāma pratyaya*. The commentators named this "intervening state" as *asaṁprajñāta samādhi*, a state beyond *saṁprajñāta*. However, this intermediate stage cannot be a *nirbīja* because Patañjali mentions about *nirbīja* in two *sūtra*, one in *Samādhi Pāda; tasyāpi nirodhe sarvanirodhāt nirbījaḥ samādhiḥ (Y.S.*, I.51) – this has also to be relinquished to experience the seedless state of *samādhi (nirbīja samādhi)*, and in *Vibhūti Pāda; tadeva arthamātranirbhāsaṁ svarūpaśūnyam iva samādhiḥ (Y.S.*, III.3) – the merging of the meditator and the object of meditation is absorption *(samādhi)*. *Nirbīja samādhi* is the ultimate which is recognised as *dharmamegha samādhi* in *Kaivalya Pāda; prasaṁkhyāne api akusīdasya sarvathā vivekakhyāteḥ dharmameghaḥ samādhiḥ (Y.S.*, IV.29) – by this acquisition, virtue pours forth, washing away all subliminal impressions and afflictions in the consciousness. From then on, a seedless state of cleanliness and clarity is experienced.

For me it appears that this *virāma pratyaya* is a penultimate state of *nirbīja samādhi*, which some commentators name as *asaṁprajñāta samādhi* or *nirbīja samādhi*. It is interesting to observe this *virāma* state in *aṣṭadaḷa yoga*. Between *yama, niyama, āsana* and *prāṇāyāma* and *dhāraṇā, dhyāna* and *samādhi, pratyāhāra* is a stage to stabilise the acquired state of attention. It acts as a consolidating state to proceed towards the inner most *sādhanā*. Hence it is the place for the role of "building up state" like *virāma pratyaya*, which is a bridge to cross from *sabīja samādhi* over to *nirbīja samādhi*.

According to Patañjali *virāma pratyaya* is between *saṁprajñāta samādhi* or *sabīja samādhi* and *nirbīja samādhi* or so called *asaṁprajñāta*.

Patañjali says, *tā eva sabījaḥ samādhiḥ* (*Y.S.*, I.46). It means the states of *samādhi* described in the previous *sūtra* are supported and hence he used the word *sabīja*. *Virāma pratyaya* being a threshold between *sabīja* and *nirbīja samādhi*, the *sādhaka* may fail to remove the residual *saṁskāra* and end up as *prakṛtilayin* or *videhin*. *Videhin* means bodiless and *prakṛtilayin* means one merged in nature (*mūla prakṛti*). If he is caught in this state, he may not be able to reach *prakṛti jaya* nor enter the province of *ātman* (*ātmānandamaya kośa*).[1] In this state, he realises *prakṛti* but he does not realise the Self.

Vācaspati Miśra in his commentary *Tattvavaiśāradi* has explained eight steps of *sabīja samādhi*, namely, *savitarka, nirvitarka, savicāra, nirvicāra, sānanda, nirānanda, sāsmita* and *nirāsmita*. For me, *nirāsmita* reads like *nirbīja*, which is the one and only one.

Śankarācārya has mentioned *sabīja* and *nirbīja* as *savikalpa* and *nirvikalpa*, whereas Rāmānujācārya has explained these two as *dharma-bhūta samādhi* and *dharmī-bhūta samādhi*. *Dharma* is the *prakṛti* and *dharmī* is the soul. *Sabīja samādhi* is also known as *sālamba samādhi* and *nirbīja samādhi* as *nirālamba samādhi*.

Samādhi is a fascinating word and many have discussed it as a topic. But rare are those who have experienced *nirbīja samādhi*. The differences between the stages of *samādhi* are so subtle and transparent that one may find it hard to differentiate distinctly.

Bīja means a seed. Hence *sabīja* means an auspicious seed as support whereas *nirbīja* has no seed or support.

Prakṛti is made of five gross elements and five subtle qualitative elements along with organs of action, senses of perception, mind, intelligence, ego or 'I'. In each state of *samādhi* one reaches an evolutionary growth with refinement. For instance, in *savitarka samādhi* the five gross elements (earth, water, fire, air and ether), and the organs of action (arms, legs, speech, genital and excretory organs), get refined, which has a bearing on *citta*. In *nirvitarka* the senses of perception (eyes, ears, nose, tongue and skin), are purified causing further refinement in *citta*. In *savicāra* and *nirvicāra* mind, intelligence and five subtle elements (sound, touch, form, taste and smell) become crystal clear for the consciousness to refine further. In *ānanda* (*sānanda* or auspiciousness), the intelligence is purified bringing wisdom. In *asmitā saṁprajñāta* the 'I' consciousness gets maturity and refines the consciousness. When all these evolutes reach purity, the consciousness reflects in pure form.

---

[1] Not to be confused with *ānandamaya kośa*. This is a special sheath realised by the *sādhaka* at *ānanda* and *asmitā* levels.

In *sabīja samādhi* the subject – the seer – and the object – the seen – exist. In *nirbīja samādhi*, the seen and the seer unite and remain in the province of *nirbīja*. Here the *jīvātman* (small self) is as clear as crystal. Then in this crystal-clear state the so called world of the seen makes the seen merge in the seer. From then on the seer alone exists and nothing else. This is *nirbīja samādhi*.

In *sabīja*, *dhāraṇā*, *dhyāna* and *samādhi* work as an integrated force. For this, the vehicles of nature are essentially required. In *nirbīja* the vehicles of nature *(prakṛti)* cease to function and the seer alone shines. The seer uses this *prakṛti* as seed for evolution and drops them all in *nirbīja samādhi*, Hence, it is called seedless *samādhi*.

Patañjali has defined *samādhi* in *Samādhi Pāda* as well as in *Vibhūti Pāda*. In *Samādhi Pāda* it is dealt practicality, while in *Vibhūti Pāda* it is explained theoretically.

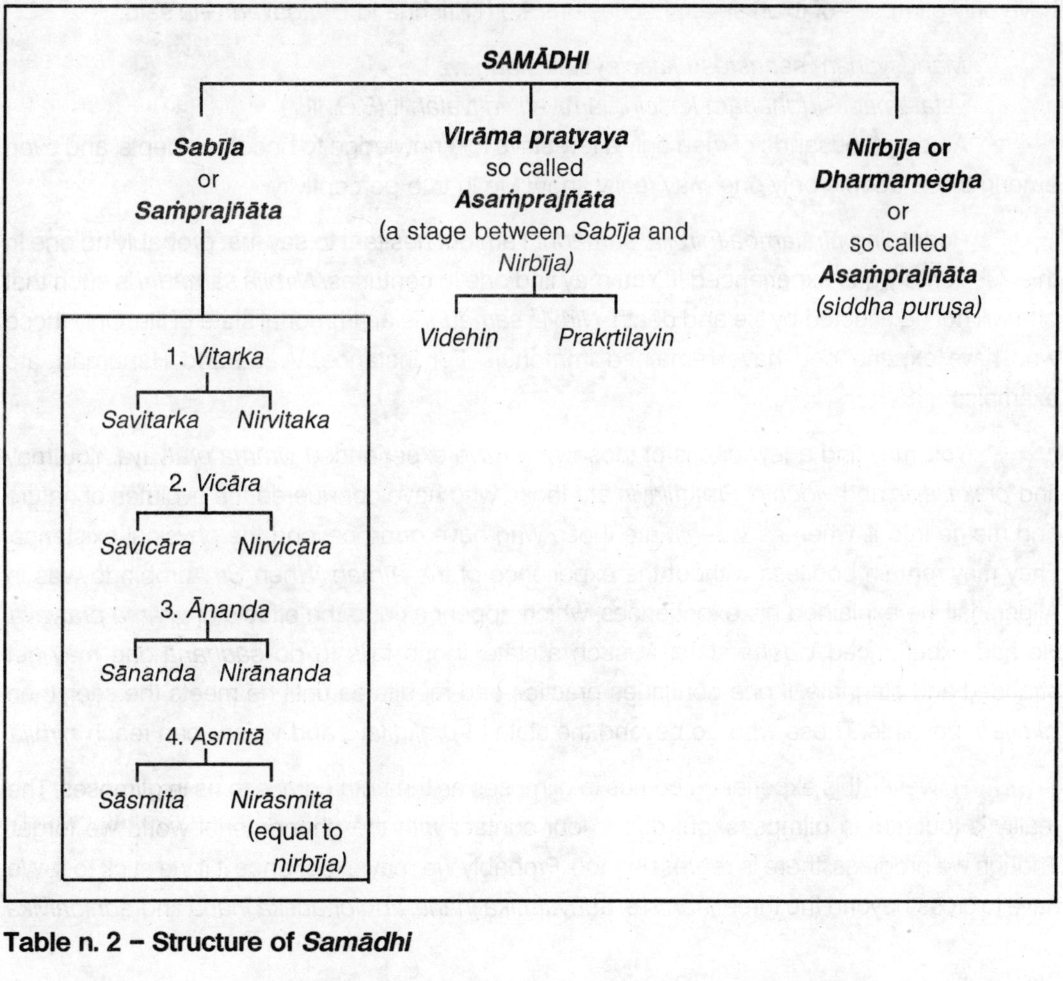

Table n. 2 – Structure of *Samādhi*

In *Vibhūti Pāda* he says: *Tadeva arthamātranirbhāsam svarūpaśūnyam iva samādhiḥ* (III.3) – when the object of meditation engulfs the meditator appearing as the subject, self-awareness is lost. This is a state of *samādhi*. For a meditator, when the object of contemplation itself transforms as "himself", he experiences *samādhi* devoid of his form. In *sabīja samādhi* he reaches the state as if he is *svarūpaśūnya*. At this stage his existence and attentiveness is totally given to the object that he is meditating upon. Whereas, in *nirbīja samādhi* there is no *svarūpaśūnyatā* but *svarūpapratiṣṭhā*. The soul reveals the soul. The seer sees the seer and the seer establishes in his own nature; *tadā draṣṭuḥ svarūpe avasthānam* (I.3).The state of *samādhi* is such that first the aspirant masters his own servants who supply him the knowledge (organs of action and senses of perception). Then he conquers the mind and intelligence, which collect and filter the knowledge from the known. When the known is fully known, he abandons all, savouring the knower of the known. Regarding myself, whether I have experienced or not, I have only glimpses of it, on several occasions. Lord Krishna in *Bhagavad Gītā* said:

Manuṣyāṇām sahasreṣu kaścidyatati siddhaye I
yatatāmapi siddhānām kaścinmām vetti tattvataḥ II (*B.G.*, III.7)

Among thousands of men only a few strive for knowledge to become adepts, and even among those adepts only one may really know Me in true perceptivity.

Regarding *nirālamba (nirbīja) samādhi*, I am not hesitant to say that probably no one in this 20th century has experienced it. You may find one in centuries. *Nirbīja samādhi* is such that one will not be affected by life and death. *Nirbīja samādhi* is an immortal state of life. Only those who have experienced have remained immortals. For instance, Vyāsa and Hanumān, are examples.

You may find a few cases of those who have experienced *virāma pratyaya*. You may find *prakṛtilayin* and *videhin*. *Prakṛtilayin* are those who have conquered the evolutes of nature and merge into it, whereas *videhin* are those who have gone beyond the physical existence. They may remain bodiless without the experience of the *ātman*. When *Śrī* Aurobindo was in Alipore jail, he explained his experiences, which appear akin to the effects of *virāma pratyaya*. He had experienced *videha* state. At such a state, if one fails to do *sādhanā* one may get stranded and stagnate. If one continues practice and meditates until he meets the seer, then *nirbīja* is possible. Those who go beyond the state of *prakṛtilaya* and *videha* can reach *nirbīja*.

However, this experience comes in glimpses as the truth comes to us in glimpses. The reality is touched in glimpses, but due to our contact with the phenomenal world we forget. Though we progress, there is regression too. Probably we may experience it if we stick to it. We have to cross beyond the three *jñāna* i.e. *adhyātmika jñāna*, *ādhibhautika jñāna* and *ādhidaivika jñāna*. But *jñāna* – knowledge – itself is a barrier. We can't give up *jñāna* as it is like hoarded wealth. As some can't give up wealth, so it is with knowledge. First one has to cross the objective knowledge and then move towards subjective wisdom. Subjective wisdom is to know the Self. For this all the three states of knowledge has to be dropped as they act as a barrier between these two *samādhi*. Let me tell you that Self is devoid of the three *jñāna*.

Having said this, I do not mean that *sabīja* is easy. If one sees in *the veda* and *purāṇa* that great *yogi*, who had experienced the truth, were coming back to the planes to share their knowledge with people. They were getting polluted while coming in contact with people. As their minds used to get polluted they were retiring to the forests to begin *tapas* again. They were staying in seclusion to remove all the impurities and reach *samādhi*. Out of compassion they would come back to the planes to uplift people towards spiritual life. They did not live in the state of *nirbīja* or *nirvikalpa samādhi* forever. So this experience is really difficult to live in a continuous state. One can only have glimpses. There is no return journey since *nirbīja* is ultimate.

Saṁprajñāta samādhi refines the *sādhaka* to enrich the stage of purity. It occurs step-by-step or layer-by-layer as the seer is in association with his layers. In *savitarka* and *nirvitarka* the *annamaya* and *prāṇamaya kośa* (sheaths) are purified. In *savicāra* and *nirvicāra* the *manōmaya kośa* is purified. In *ānanda* the *vijñānamaya kośa* is purified. In *asmitā samādhi*, and in the state of *virāma pratyaya, ānandamaya kośa* is felt. Here the *cittamaya kośa* or *mahat* gets purified. From this stage he moves towards *nirbīja samādhi*. Then he is no more a seeker, but a seer (soul). He is an *ātmamayan*.

While practising or imparting knowledge I lose my identity and I am beyond the *pañca kośa* experiencing the existence without 'I' or 'Me'. I have experienced this state is my honest acknowledgement. As far as *nirbīja samādhi* is concerned, the *vairāgya* or desirelessness has to reach the highest state, where one abandons this transient world and goes beyond. If Rāmakrishna Paramahamsa had not returned from *nirvikalpa samādhi* we would not have heard of Swami Vivekānanda, as Śri Rāmakrishna transferred all his experiences to Swami Vivekānanda.

Saint Jñāneśvara went to *nirbīja samādhi*, but did not return to relate his experiences to those who were near him. At the stage of *nirbīja*, the words end, the cycle of life and death ends, the *karma* ends as the aims of life end. Desire ends and nothing remains. The *yogi* reaches the goal – the soul. The soul is the goal. The soul and goal become one.

III.8.2. – *Kaivalya*

Nirbīja samādhi is identical to kaivalya. *Nirbīja samādhi* stand for a state of ALONENESS (*kevela*), where the soul is free from the taints and alloy of *prakṛti*.

At the end of the text Patañjali says that when the fourfold aims of life are fulfilled and transcends the qualities of nature (*guṇa*), they return to *mūla prakṛti* and then the *puruṣa* – the Soul, installs Himself in his own nature, free from all establishments and qualities.

Thus, yoga begins with discipline and ends in establishing in his own splendour.

This is yoga real and true.

SECTION IV

ON *HAṬHA* YOGA

bhakti. *Bhakti* helps in dissolving the ego a great deal. Ego cannot be conquered without *bhakti*. *Bhakti* is impossible without *jñāna* and *jñāna* cannot be acquired without right *karma*.

Through profound meditation the knower, knowledge and the known become one. The seer, the sight and the seeing have no separate existence. When a musician becomes one with his instrument, music emanates from it. Similarly, meditation is not created, it just happens. It is entered into.

Therefore, courses on *dhyāna* are brain-washing and an eye-wash. When the tree has grown from the best of seeds, nurtured and nourished, it bears healthy fruit. One has to wait until the tree grows for it to give those fruit. But people have become immature and impatient; they want everything ready-made. They want the fruits before the tree grows. Without proper nurturing and maturing of all aspects of *sādhana* and *anuṣṭhāna*, people want to jump to meditation, which takes them nowhere. Momentary sensual peace is neither real peace nor to be considered as meditation.

III.7.6. – Is meditation isolating

Isolation means to cut off from everything and to live a dejected lonely life. It is a self-abnegating and nihilistic approach. Isolation is not meditation.

Isolation (*kevala*) means isolating the agents or the tributaries of the sea of the Self and to experience the state of self-aloneness. This aloneness stands for the establishment of the Self, or explicitness of the Self (*swami svarūpa*), this is what commentators mean.

Look at myself and my life.

Am I isolated from society? Am I morose and lonely or am I full of energy? Do I not practise and do I not teach? Do I not look after all those who come to this Institute, for their well being? I am doing all this as an offering to that Unlimited Force and that is my meditation. I am not sitting in a lonely place, but see all the faces of life! I am enjoying the joy that comes from my *sādhana* and at once share with all what I experience for them to feel that auspicious joy. Is it not for me total involvment and absorption in what I do that I share the good with all?

SECTION IV – ON *HAṬHA YOGA*

IV.1. – *Yama* and *niyama* in *haṭha yoga*

Haṭha yoga is considered as *ṣaḍāṅga yoga* because it begins with *āsana* as its first limb. This does not mean that Svātmārāma has no respect for *yama* and *niyama.*

Yoga Sūtra defines in clear terms the ethical discipline in the form of *yama* and *niyama. Haṭhayoga Pradīpikā* touches ten principles of *yama* and ten principles of *niyama* in one stanza,[1] before *āsana,* without defining them in depth. Hence, many think that *Haṭhayoga Pradīpikā* has not dealt with ethical disciplines. Perhaps the ethical principles of *yama* and *niyama* were assumed to have been already part of life in that era.

Svātmārāma certainly indicates that the *sādhaka* should stay and practise at a place where the dutiful king rules with *dharma.* This is the sign to show that he wanted the *sādhaka* to practise in a country, which was ruled by ethics. Then he can be stress free, disturbance free and botheration free for practice. Once the practitioner is free from all worries and day-to-day problems of life, there is less chance of committing anything wrong. Here, he involves social ethics besides individual ethics. Patañjali demands *yama* and *niyama* irrespective of whether they are difficult or easy, but Svātmārāma explains their contents.

Today we are caught up in the world of intellectual competition. We think of how to be non-violent when the world is violent, or how to hold on to the truth when the world speaks untruth. Such questions do bother us. Knowing such tendencies of the world, Svātmārāma brings to our attention to follow as far as possible, the ten principles of *yama* and ten principles of *niyama.*

---

1 The ten principles of *yama* are; non-violence (*ahiṁsā*), truthfulness (*satya*), non-stealing (*asteya*), celibacy (*brahmacarya*), forbearance (*kṣamā*), fortitude (*dhṛti*), mercifulness (*dayā*), straight-forwardness (*ārjava*), moderation in food (*mitāhāra*) and purity or cleanliness (*śauca*).

Similarly, the ten principles of *niyama* are austerity or zeal (*tapas*), contentment (*santoṣa*), belief in God (*āstikya*), charity (*dāna*), worshiping of God (*Īśvara pūjana*), listening to the study of scriptures (*siddhānta vākya ravaṇa*), modesty (*hṛi*), discerning mind (*mati*), prayer (*japa*) and sacrifice (*huta*).

While explaining *Siddhāsana,* Svātmārāma says that one has to contemplate on *ātmā* to be an *ātmadhyāyi.* Does this not suggest that one has to reach the soul in an *āsana,* and question whether it is possible to reach the soul without *yama* and *niyama?*

Patañjali brings the quintessence of *yama* and *niyama* in one *sūtra: śraddhā vīrya smṛti samādhiprajñā pūrvaka itareṣām* (*Y.S.,* I.20). One has to practise yoga with faith *(śraddhā),* courage *(vīrya),* memory *(smṛti)* and awareness of equanimity *(samādhi prajñā).* One has to use each day's practice as a springboard to proceed for perfection in *sādhanā.* Svātmārāma also speaks of the needed aspiration: *Utsāha sāhasāt dhairyāt tatvajñānāt ca niṣcayāt janasaṅga parityāgāt ṣadbhiryogaḥ prasidhyati (I.16)*

He says that the *sādhaka* succeeds in yoga by following cheerfulness, perseverance, courage, true knowledge, firm faith in the words of the *guru* and by abandoning the company of people,

The qualities for the practice of yoga are love, affection, zeal, willpower, courage, strength, vigour and vitality.

Thus it is clear that both *Haṭha yoga* and Pātañjala yoga establish that *yama* and *niyama* irrespective of caste, creed, class, gender or religion are a must in the pursuit of yoga *sādhanā.*

IV.2. – Is not *Haṭha yoga* a physical yoga

I have covered this aspect many times in these volumes, yet such questions arise. It is beyond my comprehension.

Ha represents the never fading Sun – the Soul, and *ṭha,* the waning and waxing moon – the consciousness. The union of these two is *haṭha yoga.* Also *ha* stands for the right side and *ṭha* the left side of the body. The proper alignment and balance of the two sides of the body, mind and intelligence is *haṭha yoga.*

The earth element is the foundation for other elements to function. Svātmārāma begins with the *annamaya kośa,* the base of the body. He wants the practitioner to be honest to himself in his practices. Then he explains various types of *prāṇāyāma* for the healthy function of cellular, nervous and glandular systems, which belong to *prāṇamaya kośa.* Afterwards he speaks on *kuṇḍalinī.* Patañjali uses *prakṛti-śakti* or *sva-śakti* for *kuṇḍalinī. Svāmi-śakti* is *puruṣa-śakti* and *sva-śakti* is *prakṛti-śakti. Prakṛti śakti* is necessary to know the *puruṣa-śakti* and *puruṣa* is needed to evolve by using *prakṛti śakti. Śakti* is a power that processes filtration and purification of *prakṛti.* This *śakti* is pure energy or *prāṇa.*

With the regular practice of *āsana* and *prāṇāyāma,* the respiratory system (the gates of health), the blood vessels, nerves and the organic body, are purified and toxins eradicated. The root cause of most diseases lies in the track of the digestive-excretory systems, from the mouth cavity to anus, which is called *mahā nāḍī* (major tubular organ of the body). If these two systems function rightly, then the other systems follow. Therefore the importance of food is given as conducive to health.

Then for an intense practitioner *(tīvrasaṁvegin),* the focus is on *mudrā* and *bandha,* as well as the inverted *āsana (viparīta sthiti),* balancing *āsana (bhujatolana sthiti)* and back bendings *(pūrva pratana sthiti).*

The physical power *(śarīra śakti)* surfaces through *āsana sādhanā. Nāḍī śakti* and *manas śakti* emerge from *prāṇāyāma* and *pratyāhāra,* will-power or intellectual power *(buddhi śakti)* through *dhāraṇā* and *dhyāna, icchāśakti* from spiritual power, and cosmic power *(mahat)* from *kuṇḍalinī* or *prakṛti-śakti.* The union of the energy of nature *(prakṛti-śakti)* with the energy of *ātman (puruṣa-śakti)* is yoga. This union is nothing but the awakening of that divine power *(divya śakti).* This is known as *kuṇḍalinī.*

Later Svatmārāma covers the other aspects of yoga, namely *pratyāhāra, dhāraṇā, dhyāna* and *samādhi.* As Patañjali explains the effect of yoga is for *kleśa karma nivṛtti* as the end of afflictions and of *karma* (*Y.S.,* IV.30), Svātmārāma explains *prāṇa vṛtti, manō nivṛtti* and *vāsanā nivṛtti,* and advises to control them so that energy *(prāṇa)* flows inside *suṣumṇā,* the central path: When the *prāṇa* is without any movement (in *kuṁbhaka*), and the mind is absorbed in the Soul, then that state of harmony is called *samādhi* (*H.Y.P.,* IV.6). If one understands my favourite word "measured alignment", one will be able to understand that the nervous system has to align with body, mind and soul. Grossly, one may equate *suṣumṇā* with the central nervous system and *piṅgaḷā* and *iḍā* with the sympathetic and parasympathetic nervous systems.

Svātmārāma devotes the last chapter on *samādhi* saying, "As long as *prāṇa* does not enter the centre of *suṣumṇā* and pierce the *brahmarandhra* which is in the crown of the head, and as long as the *bindu*[1] is not firm, *citta* does not transform to the nature of the *ātman*".[2] Those who only talk of *dhyāna* are vain talkers.

[1] *Bindu* means 'drop' or 'dot' in *tantric* and *haṭha yogic* texts means semen or *retas,* but it stands also for *brahman* (*Varāha Upaniṣad,* 50).

[2] *Viśeṣadarśinaḥ ātmabhāva bhāvanānivṛttiḥ* (*Y.S.,* IV.25) – for one who realises the distinction between *citta* and *ātmā,* the sense of separation between the two disappears.

The concluding stanza of *Haṭhayoga Pradīpikā* clearly throws light on the state of *samādhi* which is experienceable but not explainable. The light of that cannot be taught or forced. When the maturity in *sādhanā* and ripe wisdom is attained, then this state is experienced. It dawns only by one's own *sādhanā* and God's grace.

Hence, *haṭha yoga* starts from physical (*annamaya-kośa)* and leads towards spiritual state (*ātmānandamaya kośa*), cleansing the intermediate sheaths namely, *prāṇamaya kośa, manōmaya kośa, vijñāmaya kośa* and *ānandamaya kośa.*

IV.3. – *Ṣaṭkarma* (six cleansing actions)

Neti, dhauti, basti, kapālabhāti, nauli and *trāṭaka* are the six cleansing methods dealt in *Haṭha vidyā Pradīpikā.* The view today is that those who do not do these cleansing processes are non-yogic *sādhaka.* The techniques like *trāṭaka* are equated with spiritual yoga and *āsana* is relegated to physical yoga.

Ṣaṭkarma was not used at the time of Patañjali, but introduced later as new diseases surfaced. We know that modern amenities and comforts have brought lots of new diseases with new treatments. Similarly, at the time of treating certain new diseases, yogis of those days studied and discovered drastic remedies like *ṣaṭkarma* and introduced them in their yogic texts.

Today we have physicians and surgeons. Physicians prefer medicinal therapy while surgeons prefer surgery. In yoga too, yogis followed conventional treatment and the drastic treatment. Physicians like to postpone drastic treatment whereas surgeons advise surgery immediately. The patient with a discrete mind decides either one of them and goes for it. Some with oscillating minds like to go in for the third option, alternative medicine like *āsana* and *prāṇāyāma.*

Today's treatment on health has become a money-earning project. Sometimes it is this money-earning motivation that encourages unnecessary surgery, although it is true that it has proven to be a boon to deal with diseases.

Please note that there are conventional treatments and non-conventional treatments which we find in *haṭha yoga* texts.

The first chapter of *Haṭhayoga Pradīpikā* speaks of *āsana* and Svātmārāma says that the correct practice of *āsana* cleanses the nerves like cleaning a drainage system. *Āsana* throw out the toxins and the waste matter by natural available means and eradicate the diseases: *kuryāttadāsanaṁ sthairyamārogyaṁ cāṅgalāghavam* (*H.Y.P.*, I.17) – *āsana* brings (physical and mental) steadiness, freedom from diseases and lightness of limbs.

In the second chapter Svātmārāma speaks about *prāṇāyāma*. He begins with *Nāḍī Śodhana prāṇāyāma* – the most advanced and subtle *prāṇāyāma*. He says that by practising wrong *prāṇāyāma* one invites various problems and diseases. He insists on correct practice of *prāṇāyāma*. Only when he comes to the point of excess of fat, phlegm and mucus does he advise *ṣaṭkarma*. He clearly says *ghaṭaśodhanankāraka* (*H.Y.P.*, II.23), which means "that which purifies the body". The *Gheraṇḍa Saṁhitā* also calls it *ghaṭaśuddhi* (*G.S.*, I.8). *Ghaṭa śuddhi* means body purification. Does *aṣṭāṅga yoga* cleanse or not? Are *āsana* and *prāṇāyāma* not internal cleansers? *Āsana* and *prāṇāyāma* are traditional methods, *ṣaṭkarma* are drastic methods.

Haṭhayoga Pradīpikā says:

Medaḥ śleṣmādhikaḥ pūrvam ṣaṭkarmāṇi samācaret I
anyastu nācarettāni doṣāṇam samabhāvataḥ II (*H.Y.P.*, II.21)

Those having an excess of fat, mucus or phlegm must practise the six cleansing acts first (i.e., before the practice of *prāṇāyāma*). Those in whom the three *doṣa* (humours) are in a balanced state need not practise them.

It clearly says that those who are tremendously obese and are choked in nose, mouth, stomach and excretory canal should practise these, but certainly not others. According to him, these are meant for those who are abnormally unhealthy, with excessive fat, phlegm and cold or those in whom the humours of the body, viz. *vāta, pitta* and *kapha,* are in maximum, totally aggravated and vitiated.

Āyurveda too explains the *śodhana kriyā*, which includes emission (*vamana*), enemata (*virecana*), purging (*basti),* enema to head (*śirovirecana*) and blood letting (*rakta mokṣaṇa*). In the same way, Svātmārāma too advises one to go for such treatment if needed. Hence, it is purely a treatment. Then he switches over to *prāṇāyāma.* He says that some *ācārya* do not agree with treatments like *ṣaṭkarma* but insist on the practice of *prāṇāyāma* to balance the *tridoṣa* and *saptadhātu.*

Prāṇāyāmaireva sarve praśuṣyanti malā iti I
ācāryāṇāṁ tu keṣāñcidanyat karma na saṁmatam II (*H.Y.P.*, II.37).

Some teachers are of the opinion that practice of *prāṇāyāma* alone removes all impurities (of the *nāḍī*) and do not accept other means (i.e., six cleansing acts).

Even some *ācārya* prior to Svātmārāma have established the fact that the *ṣaṭkarma* are not necessary. For instance *Yogayājñavalkya Samhitā* advises the practice of *prāṇāyāma* for the purpose of *nāḍī śuddhi* (V.19-20).

Some of these cleansing techniques can even be harmful. Many have suffered with infection on account of cleansing nostrils with *jalaneti* and *sūtraneti.* One of my doctor students, Dr. Ginde, in 1970 said that he had to operate on practitioners to remove the thread which remained in the food pipe.

In my practice, I stuck to Patañjali, stuck to *āsana* and *prāṇāyāma* and began finding means to eradicate diseases through *āsana* and *prāṇāyāma*, rather than through drastic means.

Search and research are ongoing processes. We have to practise to introduce deep penetrative actions in the same *āsana* and *prāṇāyāma* so that new ideas and approaches are introduced to increase the defensive energy, and diseases and suffering are kept at bay.

Whatever I have to say on *ṣaṭkarma,* I have said it. To do or not to do is left to one's own sweet will.

IV.4. – *Haṭha yoga* and *samādhi*

The fourth chapter of *Haṭhayoga Pradīpikā* speaks thoroughly on *samādhi.* It is named as *samādhi nirupaṇam.* Svātmārāma explains the state of *samādhi* in simple words even for a common man or average intellect to understand. In IV.5., he gives the example of salt. As the salt dissolves in water and becomes one with it and water has one taste, salty, at all levels, so in *samādhi* the mind[1] dissolves completely in the Soul.

Prāṇa and mind have a close connection. For example, when the mind fluctuates, *prāṇa* fluctuates. Watch the breath. When it moves rhythmically soft and smooth, the mind too remains steady and stable. The moment the mind wanders; the breath pattern changes.

Prāṇa is in every cell of the body. If each cell is stabilised, *citta* is stabilised. When *prāṇa* is quietened or dissolved, mind too is dissolved. This is the state where breath and mind feel as

[1] Svātmārāma does not use the word *citta* as Patañjali. Probably at the time of Patañjali, *citta* was more in vogue than mind. *Citta* covers mind, intelligence and I, and therefore the people of that time were referring to *citta.*

At the time of Svātmārāma the intellectual calibre must have been lost, and the word mind occupied the place of *citta.*

if they are one and maintain harmony *(samarasatvam)*. When *jīvātmā* and *paramātmā* have this state of equilibrium, it is *samādhi*.

In order to reach this state one needs to study both the container of the mind, the body, and desires *(vāsanā)*. Svātmārāma refers to *citta* as mind and this mind has an affinity to *prāṇa* as well as *vāsanā*. It is activated by either one of these or both. Mind is the house of *vāsanā* and *prāṇa* is the vehicle of *vāsanā*. *Vāsanā* in one sense are eternal, hence human beings are full of desires, hopes and ambitions. As milk and water become one when mixed, mind and *prāṇa* become one even if one of them is restrained.

Svātmārāma and Patañjali agree with each other, though they use a different words on this spiritual aspect. *Haṭhayoga Pradīpikā* gives the clear indication of the relation between the body and the mind:

Manaḥ sthairye sthiro vāyuḥ tato binduḥ sthiro bhavet I
Bindusthairyāt sadā sattvam piṇḍasthairyaṁ prajāyate II (*H.Y.P.*, IV.28)

It means that when mind is stable, *prāṇa* becomes stable, if *prāṇa* is stable, the semen is stable; if semen is stable, *sattva guṇa* is stable; if *sattva guṇa* is stable, body is stable. *Yoga Sūtra* says: *sthira sukham āsanam* (*Y.S.*, II.46) – perfection in *āsana* brings firmness in body and benevolence in mind.

In *āsana*, one needs to become stable by keeping out desires and *prāṇa* stable. Patañjali speaks in a philosophical language and Svātmārāma speaks with practical references. For him, stability of body *(dehasthairya)* is stability of semen *(bindusthairya)*. Semen is the essence of the seven ingredients of the body *(sapta dhātu)*. The product of semen is *ojas* and *tejas*, which is essential to tread on the spiritual path. Semen is meant for *bhoga* as well as yoga. Svātmārāma connects the purity of body with the pure state of consciousness. I have often said that people often come to yoga for a sense satisfaction *(bhoga)*, very few for religiousness in practice *(yoga)*.

Samādhi is purity of *citta*. It is a state of *samādhāna*, or the attainment of *samarasatva*. In *samādhi* one needs to have *dehasthairya, bindusthairya, manasthairya, prāṇasthairya, buddhisthairya, sattvasthairya, cittasthairya* along with their purity – *śuddhi*.

This is the essence of *Svātmārāma yoga* as well as *Pātañjala yoga*.

IV.5. – *Haṭha Yoga* and *Pātañjala Yoga*

It is unfortunate that many with wrong notions misrepresent *Haṭha yoga* and *Pātañjala yoga* without proper reading, which pains many aspirants. *Ha* in the *Haṭhayoga Pradīpikā* means the sun or the Soul and *ṭha* means the moon or the consciousness. Patañjali wants the *citta* (part of *prakṛti*) to merge in *puruṣa*, Svātmārāma too advises to dissolve the *citta* (moon) in the Soul (sun).

In *Haṭha Yoga ṭha* stands for consciousness while in *Pātañjala Yoga citta* is said to be the sprout of the soul. Consciousness *(citta)* as moon, wanes and waxes. Patañjali advises restraint *(nirodha)* or suspension *(stambha)*, to put an end to the waxing and waning of consciousness so that it reaches the state of steadiness like the sun. Like the never fading sun, the soul never fades, but shining ever fresh.

The moon waxes for fourteen days, and wanes for fourteen days. The thought waves in consciousness wax and wane every now and then. Whether it is the yoga of Patañjali or Svātmārāma, the aim of both is to stop the waning and waxing of the consciousness.

Patañjali begins the *Yoga Sūtra* with *samādhi* whereas the *Haṭhayoga Pradīpikā* explains it at the end. Armchair yogis brainwash the aspirants with the notion that Svātmārāma's yoga is physical. See what Patañjali says in *Sādhana Pāda*. If Svātmārāma begins addressing the subject from the periphery towards the causal body, Patañjali starts from the causal body and then moves towards the peripheral body and returns to conclude at the causal body.

The first chapter of *Haṭhayoga Pradīpikā*, deals with *āsana*, the second on *prāṇāyāma*, the third on *mudrā* and the last on *samādhi*.

My advice to all would be to read Patañjali's second chapter *(Sādhana Pāda)* first, then read the first chapter *(Samādhi Pāda)*. As he combines the essence of the first and second and chapters in *Vibhūti Pāda*, one can easily grasp the subject matter.

As one acquires powers through yogic *sādhanā*, Patañjali cautions in the later part of *Vibhūti Pāda* not to pay attention to the *siddhi* but to proceed to establish the soul *(puruṣa)*. He explains in this chapter how intuitive wisdom surfaces, whereas in the fourth chapter *(Kaivalya Pāda)* he proceeds showing what actions are to be done after emancipation. Hence, I say with confidence and courage that I see no difference between the two texts. Both are *mokṣa śāstra*.

The mistaken knowledge superficially has arisen in the minds of intellectuals that *haṭha yoga* is physical because thirteen or fourteen *āsana* are explained about which one does not find any reference in Pātañjala text, except the names of *āsana* described by Vyāsa while commenting on *āsana*. Besides *āsana* and *prāṇāyāma Haṭhayoga Pradīpikā* covers *ṣatkarma* and *mudrā*. Patañjali's approach is to define the characteristic or substratum *(dharmi)* of the *āsana* and not the character *(dharma)* for the practitioner to get totally absorbed and meditate in each *āsana*.

Each *āsana* is a meditation as one has to involve oneself in it to calibrate from the body to the self and from the self to the body. He wants the mind to be drawn towards the self in each *āsana*. While commenting on this *sūtra*, Vyāsa gives a list of *āsana* such as *Uṣtraniṣadanāsana, Krauñcaniṣadanāsana, Hastiniṣadanāsana, Padmāsana, Vīrāsana, Bhadrāsana, Swastikāsana, Daṇḍāsana, Sopāśrayāsana, Paryaṅkāsana, Samasaṁsthāsana* and so forth. If one thinks that Patañjali speaks of only one *āsana*, then he is in want of knowledge and understanding. If so he would have to refute Vyāsa.

There is another connotation for *Haṭha*. *Haṭha* means "force" and *haṭha yoga* is to force the mind precipitating one to abstain from external objects. This means, that *haṭha yoga* is a yoga of will-power. The author of *Haṭha Vidya Pradīpikā* now called as the *Haṭhayoga Pradīpikā* is Svātmārāma. The very name of the author signifies what he derived from the practice of *haṭha yoga*. *Sva* means "ones own", *ātmā* means "Self" and *rāma* means "one who is dwelling and living in the abode of the soul".

Whatever way one may name yoga, it is an essential requirement in this modern age that is becoming inactive, slow, dull, lazy, abiding in worldly pleasures.

Haṭhayoga does not deal only with *āsana*. The text speaks of *āsana, prāṇāyāma, ṣaṭkarma, bandha, mudrā, cakra* and *samādhi*. If one reads the stanzas in the chapter on *samādhi*, of the *Haṭhayoga Pradīpikā* then I am sure the reader changes his thoughts on this text.

People think that *cakra* have no place in *Pātañjala Yoga*. Patañjali refers to *cakra* by different names. He calls *maṇipūraka* as *nābhicakra, anāhata* as *hṛdcakra* (*hṛd* means heart), *viśuddhi* as *kaṇṭhakūpam, svādhiṣṭhāna* as *kūrmanāḍi* (epigastric region), *ājñā* as *mūrdhajyoti* and so forth. Besides *cakra Haṭhayoga Pradīpikā* speaks on *nāḍi, nāda, kalā* and *bindu*.[1]

Vibhūti Pāda of *Yoga Sūtra* guides in the conquest of *prakṛti*, then *Kaivalya Pāda* explains the consecration of the *puruṣa*.

---

1 *Nāḍī* means blood vessels in the body, *nāda* is sound. The arteries and veins make a sound. When disturbed the sound of it becomes unrhythmic and when undisturbed it is rhythmic. Even the organs of the body while pumping or vibrating make sound. Especially, *dhamani* makes a very strong sound. From *nāḍī* comes *nāda*. Through this *nāda* the *dhāraṇā* is done on the part or section of the body, so that the inner sound becomes audible. *Kalā* is a part. *Bindu* indicates the end of sound. *(H.Y.P.,* IV.1)

Both texts deal with body, mind, intelligence and soul. They touch all aspects of the human being, and therefore let us study all aspects of yoga from both the books and judge impartially.

Yoga is a way of life. It is a discipline. Freedom from afflictions being the goal, it needs discipline. As we are entangled in the net of body, mind, ego and intellect, we have to come out from this net through all aspects of yogic practice. One cannot take one aspect and neglect the other. Let us take all good points from yogic textbooks and use them for our progress in our *sādhanā*.

SECTION V

KUṆḌALINĪ

In *Vibhūti Pāda* he says, *Tadeva arthamātranirbhāsam svarūpaśūnyam iva samādhiḥ* (III.3) – when the object of meditation engulfs the meditator appearing as the subject, self-awareness is lost. This is a state of *samādhi*. For a meditator, when the object of contemplation itself transforms as "himself", he experiences *samādhi* devoid of his form. In *sabīja samādhi* he reaches the state as if he is *svarūpaśūnya*. At this stage his existence and attentiveness is totally given to the object that he is meditating upon. Whereas, in *nirbīja samādhi* there is no *svarūpaśūnyatā* but *svarūpapratiṣṭhā*. The soul reveals the soul. The seer sees the seer and the seer establishes in his own nature; *tadā draṣṭuḥ svarūpe avasthānam* (I.3). The state of *samādhi* is such that first the aspirant masters his own servants who supply him the knowledge (organs of action and senses of perception). Then he conquers the mind and intelligence, which collect and filter the knowledge from the known. When the known is fully known, he abandons all, savouring the knower of the known. Regarding myself, whether I have experienced or not, I have only glimpses of it, on several occasions. Lord Krishna in *Bhagavad Gītā* said:

Manuṣyāṇām sahasreṣu kaścidyatati siddhaye I
yatatāmapi siddhānām kaścinmām vetti tattvataḥ II *(B.G., III.7)*

Among thousands of men only a few strive for knowledge to become adepts, and even among those adepts only one may really know Me in true perceptivity.

Regarding *nirālamba (nirbīja) samādhi*, I am not hesitant to say that probably no one in this 20th century has experienced it. You may find one in centuries. *Nirbīja samādhi* is such that one will not be affected by life and death. *Nirbīja samādhi* is an immortal state of life. Only those who have experienced have remained immortals. For instance, Vyāsa and Hanumān, are examples.

You may find a few cases of those who have experienced *virāma pratyaya*. You may find *prakṛtilayin* and *videhin*. *Prakṛtilayin* are those who have conquered the evolutes of nature and merge into it, whereas *videhin* are those who have gone beyond the physical existence. They may remain bodiless without the experience of the *ātman*. When *Śrī* Aurobindo was in Alipore jail, he explained his experiences, which appear akin to the effects of *virāma pratyaya*. He had experienced *videha* state. At such a state, if one fails to do *sādhanā* one may get stranded and stagnate. If one continues practice and meditates until he meets the seer, then *nirbīja* is possible. Those who go beyond the state of *prakṛtilaya* and *videha* can reach *nirbīja*.

However, this experience comes in glimpses as the truth comes to us in glimpses. The reality is touched in glimpses, but due to our contact with the phenomenal world we forget. Though we progress, there is regression too. Probably we may experience it if we stick to it. We have to cross beyond the three *jñāna* i.e. *adhyātmika jñāna*, *ādhibhautika jñāna* and *ādhidaivika*

SECTION V – *KUṆḌALINĪ*

V.I. – What is *kuṇḍalinī*

Kuṇḍalinī is a divine cosmic energy *(divya śakti),* which is present in a latent form in every human being. It is considered to be like a serpent with its face downwards indicating bondage. Man has two-faced desires. One is to go with worldly pleasures *(laukika jñāna)* and other is toward spiritual knowledge and bliss *(vaidika* or *adhyātmika jñāna).* It is natural for a human being to go with the current of *laukika jñāna* but to go with *vaidika jñāna* is against the current and natural tendencies. This requires a blazing fire of will-power and great effort to turn natural tendencies towards spiritual aspects.

In the early days *kuṇḍalinī* was known as *agni.* According to Patañjali, it is the strength of *prakṛti* that has this divine power *(śakti).* For most of us it is covered with *vikṛti-śakti* such as disease, sickness, emotions of anger, wrath, fear, disgust, aversion and so forth.

This dormant divine energy has to be uncovered and then to be awakened. When one is purified and sanctified in body, mind, intelligence and consciousness, then it paves its avenue in its own inner royal path. This royal path is in the centre axis of the human being called *citrā.* This runs within the *suṣumnā nāḍī.* As the wires are connected to the main source of electrical energy, *prāṇa* in the form of physical, mental, intellectual, spiritual and cosmic energy is connected to this divine force. The *prakṛti-śakti* from body to the conscience has to flow towards the principal stream – *ātma-śakti.*

Kuṇḍalinī is symbolised as a coiled energy *kuṇḍalākāra,* which has to be uncoiled and straightened to move into the subtle *citrā nāḍī,* which is within the *suṣumṇa.* Many do not know how to keep the gross spine erect and have no intellectual sensitivity of the tailbone, yet think of playing with *kuṇḍalinī.* When one does not know the body with its constituents, how can one think of awakening this divine energy that is hidden deep within?

Inquisitiveness is a part of human intelligence. First one has to make an inquiry of the gross body, which remains unknown before going into the query of the subtle body.

In the chapter XI, of the *Bhagavad Gītā*, Lord Krishna tells Arjuna, "Now I offer you to see my real form, the *viśvarūpa darśana*. Before this I bless you with divine eyes as you cannot see my form with your normal eyes". But in spite of having divine eyes Arjuna could not bear the sight of Lord Krishna in his Cosmic Form, and hence he requested the Lord to appear in his natural form. This grace from Lord Krishna is the Divine *Śakti* or *kuṇḍalinī śakti*.

There are two types of living. One is in learning worldly ways of living *(laukika)* and the other way of learning is the spiritual ways of living *(vaidika* or *adhyātmika)*. They do not go together. Unless and until we discipline our entire system to become divine, we will not experience this *kuṇḍalinī śakti*. For this, the divinity of the body is very essential for this divine *prakṛti* to unite with the divinity of the soul. We have a huge gulf between body and mind, mind and soul. Let us work to bring them closer to each other. Then I think I shall not have to explain *kuṇḍalinī* power, because one experiences it for oneself.

V.2. – *Nāḍī* and its function

The word *nāḍī* is derived from the *Sanskṛt* verb *nāḍ*. It means a hollow stalk or tube. It means vibration or resonance indicating the sound element. I consider the *nāḍī* as a bridge between the physical, physiological, mental, intellectual and spiritual bodies.

We have several physiological systems working in the body with their allotted jobs. Our movements, mobility, thinking and imaginative process depend on these systems. There are several tubes, vessels and fibres functioning in these systems.

Just think of the digestive and excretory systems. They make one single tube that begins from the mouth cavity and ends at the anus. It is called the major middle path *(mahānāḍī*, or *madhyanāḍī)*. There are salivary duct glands, oesophagus, stomach, a tube like ileum, duodenum and small and large intestines. For digestion the liver, gallbladder, spleen and pancreas pour their juicy essence to help digestion.

Now think of the circulatory and nervous systems along with the lymph vessels. What a network the body has! The whole body is connected with *nāḍī*, from one end to the other, covering the remotest corners of the body!

Basically the *nāḍī* is a tubular shaped conduit, which carries food, water, air, energy, sensory and motor messages. It carries blood, lymph, semen, ovum, waste matter and so forth. Muscles spindles, ligaments and tendons carry energy to keep the muscles and bone-joints in order to function properly. We have the ductless glands that secrete hormones directly into the blood stream.

The Science of yoga found the *nāḍī* to be non-perceivable as well as perceivable. Some pathways are seen or felt, and some are not seen or felt.

Modern science has discovered and explored the sound vibration, which can be recorded and mapped to know the inner activities. Sonography reveals many facts which otherwise would not be possible to know. The *āyurvedic ācārya* had developed the *nāḍī-parikṣā* to such an extent that through the pulse they could make out whether *vāta-nāḍī* or *pitta-nāḍī* or *kapha-nāḍī* is active. They could make out whether the food is digested or not. They could diagnose diseases, make out whether a woman is pregnant or not and if pregnant, whether she carries a baby boy or a baby girl. They could check the blood pressure or evaluate the cholesterol by the sound of *nāḍī*. They could make out the behavioural pattern and the mental state of a person. Some *āyurvedic ācārya* of today read the past and future of their patients by just taking their pulse. This examination of pulse *(nāḍī-parikṣā)* was an advanced science in India.

The central nervous system is composed of the brain, the spinal cord and the nerves extended from it. The nerves are connected to the brain and the body. They have two functions; a) to receive the impulses coming in over the afferent or sensory nerves and b) sending impulses out over the efferent or motor nerves.

The brain and spinal cord come under the central nervous system, and the part of the nervous system that connects and links the internal organs of the body is the autonomous nervous system. The autonomous nervous system has two major functions, a) the function of internal organs and, b) emotional behaviour. The autonomous nervous system is divided as the sympathetic and parasympathetic nervous systems.

In yogic terminology these three main *nāḍī* are called *iḍā*, *piṅgaḷā* and *suṣumṇā*. These are close to parasympathetic, sympathetic and central nervous systems. The afferent nerves are *jñāna-nāḍī* and efferent nerves, *karma-nāḍī*. The central nervous system is *buddhi-nāḍī*. The afferent nerves receive the message and hence they are *jñāna-nāḍī*, efferent nerves act and hence they are *karma-nāḍī*.

The right vagus nerve and the left vagus nerve can be equated with *puṣā* and *yaśasvinī*. *Puṣā* is on the right ear behind *piṅgaḷā* and *yaśasvinī* is on the left ear behind *piṅgaḷā*.

According to the yogic texts, there are thousands of *nāḍī* in the body, which spread like a vast web. There are 72,000 *nāḍī* originating from *kandasthāna* (*kanda*, bulb-root, *sthāna*, position or seat) below the navel, each of them branching off with 72,000 *nāḍī*. In the same way 101 *nāḍī* originate from the seat of the Soul *(ātmasthāna* or *hṛdayasthāna)* branching each into 72,000 *nāḍī*, except one known as *citrā nāḍī* which has no branch but connects the *ātmasthāna* to *brahmarandhra* (the seat of Brahma, at the top of the head) through *suṣumṇā*.

Patañjali mentions, *nābhicakre kāyavyūhajñānam* (*Y.S.*, III.30) knowing the functions of the navel, the yogi acquires perfect knowledge of the disposition of the human body. This is very close to the net of *nāḍī* that spreads from *kanda* below the navel.

Iḍā is on the left and *piṅgaḷā* is on the right of *suṣumṇā* and *suṣumṇā* is in the centre of the spine. They control our *sāttvic, rājasic* and *tāmasic* nature. These three *nāḍī* suggest that they are beyond physical existence having intangible and invisible influence. Apart from these three major *nāḍī*, *gāndhārī* and *hastijihvā* are connected to the left and right eyes, aiding seeing whereas *yaśasvinī* and *pūṣā* represent the left and right ears aiding hearing. *Sarasvati nāḍī* controls the tongue (speech as well as intake of food). Food and speech having close connections, controls the functions of the abdominal organs to maintain their health. *Śūrā nāḍī* begins from the navel and ends at the base of the brain between the eyebrows. It connects *nābhi cakra* to *ājñā cakra* but its function is not mentioned in the texts. The *rākā nāḍī* creates hunger and thirst whereas *viśvodari* does the function of absorption. The *ālambusā nāḍī* bifurcates mouth and anus - forming the *mahānāḍī*. The *śaṁkhinī nāḍī* terminates at the genital organs carrying the essence of food. *Ālambusā* helps in taking the food, *rākā* instigates, and *śaṁkhinī* absorbs. *Śukra* or semen is used either for reproduction *(adhogati)*, or for making it to move upwards *(ūrdhvagati)*. When the semen ascends, it is called *ūrdhvaretas (ūrdhva* means semen and *retas* means seed, fortitude and radiance).

Rākā starts from *kandasthāna* but as it proceeds towards the mouth it gets connected with the oesophagus as well as the trachea. It also collects sinus to clear the passage of respiration and provoke hunger and thirst. The evacuation is done by *kuhū* and *vāruṇi*. *Kuhū* evacuates and *vāruṇi* controls the bladder. When the energy enters *suṣumṇā* from *iḍā* and *piṅgaḷā*, the hunger, thirst and evacuation are conquered. *Kūrmanāḍī* connects the navel to the pit of the throat and stabilises the body and mind.

The *nāḍī* that starts from the heart works on the network of arteries, capillaries and veins. This heart *nāḍī* has a great importance from the yogic point of view. Though the heart is known as a physiological organ, it is also considered as the abode of the soul. It is called *hṛdayam* or the spiritual heart. It is the seat of *prāṇa*. As the blood vessels originate and end in the physiological heart, the subtle *nāḍī* carrying energy *(prāṇa)*, intelligence *(prajñā)*, emotions, feelings and the source of consciousness and conscience *(viveka)* originate in the heart. It is also the origin of desire *(vāsanā)*, as well as aspiration for self-realisation *(ātma sakṣātkāra)*.

Citrā is a subtle divine *nāḍī* and not a physical *nāḍī*. Though its place is said to be in the heart, it decides our fate. It splits into two at the base – one going downwards towards the generative organ and the other going upwards towards the crown of the head.

I have often said that the heart is the *ātmasthāna*. The *antarātman* exists in the heart. When *suṣumṇā* takes the divine energy up, it is called *nādarūpiṇi*.

The *vijñāna nāḍī* originates at the navel and connects the gross *nāḍī* to the subtle *nāḍī* for our inner journey. *Vijñāna nāḍī* is the channel of consciousness. *Vi* means special or *viśeṣa* and *jñāna* means knowledge. Only through the development of this special knowledge, it is possible for the consciousness to reach the state of purity *(sattva śuddhi)*, as consciousness alone takes one towards *ātman*, uniting *prakṛti śakti* with *puruṣa śakti* and then making *puruṣa śakti* to move towards *paramātmā śakti*.

V.3. – *Cakra*

The human body functions like an automatic machine. Anatomical study reveals that each one of us has the same organs, flesh and bones. Nowadays sonography, X-ray or CT scan confirm these observations. The only thing that cannot be scanned or X-rayed is the mind and consciousness. Psychoanalysis reveals only the outer mind (the mind which is close to the peripheral body), similar to the iceberg where only 1/11th of the ice is seen whereas the rest of it remains under water.

If a man was made up of only flesh, bones, joints and muscles, we would have all been alike and life would have been monotonous. The real stuff between the skin and the soul is not only the flesh and organs of the body but also the other vehicles of the self, namely mind, intellect, emotions, vital energy, sense of I, will-power, discriminating consciousness and conscience. These inner vehicles of the self change the nature, texture, behaviour and character from one person to another.

Prakṛti-śakti is like the river water or the electrical current of a live wire, running constantly. This *prakṛti-śakti* leads man either towards worldly pleasures or spiritual emancipation *(puruṣa-śakti*.

In yogic terminology the above mentioned stuff between the skin and the soul is *prakṛti-śakti,* and the soul is *puruṣa-śakti* or *parāśakti.*

This energy of nature *(prakṛti-śakti)* was known originally as fire *(agni).* Later, yogis called this *agni* as *kuṇḍalinī. Kuṇḍalinī* is a divine cosmic energy that exists in each one in a latent state. Due to ignition of *prakṛti śakti* and its sprouting, man is encouraged to gravitate either towards the self or towards the pleasures of the world. But, as the flame of the fire moves upwards, the *prakṛti śakti* aspires to move upwards towards the seat of the soul *(ātman).* This fire remains un-ignited in its dormant state, facing downwards, as if hidden in ashes. A yogi or a yogini ignites it with the fire of yoga *(yogāgni śakti)* and makes it to move upwards towards the *puruṣa.*

The vehicles of the self are covered with *rajas* and *tamas* qualities of nature. These qualities are vibrancy and inertia. The *rajas* and *tamas* express themselves in the form of hindrances, like disease, laziness and doubt. These hindrances cloud the divine energy. Many a time, we experience its presence but we cannot hold on to it because we go back to our old ways of thinking and living. It is like the fire when extinguished, the remaining wood gets covered with ashes, so it is with the *ātman* that is covered with the ashes of the fire of knowledge *(jñānāgni).*

Everyone knows that if the spine, brain, central, autonomous and peripheral nervous systems are healthy, the human being is healthy. Medical science admits that health of the body depends upon the health of the mind and vice-versa. The scientists have started understanding the relationship between psyche and soma. Yoga knew this from time immemorial and excavated the depth of the mind, recognising the concept of spiritual health. In order to have spiritual health, there is a system in the spine, beyond the physical body. The centres of this system are called *cakra.* In other words if the *cakra* are healthy, then he is certainly healthy physically as well as spiritually.

Cakra, which are said to be inside the spine, rule and govern the gross and subtle elements of the body leading us on the path of divinity. *Cakra* is a wheel or a ring. They are located at tne vital centres of the spinal canal. Like the nerves *(nāḍī)* connecting the brain and the body, the *cakra* connect the body to the self through the triune of gross (*sthūla),* subtle (*sūkṣma)* and cause (*kāraṇa śarīra)* bodies, and five sheaths *(kośa),* the anatomical, physiological, psychological, intellectual and spiritual.

Sthūla śarīra is the anatomical body *(annamaya kośa).* The organic body including all the physiological systems is *prāṇamaya kośa.* The psychological and emotional body that influences the faculty of awareness, feeling and motivation is *manomaya kośa.* The intellectual sheath that controls and supervises the process of analysing, reasoning, judgement and wisdom is *vijñānamaya kośa*. *Prāṇamaya, manomaya* and *vijñānamaya kośa* come under the regime of *sūkṣma śarīra* or subtle body.

Ānandamaya and *ātmānandamaya kośa* are the innermost sheaths around the throne of the soul, and comes under the regime of *kāraṇa śarīra*. The *kāraṇa śarīra* is the inner rudiment or the causal frame of the body. The feel of all *kośa* fades in *samādhi* (*Y.S.*, III.3). Beyond *ānanda*, only the Soul exists which is free from all complementary and supplementary actions and reactions.

The brain functions at physical, mental and intellectual levels through its connecting vehicle, the neurons or the nerve cells. Similarly, the *cakra* function with the vital energy *(prāṇa)*. *Prāṇa* is the vibrating energy existing in the form of physical, physiological, mental, intellectual, spiritual and cosmic energies. The *cakra* pick up the cosmic energy *(mahat-prāṇa)* and distributes it throughout the body via the connecting channels *(nāḍī)*. As an antenna picks up the radio waves and transforms them into sound, *cakra* too receive the cosmic energy and transform it into the subtle, secret, silent, sublime inner mystical energy. The *cakra* fuse splendour *(tejas)* and lustre and light *(ojas)*, and convert the cosmic energy into spiritual energy and make them to circulate in the human system through vibration via the circuit of the *nāḍī*.

Since *cakra* are not visible, they remain inaccessible. They are tangible only through their effective activities and functions. The aspirant has to find their functioning's only by adopting and practising with zeal the eight aspects of yoga till he has realised the divine Soul in him.

There are in all eleven main *cakra*. Among them six are most important. The other five *cakra* are partially dependent on the main six *cakra*. The eleven *cakra* are: 1) *mūlādhāra*, 2) *svādhiṣṭhāna*, 3) *maṇipūraka*, 4) *sūrya*, 5) *manas*, 6) *anāhata*, 7) *viśuddhi*, 8) *ājñā*, 9) *soma*, 10) *lalāṭa*, and 11) *sahasrāra*. The six most important *cakra* are *mūlādhāra, svādhiṣṭhāna, maṇipūraka, anāhata, viśuddhi* and *ājñā*. And the topmost *cakra* is *sahasrāra*. It is in this *cakra* that *prakṛti śakti* or *kuṇḍalinī śakti* unites and merges in pure, sacred and sublime form with the soul *(puruṣa śakti)*.

These *cakra* are not plexus. Plexus are outside the spinal column while the *cakra* are inside the spine. The *cakra* may be running parallel to the plexus.

1. *Mūlādhāra cakra* – It is located above the anus between the anal mouth and genitals. It is parallel to the sacral or genital plexus. It governs the *apāna vāyu* and *dhanaṁjaya*

upavāyu[1] as well as the earth element *(pṛthvi tattva)* with odour *(gandha).* It is the base of the anatomical sheath *(annamaya kośa),* which results in the integration of body *(śarīra saṁyama)* through yogic practices. The person under the influence of this *cakra* is caught in the worldly pleasures. On the other hand, when this *cakra* comes under control, one conquers the anatomical and physiological bodies and reaches the state of *ūrdhvaretas.* The sexual energy begins to sublimate. He becomes vitally firm, but free from sexual desire. The presiding deity of this *cakra* is Gaṇapati.

2. *Svādhiṣṭhāna cakra* – This is situated between genitals and hypogastric plexus. It governs the same *vāyu* that come under the control of *mūlādhāra* as well as *āp-tattva* and its subtle quality is taste *(svāda).* This *cakra* rules over *annamaya* and *prāṇamaya kośa.* Man under the influence of this *cakra* remains satisfied with worldly wishes such as food, money and family life. He remains self-centred. He is under the influence of lust and anger. He has a strong attachment for life and fear of losing it. When conquered he is not only free from disease and fatigue but also acquires vibrant health. A self-centred person begins to feel the change in his attitude and becomes friendly and compassionate. He gets control over the senses *(indriya-saṁyama).* The presiding deity of this *cakra* is *Brahmā.*
3. *Maṇipūraka cakra* – This is situated slightly below the navel region called solar plexus. It governs *samāna* and *kṛkara vāyu* as well as the fire element *(tejas-tattva).* It is a foundation of the physiological sheath *(prāṇamaya kośa).* Man under the influence of this *cakra* has constant fears. The mind being feeble remains confused and shattered. When activated and controlled, one remains calm and quiet even in adverse circumstances. One has to work through yoga to get integration of energy *(prāṇa-saṁyama).* The yogic texts say that just below the navel, there is an egg-shaped bulb called *kanda.* From here 72,000 *nāḍī* are said to spread throughout the body, each one branching off again into another 72,000, which have countless outlets and functions. The energy from these *nāḍī* is reversed by creating inlets that make the person tremendously powerful and courageous. The presiding deity of this *cakra* is Vishnu.
4. *Sūrya cakra* – It is between the navel and the diaphragm. It governs the *samāna* and *kṛkara vāyu* as well as the fire element *(tejas-tattva)* and *prāṇamaya kośa.* By conquering this *cakra* one conquers hunger, fear, greed and passion, which in turn keeps the abdominal organs healthy and increases the life span.

---

[1] *Dhanaṁjaya,* litterally, "the conquest of wealth", is one of the five subsidiary *vāyu.* It pervades the entire body and does not leave it even after death. The texts of yoga, specially the *Yogopaniṣad* talks a lot about its functions. It is believed that *dhanaṁjaya* is responsible for transformations of the body after death. The shining appearance of the body of a yogi after death is on account of *dhanaṁjaya*'s activity. *Śāṇḍilyopaniṣad* (I.4.13) considers the production of phlegm as a function of this *vāyu.*

5. *Manas cakra* – It is situated between the diaphragm and the heart, presiding over the fire element *(tejas tattva)*. It is the foundation of the mental sheath *(manōmaya kośa)*. It is the seat of emotions. When conquered, that person is full of love and compassion. It ignites the power of imagination and creativity.
6. *Anāhata cakra* – It is situated in the heart region, the abode of the soul between physical and spiritual heart. It rules over the *prāṇa* and *devadatta vāyu* as well as *manōmaya kośa*. The element of air (*vāyu-tattva*) presides, and its subtle element is touch. The man under the influence of this *cakra* is full of aversion, jealousy and hatred. When conquered, it strengthens the emotional heart, develops adoration and knowledge. The aspirant becomes free from sensual pleasures and aversions and follows the spiritual path. It is the source of faith, reverence, love and devotion. One gets the integration of mind *(manō-saṁyama)*. The presiding deity of this *cakra* is Shiva.
7. *Viśuddhi cakra* – It is situated near the throat at the base of the neck, at pharyngeal plexus, and presides over the element of ether *(ākāśa-tattva)* and *udāna* as well as *kūrma vāyu*. It rules over the intellectual sheath *(vijñānamaya kośa)*. When activated, pierced and conquered one develops the power of grasping and understanding knowledge. The attachments towards worldly pleasures shed away and one proceeds towards the self. The aspirant becomes intellectually alert and clear. Speech becomes distinct and fluent. One gets integration of intelligence *(buddhi saṁyama)*. The presiding deity is the individual soul *(jīvātman)*. According to Patañjali, *jivātman* is *drastā* (*Y.S.*, I.3, II.17).
8. *Ājñā cakra* – This is situated between the two eyebrows at the base of the brain. It is recognised as the seat of command. It also has control over *ākāśa-tattva*. It rules over *ānandamaya kośa (kāraṇa śarīra)* and controls *prāṇa* and *devadatta*. One develops pride, ego and lust. A person becomes self-conscious and ego pervades his intelligence. When the *cakra* opens, command over the body takes place. The *sādhaka* develops a spiritual aura and the ego begins to dissolve. The affliction or *asmitā kleśa* fades out. The presiding deity is the individual self.
9. *Soma cakra* – It is situated at the base of the brain, near the hypothalamus. It rules over *ākāśa-tattva* and *ānandamaya kośa* as well as *vyāna* and *nāga vāyu*. When conquered, he becomes free from excitement, anger, worry and animosity, and remains cool and quiet. He develops himself to surrender to the Supreme as the fire of ego gets extinguished. This *cakra* controls the temperature of the body and the temper of mind. The mind doesn't hanker any more for food.
10. *Lalāṭa cakra* – This is situated slightly above the hypothalamus. It rules over *cittamaya kośa*. By conquering it the *citta* gets purified and ego is sublimated. No more does he

indulge in enjoying the fruits of action. In other words, he becomes the master of his destiny. The seat of individuality, which is at the top of the brain, gets quietened and the feeling of 'I' and 'Me' dissolves. Thus, comes the conquest of *citta* or integration of consciousness (*citta saṁyama*).

11. *Sahasrāra cakra* – It is situated at the upper most cerebral centre, which is above the elemental world. It is the seat of *Parabrahman* (*puruṣa viśeṣa* as named by Patañjali). This *cakra* rules over *ātmamaya*. It is conquered only through intuitive knowledge that expresses itself when the conscience is cleansed, purified and consecrated. The *sādhaka* crosses the barriers of the body, mind, intelligence, emotions, memory, imprints and reaches emancipation (see table n. 3 & 4 on following pages).

Practice of *aṣṭāṅga yoga* awakens the divine energy which is hidden within man. *Āsana, prāṇāyāma, bandha* and *mudrā* is practised in order to open and alert the *cakra* to receive the awakened divine power, and to close all the outlets so that he finds the inlets and pierces the energy *(śakti)* to move towards *sahasrāra*. Often, the subtle elaborative and penetrative techniques in each *āsana* and *prāṇāyāma* play a major role, enabling the practitioner to have access to these *cakra*. In the process of performing the *āsana* and *prāṇāyāma*, the muscles, bones and joints are activated and mobilised. Similarly with the help of five gross and subtle elements, *pañca vāyu (prāṇa, apāna, vyāna, udāna* and *samāna)* and *upavāyu (dhanaṁjaya, kṛkara, nāga, devadatta* and *kūrma),* the consciousness becomes free from *vṛtti* and gets stabilised. The practice of *āsana* and *prāṇāyāma* opens the *nāḍī* that have to reach the *cakra*. In turn, the *cakra* vibrate and generate energy, which is relayed all over the body and all the sheaths. The glands that are under the control of the *cakra* are revitalised. The organs are rejuvenated. The emotions are stabilised. This way, *prakṛti śakti* gets nurtured, revitalised, purified, sanctified and revitalised towards the divine state in the cause body (*kāraṇa śarīra*), where *prakṛti śakti* becomes one with *puruṣa śakti*.

This divine union of *prakṛti* or *kuṇḍalinī* and *puruṣa* via the *cakra* is the aim and the end of *aṣṭāṅga yoga*.

V.4. – Does *Yoga Sūtra* mention *kuṇḍalinī*

The divine force of nature *(kuṇḍalinī)* flows without interception once the path is cleansed. Patañjali mentions about *kuṇḍalinī* in the fourth chapter but the word is different: *jātyantara*

	Name of *cakra*	Location in the body	Connection with Physiological system	Endocrine glands coming under control	Control over *Kośa*
1	*mūlādhāra*	above anus – between the anal mouth and the genitals (in the pelvis above anus)	skeleto-muscular, reproductive	testes, ovaries	*annamaya*
2	*svādhisṭhāna*	between genitals and hypo gastric plexus (above the organs of generation)	excretory		*prāṇamaya*
3	*Maṇipuraka*	situated below the navel	gastric, digestive	pancreas/islets of langerhans	*prāṇamaya*
4	*Sūrya*	between navel and diaphragm	gastric, digestive	pancreas/islets of langerhans	*prāṇamaya*
5	*manas*	between diaphragm and heart (between the navel and the heart)	respiratory, circulatory	adrenals	*manōmaya*
6	*anāhata*	heart region	respiratory, circulatory		*manōmaya*
7	*viśuddhi*	above the chest near the throat at the base of the neck	respiratory, organs of speech	thyroid / parathyroid	*vijñānamaya*
8	*ājnā*	between the two eyebrows at the base of the brain	nervous, glandular	pineal /pituitary	*ānandamaya*
9	*soma*	at the base of the brain above the hypothalamus	nervous, glandular	pineal /pituitary	*ānandamaya*
10	*lalāta*	slightly above hypothalamus			*cittamaya*
11	*sahasrāra*	at the uppermost cerebral centre			*ātmamaya*

Table n. 3 –The dominion of the *cakra*

	Name of *cakra*	*Bīja mantra*	Colour	No. of petals	Letters	Presiding deity	Elements	Subtle quality	*Vāyu*	*Upvāyu*	*Saṁ-yama*
1	*mūlādhāra*	*laṁ*	crimson	4	*vaṁ, śaṁ, ṣaṁ saṁ*	*Gaṇapati*	*pṛthvi* (earth)	*gandha* (smell)	*apāna*	*dhanamjaya*	*śarira*
2	*svādhisṭhāna*	*vaṁ*	vermilion	6	*baṁ, bhaṁ, maṁ, yaṁ, raṁ, laṁ*	*Brahmā*	*āp* (water)	*svāda rasa* (taste)	*apāna*	*dhanamjaya*	*indriya*
3	*maṇipūraka*	*raṁ*	dark hue	10	*ḍaṁ, ḍhaṁ, ṇaṁ, taṁ, thaṁ, daṁ, dhaṁ, naṁ, paṁ, phaṁ*	*Viṣṇu*	*tejas* (fire)	*rūpa* (shape)	*samāna*	*kṛkara*	*prāṇa*
4	*Sūrya*		colour of *bhandūka* (deep red) flower			*Viṣṇu*	*tejas* (fire)	*rūpa* (shape)	*samāna*	*kṛkara*	*prāṇa*
5	*manas*					*Viṣṇu*	*tejas* (fire)	*rūpa* (shape)			*manas*
6	*anāhata*	*yaṁ*		12	*kaṁ, khaṁ, gaṁ, ghaṁ, ṅgaṁ, caṁ, chaṁ, jaṁ, jhaṁ, jñaṁ, ṭaṁ, ṭhaṁ*	*Śiva*	*vāyu* (air)	*sparśa* (touch)	skin - *prāṇa*	*devadatta*	*manas*
7	*viśuddhi*	*haṁ*	Smoky purple	16	*aṁ, āṁ, iṁ, īṁ, uṁ, ūṁ, ṛṁ, ṝṁ, riṁ, ṝṁ, eṁ, aiṁ, oṁ, auṁ, aṁ, aḥ*	*Jivātman*	*ākāśa* (ether)	*śabda* (sound)	organ of speech - *udāna*	*kūrma*	*buddhi*
8	*ājnā*	*āuṁ*	White	2	*haṁ, kṣaṁ*	*Ātman*	*ākāśa* (ether)	*śabda* (sound)	ears - *prāṇa*	*devadatta*	*buddhi*
9	*soma*					*Ātman*	*ākāśa* (ether)	*śabda* (sound)	*vyāna*	*nāga*	*buddhi*
10	*lalāṭa*					*Ātman*	*ākāśa* (ether)	*śabda* (sound)			*citta*
11	*sahasrāra*		White with red filaments	1000	Each petal contains all letters	*Paramātman*					*ātmā*

Table n. 4 – *Cakra* and their associated properties

pariṇāmaḥ prakṛtyāpūrāt (IV.2) – the abundant flow of nature's energy brings about transformation in one's birth aiding the process of evolution. *Kuṇḍalinī* is *prakṛti śakti* according to Patañjali. Patañjali guides how one has to make use of this divine force which flows in abundance: *nimittaṁ aprayojakaṁ prakṛtīnāṁ varaṇabhedaḥ tu tataḥ kṣetrikavat* (IV.3) – he gives the analogy of a farmer: As a farmer builds embankments to regulate the flow of water to his fields, the prudent yogi channels the potential flow of this energy and divert it for spiritual development.

Today, everyone claims to practise *Kuṇḍalini Yoga* and claims to have awakened *kuṇḍalinī*. God alone knows whether they understand what they claim. *Kuṇḍalinī* is a divine energy. Divine energy cannot arise if divinity is not built up in the practitioner. It flows in a full-blown yogi and not in others. The yogi has to build dykes at various chambers of the spine for the energy to soak in, so that he may not be drawn again to the actions which create afflictions: *hānam eṣāṁ kleśavat uktam* (*Y.S.*, IV.28) – as a practitioner strives to be free from afflictions, the yogi must handle these latent impressions judiciously to extinguish them. Otherwise he has to struggle like a *sādhaka* to be freed from entanglements.

So let us not cheaply use this word *kuṇḍalinī*. I say this because Svātmārāmā speaks of *kuṇḍalinī* in the third chapter, after speaking on mastery of *āsana*, *prāṇāyāma*, *mudrā* and *bandha*. The effect of arousal of *kuṇḍalinī* is the same as explained in *Vibhūti Pāda* of the *Yoga Sūtra*.

V.5. – Awakening of *kuṇḍalinī*

I do not claim that I can awaken *kuṇḍalinī*, but yoga certainly does. Only arrogant and egoistic yogis may claim that power. *Śakti* means power or energy and *śaktipāt* means dripping of power. This indicates the course of movement of divine power, and *śaktipāt* means the pouring or dropping or passing of that divine energy. We fritter away our energy on enjoyments. If energy used for pleasures is restrained and transformed into spiritual *sādhanā*, it gets united with the Self as light or fire *(tejas)* or lustre of life *(ojas)*. Awakening of this divine energy *(divya śakti)* is *kuṇḍalinī*. Please know that this divine energy gets awakened only by divine grace. And the divine grace is something which one cannot dream of. It comes when the *sādhaka* is ripe in practice and wisdom.

There is no yoga termed as *kuṇḍalinī yoga*, but there is an *Upaniṣad* called *Kuṇḍalinyopaniṣad*. Yoga is yoga. *Haṭhayoga Pradīpikā* and other yoga texts mention the divine power as *kuṇḍalinī śakti* and not as *kuṇḍalinī yoga*.[1] Yoga texts mention the awakening of this divine energy. *Haṭhayoga Pradīpikā* says that one has to put in all efforts to awaken the sleeping or dormant energy (*H.Y.P.*, III,5). The *prakṛti* has to be brought to the realm of the soul. In reality, only true saints have their *kuṇḍalinī* awakened by divine grace.

In *Yoga Sūtra* IV.2, Patañjali terms this energy as *prakṛti śakti: jātyantara pariṇāmaḥ prakṛtyāpūrāt* – the abundant flow of nature's energy brings about a transformation in one's birth, aiding the process of evolution.

Please understand that *kuṇḍalinī* is a power of pure intelligence. If one has got that pure power, know that the divine grace has dawned on him. I see that those who claim that their *kuṇḍalinī* has been aroused do not reflect that *ojas* or lustre of life. They are emotional, whimsical and impulsive, yet they claim that their divine power has awakened in them. The only thing I can say for them is, may God bless them.

These days, many who follow the path of *kuṇḍalinī yoga* pretend that their *kuṇḍalinī* has awakened. Though these people are victims of emotional conditions claim that they can heal and cure diseases through their power. Is this divine energy that is awakened by divine grace meant to solve ordinary problems like diabetes, depression and so forth? Often, those whose bodies, mind and intelligence are not ready dabble with this *śakti* and pay the price in the form of body ailments or mental imbalances.

One may hypnotise people with words. I don't use the words to convince anyone. I am a man of action. My action is my proof. What I do and what I have achieved through my *sādhanā* are there as proof for all to see. The fact is that one does not want one's ego to get hurt. My process of imparting this knowledge is to develop one's human quality. As a teacher, I am close to all my students and I commune with all. If I sit on the dais and if members are far from me, then where is the communion between me and them? I can talk sweetly for hours and leave them to their fate. If I go on talking with flowery language on yoga, I may be called at best a good speaker. During lecture or discourse the question of ego does not arise, because we are at a distance. Talks are make-believe words, and therefore, they trick one.

People who come to me and also go to other teachers say that their *guru* remains in silence *(mauna)* and never loses their temper. How is the silence of a *guru* going to help them? Have we to think that his silence is a grace on us?

---

1 *Saśailavanadhatrīṇāṁ yathādhāro'hināyakaḥ* I
sarveṣāṁ yogatantrāṇāṁ tathādhāro hi kuṇḍalinī II (*H.Y.P.*, III.1)
Just as Ananta, the Lord of Serpents, is the support of the Earth with its mountains and forests, the *kuṇḍalinī*, verily, is the support of all the yoga practices .

Many of you have seen me correcting those who do not understand or make mistakes. How I jump on them to correct them repeatedly. By going to several *guru,* neither understanding comes, nor gain maturity in practice. One has to stick to one teacher or *guru* and get the best from him. By that time the discriminative power may dawn in him to judge whether he has to find another *guru* for his progress. Until one finds that he has got everything from his first *guru* there is no need to search for another. When one has acquired all knowledge from his first *guru* then he can decide and judge whether or not to go in search of a new *guru.* A *guru* patting one and blessing him that the grace of God will dawn in him will be mistaken compassion. When one has not climbed even the first step of yoga, how can he claim to have reached the highest level? When I teach I always give my pupils one plus. I always guide and lead my students to get something better out of my help.

Many who go to *kuṇḍalinī guru* come to me also with their physical and mental problems. I sweat to improve their health, but they say that they are improving on account of the grace of their *guru.* They come with their problems, I work and relieve their sufferings and someone else gets the credit! I do not play with such tricks. My approach is direct and subjective. Whatever secrets I get in my *sādhanā,* I share with all, with an open mind.

As it is possible to compare the intelligence of one by coming in contact with the other, so it is on *kuṇḍalinī śakti.* One whose *kuṇḍalinī* has awakened only can tell whether that power is awakened or not. Self-proclamation is ego *(ahaṁkāra) śakti* and not divine *(divya) śakti.*

Yoga is not a soft subject to be taught with soft words. Here sweet words have no value. Teaching yoga with soft words is like feeding a diabetic patient with sweets. By giving sweets, he does not give life to that person. On the contrary he is shortening his life span. Similarly, talking sweet words and saying that the *kuṇḍalinī* is awakened is like playing with life.

Let one not take advantage of innocence and the ignorant minds of the people.

Remember, yoga is meant to purify the intelligence for enlightenment. For that to be achieved one has to work himself. Patañjali only says that the grace falls on one who is a *tīvra saṁvegin,* one who is vehemently enthusiastic, supremely energetic and pure at heart. The goal of emancipation blooms in him at once.

V.6. – Is a humming sound in the ears, a sign of awakened *kuṇḍalinī*

Do not mistake the sound in the ear as a sign of awakened *kuṇḍalinī*. Ears and eyes are sensitive organs of the brain and mind. The sound in the ears may be due to weakness, hypersensitivity, perforation or injury.

However, if there is no internal injury or severe blockage of the sinus, then *ṣaṇmukhī mudrā* will be of great help. So, one should not come to the conclusion that his *kuṇḍalinī* has awakened or show anxiety about it. Inverted *āsana* minimise or stop the humming sounds. Only one has to learn from a proficient teacher the ways of placing ears in *Śīrṣāsana*, *Sarvāṅgāsana* and *Halāsana*.

Ambitious *sādhanā* blocks the understanding of reality and leads the *sādhaka* towards ambiguity. Practise with pure innocent mind and with a natural approach. Do not practice with the ambition of awakening the *kuṇḍalinī* and do not dabble in *kuṇḍalinī* until your intelligence is fully matured and emotional stability fully earned.

Let the aim of practice be to surrender the mind to God. Let Him who is the ultimate power consider whether you are a worthy practitioner *(pātra sādhaka)* to grace for this divine power *(kuṇḍalinī)* to rise.

V.7. – Danger of playing with *kuṇḍalinī*

It is true that when the body and the nerves are not strong, any excess effort, whether good or bad, affects the individual.

In chapter four, Patañjali uses the term *prakṛti śakti* (*Y.S.*, IV.2) for *kuṇḍalinī*, but before that he says: *yogāṅgānuṣṭhānāt aśuddhikṣaye jñānadīptiḥ āvivekakhyāteḥ* (*Y.S.*, II.28). First he wants the impurities that exist in the *sādhaka* to be removed through yoga and to earn knowledge and wisdom. The aim of yoga is to experience the divinity that is hidden within. *Tantra* likes to leap straight on the aim whereas *darśana* unfolds and uncovers the truth step by step. This is the difference between *tāntric* texts and *darśana śāstra*, though their aim is the same.

Patañjali explains the effect of *prāṇāyāma* in two *sūtra*, saying that it removes the veil covering the light of understanding and makes the mind fit for *dhāraṇā*. Patañjali explains that *prāṇāyāma* works as a tool leading towards knowledge and wisdom but does not say that *prāṇāyāma* awakens *kuṇḍalinī*.

Patañjali deals with *nāḍī* and *cakra* in the *Vibhūti Pāda*. He deals with the *kūrma nāḍī* that extends from the throat to geneto-excretory organs. He refers to *cakra* naming them differently to that of *tāntric* texts, with identical locations. He uses the term *nābhi cakra* for *maṇipūraka*, *hṛd cakra* for *anāhata*, *kaṇṭhakūpa* for *viṣuddhi*, *prātibhā* for *ājñā* and *mūrdha jyoti* for *sahasrāra*. The *cakra* are the storehouse of filtered vital energy and act as wells to preserve it. They are invisible and intangible chambers. When *prāṇa śakti* is allowed to pass through *suṣumṇā*, a new light on life springs out as *kuṇḍalinī śakti*. If one works, step by step to gain physical, mental and intellectual prowess, then there will be no danger for the *sādhaka* when that divine power arises. Otherwise, it swallows the *sādhaka* as hasty actions disturb his nervous system and mental equilibrium, which may endanger his life.

Let the *sādhaka* get well established in yogic *sādhanā* before jumping to savour the essence of *kuṇḍalinī śakti* when that *śakti* graces.

When *kuṇḍalinī śakti* ascends from its dormant place and moves towards *sahasrāra* he, the yogi, becomes a *Virāṭa Puruṣa*.[1] He shines brilliantly filled with brightness as a King (*Virājamān*) ruling over the root nature (*mūla prakṛti*).

---

[1] As Lord Krishna is called as *Virāṭa Visva Puruṣa*, because he initiates the creation of nature, the yogi becomes a *viraga* or *virata puruṣa* as he rules over *mūla prakṛti* and re-creates himself.

SECTION VI

ON MY PRACTICE

SECTION VI – ON MY PRACTICE

VI.1. – Face frustration in *sādhanā*

Before yoga, I was a frustrated person and that persisted throughout in my *sādhanā*. Probably frustration may come to one and all in one way or the other. Want of determination in the beginning, failure in progression, non-fulfilment and dissatisfaction play on the minds of many practitioners to get dejected. These experiences are all part and parcel of the *sādhanā* in any of the fine arts.

I faced frustration day in and day out and yet, my inner force never allowed me to stop my practice. If I had become a victim of frustration, both my practice and teaching aspects would have remained dreams. In my early days of learning and teaching it remained as a continual frustration. This lasted for years. It may be God's will or destiny that made me build up persistence and perseverance to pursue learning the subject and teaching it. For me progress was very very slow and I was facing stagnation and negativism. Often these dejections and frustrations disturbed me and made me restless. Often I wanted to give up the *sādhanā*. But something inside me was forcing me to face all these and cross the bridge from frustration to exhilaration. This inner voice not only gave me hope but made me to dig and plough the subject to trace the minutest change that was striking me and to accept in my practice or teaching. I was dull, unintelligent and non-cheerful by nature. The moment I could feel a hair-split of progress, I was cheerful in my heart and it was elating me. With all my frustration the willpower in me was not ready to accept failures but to continue with those failures I was under this determined frame of mind to attempt and re-attempt as long as my body and mind could endure. Therefore, I suggest that one has to accept the frustrations and failures as inevitable and find means to overcome them.

If one is caught in frustration, do not say good-bye to the *sādhanā* but have a determined will to accept the failures and continue to find out when they would leave you.

Build up a constructive will like me to come out from the gloomy state that happens in any *sādhanā*.

Learn to analyse the notion of frustration and see you are not caught in that veil. Sharpen the head and heart to overcome frustrations and dejections.

VI.2. – Deeper meaning of practice

When I began yoga I never knew what yoga was. My *Gurujī* was not willing to explain it to me. He only said: "Practise for your health." I took that as a *mantra*. As I was ill from birth, it took me six years of practice to experience health and a sense of well-being. As people started coming to me to learn, it opened my eyes that minimum practice and insufficient presentation would not be enough to teach in order to make them experience the feel of the subject. I began watching and studying my body and mind to look within to observe and reflect on actions and non-actions, and began learning to co-ordinate my study in each *āsana*. When body was not willing, my mind used to force the body to do the *āsana*. Fortunately, people who were coming were intelligent and their queries on yoga opened my eyes and trained my mind to judge and to get the feel of each and every part of my body in each *āsana* while practising.

No doubt, it took me years to make my body and mind move concurrently in *āsana*. After years of uninterrupted practice of *āsana* with physical and intellectual sweat pouring together, I succeeded in making the practice to be lively with the feel of exhilaration and jubilation. As my practice progressed, my intellectual eye began judging the movements of body and mind with each *āsana*. Often my physical eyes failed me but the intellectual eye never let me down. It helped me to perfect the *āsana* with discernment. My dormant state of intelligence started stirring my body and mind to reach the extension and expansion to the fullest possible state. It made me to think of *āsana* as God and I became a devotee of *āsana*. From my observation and attention I was able to eradicate the distorting and contorting movements in my body and illusive thoughts in my mind. Thus, the queries from my earlier students helped me to learn, unlearn and re-learn the *āsana*, which made me to improve my presentation of them. Thanks to my intelligent students in those early days, who lit the lamp of light in me to further my study in my practices.

This correct understanding of the *āsana* made me maintain the natural anatomical structure without contortion or distortion in presentation. I also learnt to keep the broadness of the chest of *Tāḍāsana* in *Śīrṣāsana*, *Sarvāṅgāsana*, *Ardha Matsyendrāsana* and so forth. With these thoughts I worked in all the *āsana* to bring out that natural state of anatomical structure, which made my intelligence to spread and balance evenly along with the extension and expansion of the body.

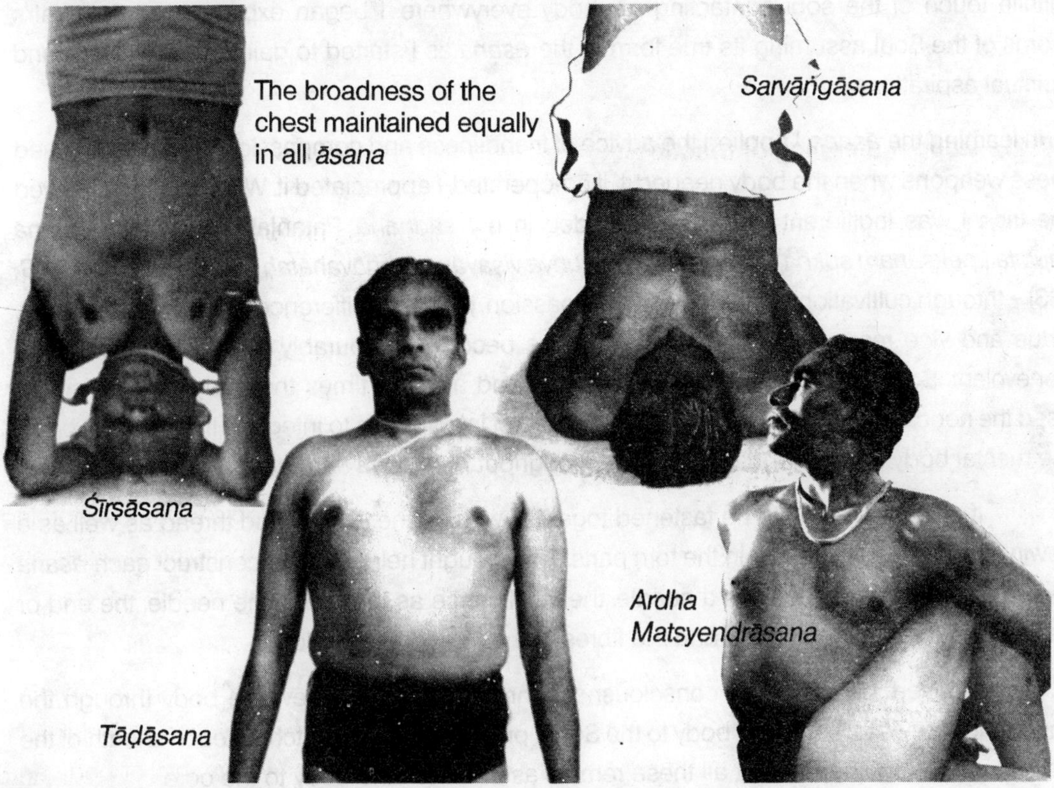

Table n. 22 – Maintaining natural anatomical structure in *āsana*

The idea of the two banks of a river made me think judiciously of the body having two banks. If one bank of the body is the skin, the other bank is the intelligence. I made this river of intelligence from its source point to flow touching evenly the inner surface of the skin. This enabled me to perform the *āsana* to bring the intelligence not only closer to the body, but the conscientiousness also. This conjunction of intelligence and consciousness made me to feel the core with its container – the body. This bringing of intelligence and consciousness in my *āsana* practice later led me to infuse awareness to unite the self and *prāṇa* (energy) within the body. The observation of this vertical intelligence of my head and the horizontal intelligence of my heart helped me to trace the middle line throughout my body from the centre of the head to the centre of the two feet and arms. This brought me to understand what right measured alignment is and what intuition means! This way I learned culturing the body, mind and intelligence. I made the self to feel its flow in my practice.

I am sure, if all of us pay attention to the entire cellular system of our body with total awareness and attention, all will experience what I am saying in their practices. This self-attention in the cells in my practice of *āsana* kept me far away from the body consciousness. I felt the infinite touch of the soul contacting my body everywhere. I began experiencing Patañjali's words of the Soul assuming its true form in the *āsana* as I started to gain spiritual health and spiritual aspirations.

In learning the *āsana*, I applied the advice of friendliness and compassion of Patañjali. I used these weapons when the body needed. If it co-operated, I appreciated it. When the mind played the trick, I was indifferent to it but proceeded in my *sādhanā*. Patañjali says: *maitrī karuṇā muditā upekṣaṇaṁ sukha duḥkha puṇya apuṇya viṣayāṇāṁ bhāvanātaḥ cittaprasādanam* (*Y.S.*, I.33) – through cultivation of friendliness, compassion, joy and indifference to pleasure and pain, virtue and vice respectively, the consciousness becomes favourably disposed, serene and benevolent. Sometimes the mind was rebelling and at other times the body was refusing. I used the needle of consciousness with the thread of intelligence to integrate the physical body, the mental body and the conscious body throughout my *āsana sādhanā*.

If a torn cloth has to be fastened together, we use the needle and thread as well as a sewing machine to stitch to join the torn parts. This thought helped me to construct each *āsana* by using the consciousness as a needle, the intelligence as the eye of the needle, the end or head of the thread as the mind and the fibres of the thread as the cloth.

I moved the needle of consciousness through its eye, to sew the body through the fibres, and sinews to fasten the body to the Soul. I practise as if I am stitching each sheath of the body to come together so that all these remain as one from the body to the core.

This way I got the deeper meaning of each *āsana* and am sure that it is possible for all to reach this state of zenith in each *āsana*.

VI.3. – How to develop the intelligence in *āsana*

Is it possible for anyone to live without a body? Can movements in the body be possible without the involvement of mind and intelligence? As we are psychosomatic beings, both body and mind have to go hand in hand involving all parts of the body, tapping it totally. This is *pramāṇa vṛtti*.

We create divisions and therefore *pramāṇa vṛtti* becomes *viparyaya* or perverse knowledge or *vikalpa* or fanciful knowledge. *Pramāṇa vṛtti* is only possible when filtered attempts prove right through experience.

About my practice (which people call the *Iyengar Method* for the sake of convenience), it has no colours. I use my body as a laboratory and my knowledge and understanding as a means to find out what my practices bring and where they lead me. Each *āsana* has its own character. The understanding dawns as one makes progress in *āsana*. Their quality in the presentation changes as re-adjustments are done with a better knowledge and understanding so they derive an optimum qualitative action with right reflection. If these imprints go on alternating, it means one has not reached that optimum level. If he reaches this state, then it is *pramāṇa vṛtti*.

For example, watch *Tāḍāsana*. One arch extends and the other does not. Either the outer or the inner foot remains firm on the floor while the other may be wobbling. If one head of the metatarsal is in line with the big toe, the other might be sliding without one's knowledge. If these are not attended to, then can one say that he knows *Tāḍāsana?* This intellectual observation and ways of using it for correct presentation is a must in the *āsana*.

Take *Trikoṇāsana* (on the right side). One may be stable on both the legs when the legs are spread apart. The moment one turns the right leg to the right side, the left foot starts "flying" in the air. It may be touching the floor but the firm sensation that was established in the intermediate stage of *Trikoṇāsana* is lost due to want of attention. If one follows the line from the outer side of the big toe up to the groin of the right leg, he can see a distorted line. Secondly one can easily observe the right leg because he can see and perceive it, but to look at the left leg he has to use his mind. If he uses his physical eyes to see, he has to move his head towards the left leg which changes the centre of gravity and the possibility of losing the direction is bound to be there. In each *āsana,* the perceivable eyes help the mind to adjust that side with ease, while on the other side the mind alone has to conceive for adjustment. It requires a qualitative mind. What one perceives, he can directly correct, and for the parts that he cannot see it takes a long time for a right adjustment, as the mind has to travel and penetrate for conception. Here, I want the mind and intelligence to feel the variations in the flow of energy and the touch of intelligence to bring a harmonious feel of sensitivity throughout the body.

All the photographs that one sees in *Light on Yoga* are the architectural icons of a human body.[1] As interior decorations differ from house to house the intelligence creates various icons in architectural shapes for the *sādhaka* in each *āsana* to acquire that ascetic quality that goes with the design.

---

[1] Please see the author's article *Anukrama Sādhanā Śreni,* and plate n. 6, in *Aṣṭadaḷa Yogamālā* vol.3.

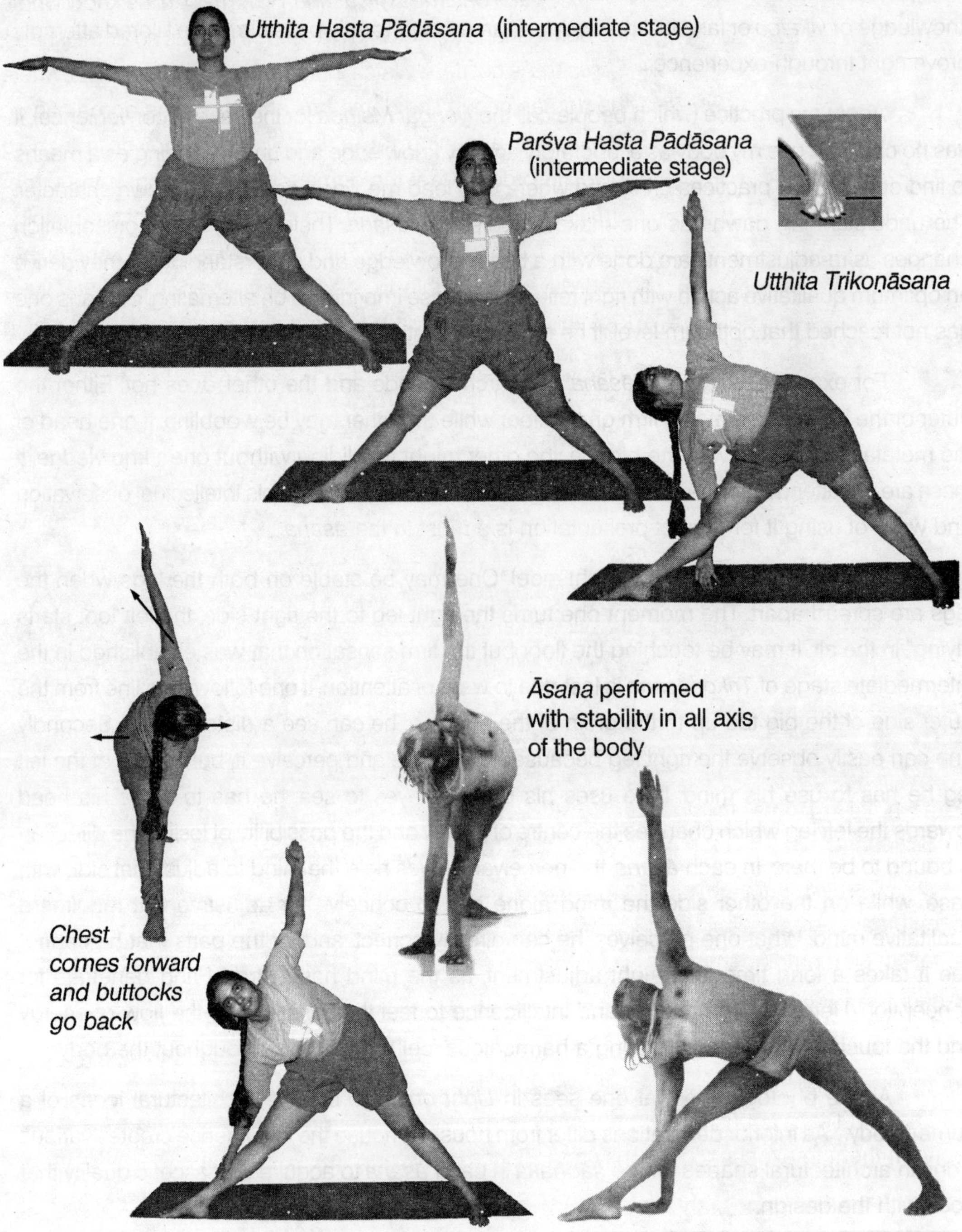

Plate n. 23 – Observation and attention in *Trikoṇāsana*

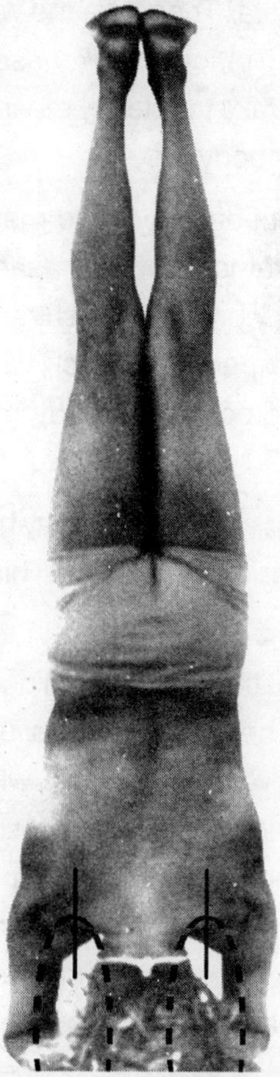

Plate n. 24 – Dome shapes in *Śīrṣāsana*

Take *Sālamba Śīrṣāsana.* How many of us know where the dome shape comes in *Śīrṣāsana*? If there is no dome shape, *Śīrṣāsana* is not right. Watch the upper arms in *Śīrṣāsana,* where the domes occur. The dome has a centre, if the dome has no centre, it is a leaning tower. Let *Śīrṣāsana* not be a leaning tower. In order to feel the dome; divide the flesh in the upper arms and the skin exactly at the middle portion of the deltoids and get a right *Śīrṣāsana.* Then the feeling is as if one is in a meditative state within. In *Śīrṣāsana,* search which parts of the legs are in contact with the mind and intelligence and which parts are not. Then tap the mind and intelligence to bring the energy to flow in these parts to feel the intelligence running in the body as if energy and intelligence are concurrently tracing and touching the inner layer of the skin from the inner body at all levels.

When we do in this way we realise what Patañjali means when he uses; *tato dvandvānabhighātaḥ* (*Y.S.,* II.48). The dualities exist even in our cellular system: fibres, cartilages, and muscles. Often one calf is thin and short while the other is thick or long. We remain insensitive at many points where our intelligence does not flow at all. If we adjust and readjust with discernment it is *kriyā yoga.* This is what Patañjali says on *sādhanā kriyā,* containing *tapas, svādhyāya* and *Īśvarapraṇidhāna.*

Tapas means passion in the art. We have to immerse ourselves in each *āsana* and in each breath. *Svādhyāya* is to study the movements that happen in the practices of *āsana,* and to reflect on them and then to remove those disintegrations that happen, and bring integration. Where the 'I' *(asmitā)* is sanctified and purified. It is *Īśvarapraṇidhāna.*

Āsana work as a principle foundation to sanctify the body, mind and soul. First we have to do the *āsana,* then study the structure to penetrate the body accurately so that we become serene and silent. Let us respect the body and treat it as a temple and *āsana* as prayers and perform them to experience serenity and silence in the practice.

Patañjali says, *pratyakṣa anumāna agamaḥ pramāṇāni.* Direct perception *(pratyakṣa),* logical thinking on doubts *(anumāna)* and to find out from the scriptural texts whether the

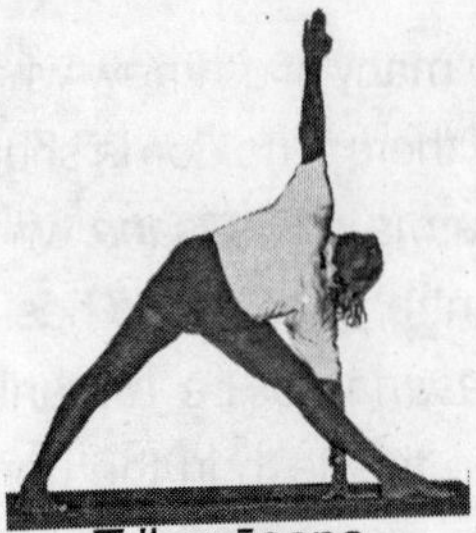

Trikoṇāsana

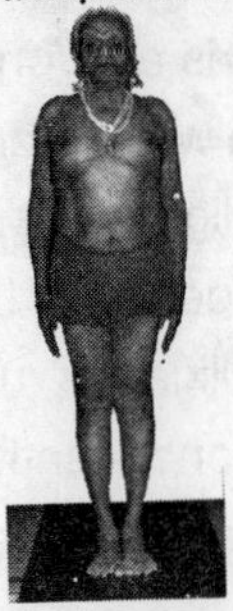

Tāḍāsana

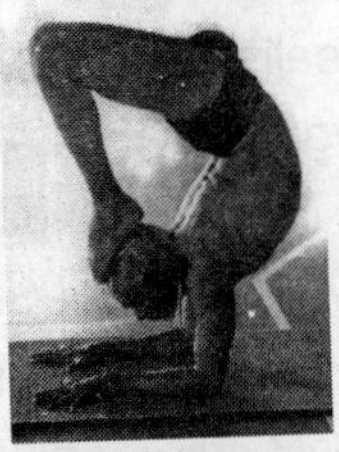

Vṛśchikāsana

Plate n. 25 – Meaning and structure in *āsana*

experiences are correct or wrong *(āgama).* These are the ways of obtaining right knowledge. When I practise *Trikoṇāsana, Tāḍāsana, Vṛśchikāsana* or any *āsana,* I take the literary meaning of each *āsana* and I structure it on my body.

This way each one has to work out ways and means to get that fineness in the architectural icon of that *āsana.* I begin to think and started alternating my practice watching the alternative experiments until the right experience struck, which was nothing but harmony, concord and balance in body, mind and self.

Though many practise *āsana* in a feeble way, they have to mould their bodies and minds for inner growth. This is hierarchy in *āsana.*

The *āsana* are so powerful that they let the intelligence sprout at every place. A beginner when he practises uses muscular strength. The muscles are covered by the skin, which has several layers. Often one uses the motor nerves aggressively to get into the *āsana.* This aggressiveness jams the skin and makes the sensory nerves of the skin insensitive. If one creates room while doing the *āsana* between the sensory nerves of the skin and the fibres of the motor nerves, then the skin receives the action for reflective action. Think and watch carefully whether the sensory nerves of the skin accept that force from flesh.

For example, if a folded letter is inserted into a small envelope, the envelope tears. In *āsana* practice, the skin acts as an envelope of the inner body. If the muscles overpower the skin, the fibres tear. The skin does not tear but the muscles tear because the skin does not give room for expansion. This is another hierarchy where one has to learn how to co-operate and co-ordinate the skin while practising. Here the attention is on the union *(saṁyoga)* of the senses of perception *(jñānendriya)* or the sensory nerves *(jñāna nāḍī)* with the organs of action *(karmendriya)* or the motor nerves *(karmanāḍī).*

Then the next hierarchy is to trace the defects in the presentation of *āsana.* For example take *Śīrṣāsana.* One will be surprised when he looks at the imprint of the head on the blanket. The imprint of the skull on one side of the blanket will be firmer but the other half of the skull's imprint may not be as firm as the other side. So, the architectural icon of the *āsana* has not been worked out by the intelligence.

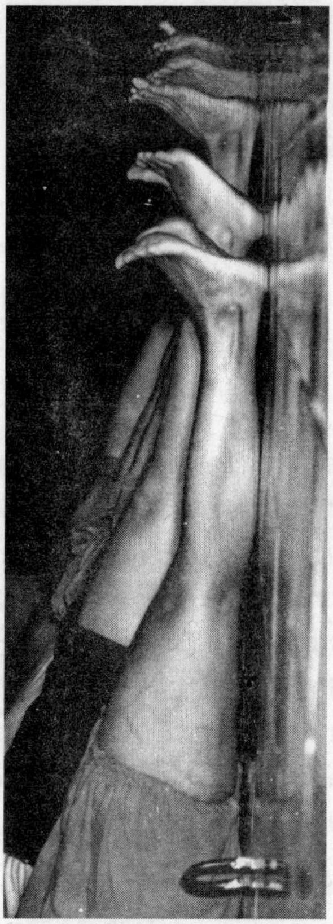

Plate n. 26 - *Pincha Mayūrāsana*

Take *Pincha Mayūrāsana*. When one tries this *āsana* he has to touch the wall with his heels. Before that he should know where to rest the heels on the wall. One will be surprised to know that he never touches the same corresponding back parts of the heels on the wall. He may be balancing but the sensations of the skin should tell him that the motor nerves extend on one leg while they are contracted on the other leg. While doing this *āsana* no one thinks this way, of touching the same spot and same parts as the other side of the body.

In *Paschimottānāsana*, the hinge of one heel remains higher than the other. When bending forward, the energy moves in one leg towards the heel, while in the other it retards from the heel. Sometimes one leg remains straight but the other bends. One has to learn to see these refractions while performing an *āsana*.

When such defects *(doṣa)*, are dissolved, one has perfected the *āsana*.

Āsana should make one like a live wire. The intelligence should be the wire. The energy should be moving in the body like the electric current. And that's the right and intelligent presentation of the *āsana*.

I observe in my practice the differences between the skin and the flesh, between the bone and the flesh, movement of energy, intellectual function and spreading the self throughout my body which makes the presentation completely different to others. What I have maintained

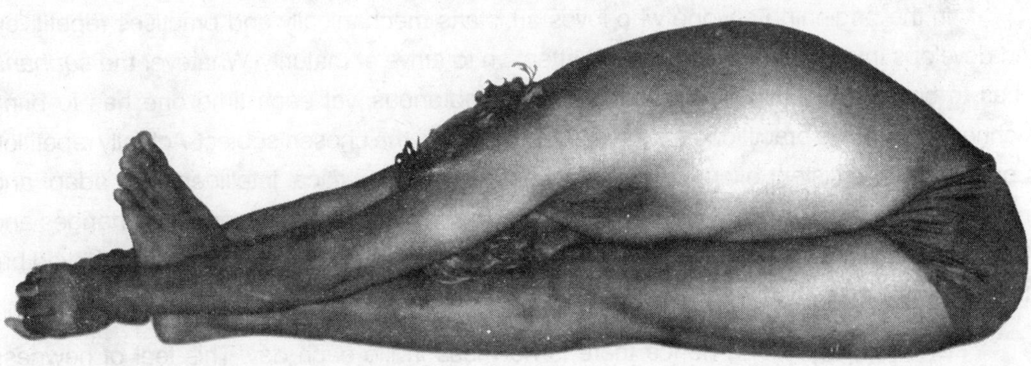

Plate n. 27 - *Paschimottānāsana*

is what others lack in their *sādhanā*. If they attend to what I have said in their practices, their *sādhanā* may not appear different to mine.

That is *āsana jaya*. Till then one should know that one has not learnt the *āsana*.

VI.4. – Is my way of yoga different

Yogic principles of my way of presentation and the methods of others may differ in their adaptation but yoga is the same. As the trunk is one but the branches are many, yoga is one but growth in adaptations may vary. Whatever the style may be, the idea of transformation remains the same. My way of practice is not different from others' except the measured alignment of the motor nerves with the sensory nerves without distortion even in the minutest part of the anatomical structure of the human body. For this one needs intellectual reflection and skilfull adjustment in the presentation of the *asana*. Here the bones, joints, muscles fibres, energy, mind and intelligence are made to function and act concurrently with balance, concord and harmony for the life force to touch and feel all the layers of the self without any division or deviation.

Measured alignment leads to precision and precision is a divine state where one experiences the cosmic force uniting with the individual force. For me, precision is the meeting point of the individual soul with the Universal Soul.

It should never be a mechanical process but it does require repetition with innovative ideas for progressive presentation of each *āsana* as it should be. One should know that all these aspects exist in the practice of all arts.

In the beginning anyone who loves art, starts mechanically and practises repetitively and develops intellectual sharpness and attention to arrive at maturity. Whatever the *sādhanā*, it has to be repetitive. No doubt repetition is monotonous, yet each time one has to bring freshness so that the practitioner does not lose interest in the chosen subject. Actually repetition is nothing but persistent effort. From these one builds up a critical intelligence to adapt and change as new ideas strike. When such subtle adjustments are introduced, new changes and alterations may strike till the trials come to an end. Then not only precise *āsana* is achieved but true creativity also sets in.

Life is dynamic and hence there is newness in life each day. This feel of newness makes one explore and monitor for innovation. The innovation and renovation act as springboard for creation. I created newness this way in my *sādhanā*. This gave space and vastness to my intelligence to explore the unreachable areas of the interior parts of the body to discover and re-model my practices. Such repeated practices alone created conditions for my intelligence to awaken the sense of creativity, freshness and newness that attracted many members from all over the world in millions to take this method of practice.

VI.5. - *Prāṇāyāma* and *dhyāna* in *āsana*

By reading the *Yoga Sūtras* of Patañjali, one may get clarity on this matter. In the second chapter Patañjali describes for beginners the first five limbs of yoga. He postulates a definite step between *āsana* and *prāṇāyāma*. Unless one has mastered the *āsana,* one cannot take up the practice of *prāṇāyāma*.

These days' people jump to *prāṇāyāma* and meditation whereas Patañjali explains that one of the effects of *prāṇāyāma* is that it trains the mind for *dhāraṇā* (concentration). Here he postulates the step for *dhāraṇā*.

One has to discipline and build up energy through *āsana* before thinking of *prāṇāyāma* or *dhyāna*. First the outer mind must be cleansed. A child going to primary school cannot straight away attend to college studies. One has to wait until maturity develops. A woman cannot deliver when she has not yet conceived. It is the same with meditation *(dhyāna)*.

Those who like to jump to *prāṇāyāma* or *dhyāna* are not keen students but fascinated students of yoga. Keenness and fascination as well as desire and aspiration do not mean the same. Fascination is like instant food while keenness is to dig into the subject. Fascination is like outer make-up or a varnish that soon vanishes. Keenness is an inner beauty, which can never fade. Desire is pleasure-seeking. It is the same for some as a kind of pleasure-seeking to jump to *prāṇāyāma* or *dhyāna;* whereas aspiration is the inner urge of the self to reach the height of the Soul.

Meditation is not just "sit quiet and be calm", but needs single uninterrupted attention *(ekatānatā)*.

Follow and practice the early preparations indicated by Patañjali from *yama* to *pratyāhāra*. Then *dhāraṇā* and *dhyāna* happens.

SECTION VII

THE PRACTICAL PSYCHOLOGY OF YOGA

SECTION VII
THE PRACTICAL PSYCHOLOGY OF YOGA

VII.1. – Is yoga pessimistic

Patañjali's yoga is not pessimistic but totally optimistic. One should not come to the conclusion that the world is sorrowful by reading his explanation about the causes of afflictions. He says that the mother of suffering is want of knowledge, as well as illusive, delusive and perverted understanding. He read the state of the mind of the people and concluded that most of us are caught in afflictions in one way or the other. But he guides us how to minimise them and build strength to endure them. After explaining the causes of affliction does he not explain the ways of conquering them? When his words of causation and conquering are so clear how can it become a pessimistic philosophy? He has not denied the world. He accepts and respects *mūlaprakṛti* – the primordial matter, as well as man's desires *(vāsanā),* which cause sorrow in him.

Patañjali explains that a practitioner of yoga has to think and cross over from the bridge of sorrow towards emancipation and bliss. As each black cloud has a silver lining, Patañjali in II.15 says that a wise man recognises this hidden tinge of sorrow in pleasures and learns to eradicate them and remain non-attached. He finds that pain is hidden in pleasure and pleasure in pain, and he does not like anyone to succumb to them. Hence he has used the word 'wise man' *(vivekin).* The wise man's conscience is stainless and hence he keeps away from temptations. He enunciates wisdom as: *ṛtaṁbharā tatra prajñā* I.48 – it means a state of seasoned intelligence or mature wisdom accompanied with insight. As we have not reached that level of matured wisdom, he suggests *aṣṭāṅga yoga sādhanā* for us.

See Patañjali's description of a wise man: *pariṇāma tāpa saṁskāra duḥkaiḥ guṇavṛtti virodhāt ca duḥkham eva sarvaṁ vivekinaḥ* II.15 – the wise man is he who keeps aloof from the qualities of nature and subliminal impressions, tinged with pleasant and sorrowful experiences. Is this not a high quality of a discriminative intelligence? Again Patañjali says that the conjunction of the seer with the seen is the cause of sorrow: *draṣṭṛdṛśyayoḥ saṁyogaḥ heyahetuḥ* (*Y.S.,* II.17) – the cause of pain is the association or identification of the seer *(ātmā)* with the seen *(prakṛti)* and the remedy lies in their dissociation.

We are caught in this cycle. Hence, he clarifies that the conjunction between the seer and the seen is meant to discover that which keeps one free from sorrows. *Sva svāmi śaktyoḥ svarūpopalabdhi hetuḥ saṁyogaḥ* II.23 – this conjunction of the seer with the seen is for the seer to discover his own true nature. Is it not for us to think and find out how we can reach this state of living with an untainted life?

VII.2. – On doubt and deliberation

The faculty of doubt is to be considered as God's gift to gain clarity. Doubt comes on account of want of knowledge and understanding. When doubt vanishes, understanding comes.

Patañjali, in the list of the obstacles, mentions doubt (*saṁśaya)* as one (*Y.S.,* I.30) and he uses the word *vitarka* for clarifying the doubts. Analytical thinking is the gateway to clear doubts. Analysis is meant for judicious thinking. If the intellect does not solve the doubts, then who else can solve them?

Doubt is an essential quality of intellect. Through doubts, one begins to consider pros and cons of each problem and come to a determined state of clarity. The philosopher Descartes proved one's very existence by saying, "I think; so I am". "I doubt, so I am". Doubt gives room to think and makes the intelligence to discriminate to develop sensitivity.

If we have no doubts, then we become heedless, and we think we are right. Patañjali classifies *vikalpa* as a *vṛtti.* Fanciful thinking can misguide, creating doubt. His idea is to churn the intelligence by doubt to verify the fact.

If doubt is taken as a shield, it refines the intellect of the head as well as the intelligence of the heart. For example, if we are doing *Vīrāsana*, the simplest of *āsana*, one leg shows that it has done well and the other leg does not feel the same. How many of us turn our heads to the right or to the left to see how the toes of right and left foot face and adjust? Why not question how it tilts? We may adjust the toes straight at the back. But we do not care to see if the inner edges of the toes of both the feet touch the floor or not, and the heads of both the metatarsals touch evenly or not. The moment we look and feel the difference, doubt compels us to think, respond and act to get clarification. If we do not look at the feet and think we are perfect in the *āsana,* who has to be blamed? When we see and do not adjust for correction, then we have no intelligence to discriminate. "Not-seeing" brings doubt, and seeing and not adjusting becomes carelessness.

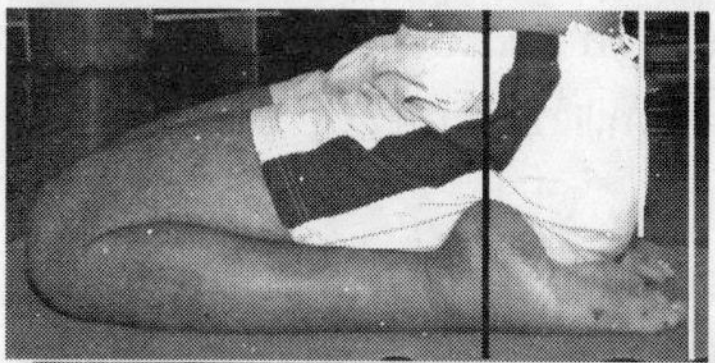

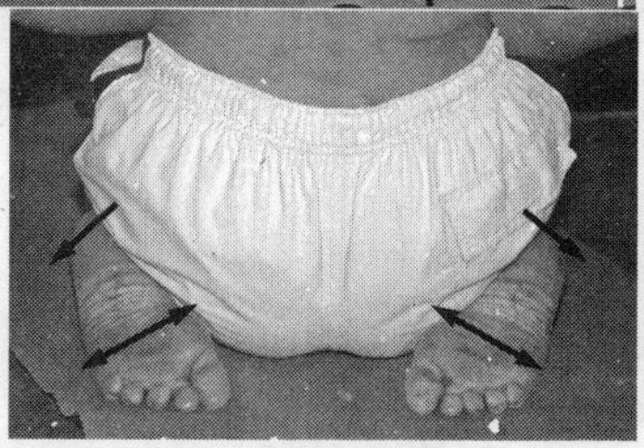

The inner edges of the feet are lifting up and are losing their length (left)

Seeing for clarification and adjustment (right)

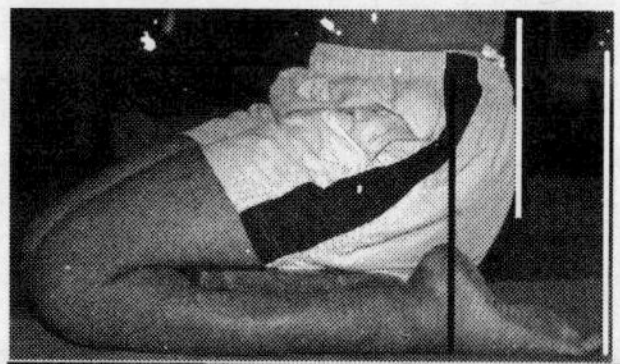

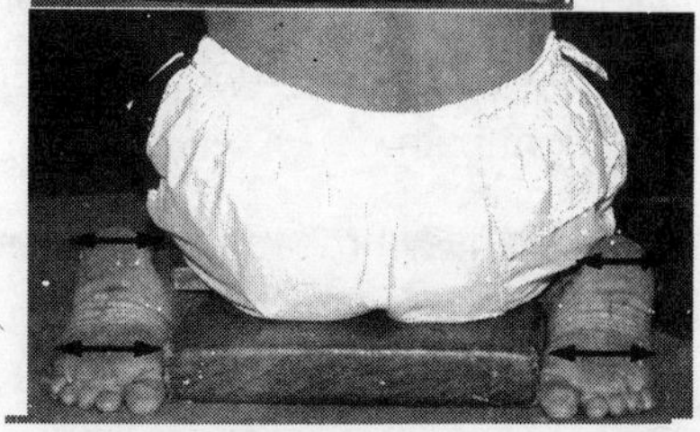

Plate n. 28 – *Vīrāsana*

Take *Pārśva Halāsana.* Though we move both the legs to the right side, how many of us observe the intelligence on both legs? Does the energy flow equally on both the legs? The right leg remains erect whereas the left leg dips to the side, or it may be vice-versa. We don't even know, though we stay in the *āsana,* which leg is acting and which is stagnating. We have to use the intellect and intelligence as a weapon and sharpen them.

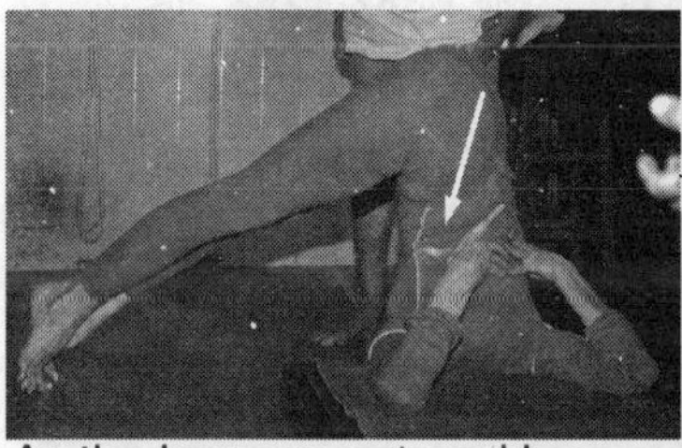

As the legs are not working evenly the hips are tilting to the right.....

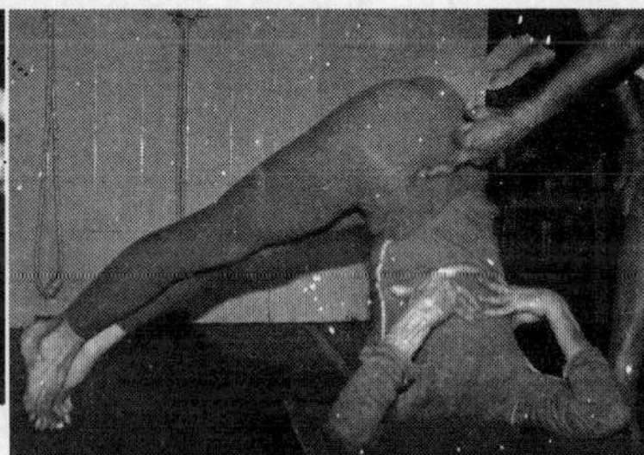

.... guidance is given .... so that the practitioner may ...

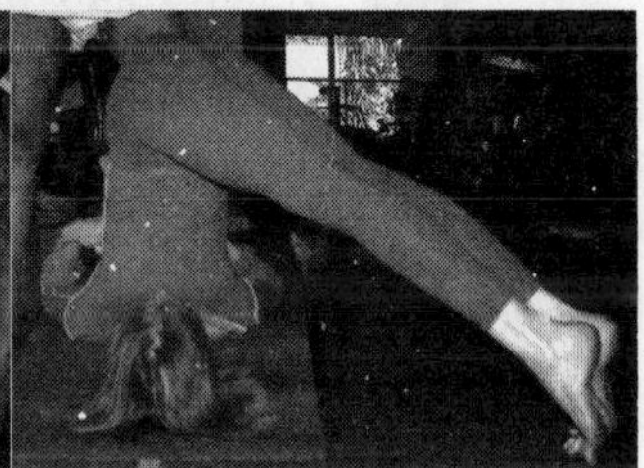

... use her intelligence to levelise the legs, hips and feet.

Plate n. 29 – *Pārśva Halāsana*

If the light is less we don't see properly, but in bright light we see clearly. Let us use our head and heart in unison in action. Clarity brings maturity. When the maturity sets in, knowledge gets well established.

Lord Krishna says that thousands among men strive for realisation and only one among thousands touches the essence:

Manuśyāṇām sahasreṣu kaścid yatati siddhaye I
Yatatām api siddhānāṁ kaścin māṁ vetti tattvataḥ II (*B.G.*, VII.3).

Among thousands of men scarcely one strives for perfection and of those who strive and succeed, scarcely one knows Me. This is the truth. I would say millions may be honest and pursue their practices without realising the perfection of the *āsana.*

There is great meaning when Patañjali mentions *pratipakṣabhāvana.* He says: *vitarkabādhane pratipakṣabhāvanam* (*Y.S.*, II.33) – when we are uncertain; when we have doubt, when we don't know what is right and what is wrong, he advises to weigh the doubts to tread on the right path.

Saṁśaya means doubt, but its right meaning is the oscillation of mind between two alternatives. *Saṁśaya* or indecision is the observation touching both ends of the question: It might be this or it might be that, we cannot decide (Vyāsa under I.30). Lord Krishna says in the fourth chapter of *Bhagavad Gītā* that with faith man obtains knowledge, and the ignorant remains unfaithful. The one having doubt is a *saṁśayātman.* He definitely perishes:

Śraddhāvāna labhate jñānam tatparaḥ samyatendriyaḥ I
Jñānam labdhvā parām śāntim acireṇādhigacchati II
Ajñascāśraddhadhānasca samśayātmā vinaśyati I
Nayam lokosti na paro na sukham saṁśayātmanaḥ II (*B.G.*, IV.39-40).

The man who is full of faith, who is devoted to it and who has subdued the senses obtains knowledge and, having obtained knowledge, goes to the supreme peace. The ignorant, the faithless, the doubting one goes to destruction. For him, there is neither this world nor the other, nor happiness nor doubting. Doubt is for our own benefit. It makes us churn *buddhi* so that we move from the doubtful mind towards a clear mind. This clear mind is the intuitive mind or the mind of the self. Patañjali advises us to trust God and meditate on God, so that the obstacles are removed: *tataḥ pratyakcetana adhigamaḥ api antarāya abhāvaḥ ca* (*Y.S.*, I.29) – meditation on God with the repetition of *āuṁ* removes obstacles to the mastery of the inner self. He also advises: *ekatattvābhyāsa: tatpratiṣedhārtham ekatattva abhyāsaḥ* (*Y.S.*, I.32) – adherence to the practice with single-minded effort to eradicate doubts. *Upaniṣad* say : *Neti Neti* – Not this, Not that. This indefinite answer is a test whether one gets satisfied with the achievement and stops acting further. *Neti Neti* is to do the *sādhanā* uninterruptedly so that we may not be caught in doubts but go deep into them to obtain clarity.

Patañjali uses doubt in the context of obstacles such as indecision, whereas deliberation is a must for cleansing intelligence. Indecision is destructive doubt and deliberation is constructive doubt.

Tasmād ajñānasambhutaṁ hṛtsthaṁ jñānāsināt manaḥ I

Chittvainaṁ saṁśayaṁ yogam ātiṣṭho'ttiṣṭha bhārata II (B.G., IV.42)

Therefore having cut asunder with the sword of wisdom this doubt in the heart that is born of ignorance, resort to yoga and so stand up, O Bhārata.

VII.3. – Can we practise with a diverse mind

Mind's character is diversion. Yoga is meant to stop this diversification of the mind. Yoga helps to restrain the modifications that do not allow the seer to remain as seer, but as a seeker *(Y.S.,* I.2 & 4). The first effect of *āsana,* by its regular practice is to get rid of, or to get healed of the chronic diseases that are incurable by medication. Only one has to structure the *āsana* according to one's capacity and they have to be done regularly. It builds up will-power and makes one live with a serene mind.

As one benefits from yoga in terms of physical balance *(śārīrika santulana),* physiological balance *(aindriyika santulana),* mental balance *(mānasika santulana),* intellectual balance *(bauddhika santulana)* and the balance of the soul *(ātmika santulana),* it can be practised even when the mind moves in varied thoughts as its aim is to still the mind.

Here, I will give an example. Sir Yehudi Menuhin realised the importance of yoga in violin playing and after the end of a session he told me: "Sir, earlier I knew what to play on the violin, after practising yoga I learnt how to play on the violin." This helped Menuhin to use his fingers and nerves with the required pressure to play violin with ease and effortlessness in a natural way. With yogic technique he enlivened music and reached perfection *(siddhi)* on his chosen path.

There are several causes for distractions and disturbances in the mind. It is not possible to pinpoint only one. In the third *sūtra* of the second chapter Patañjali describes the causes for emotional and intellectual disturbances as well as instinctive fears due to want of spiritual understanding *(avidyā),* intellectual intoxication *(asmitā),* attachment *(rāga),* aversion *(dveṣa)* and clinging to life *(abhiniveśa).* The disturbances on mind depend on lust, desire, anger, greed, infatuation, pride, jealousy or hatred. We want to be happy but if we fail in that search for happiness, then aversion *(dveṣa)* along with malice and sorrow sets in.

Patañjali says that want of spiritual understanding *(avidyā)*, is the mother of emotional, intellectual or instinctive disturbances. The mind hankers after certain objects and when these desires are not fulfilled, it diversifies, disturbs and distresses the mind of man.

Various means or methods are given by Patañjali to quieten the distracted mind and disarrayed body and to gain emotional stability. One is to surrender oneself to the circumstances and accept them, and the other is to find ways to get rid of them. His advice is: (a) surrender to God; (b) control or regularise the movement of the breath; (c) study the oscillations that go on in the mind; (d) take examples of people who have displayed tremendous forbearance to bear the upheavals of life; (e) be attentive and accept the practice of that which is appealing to one; (f) divert the mind towards a positive approach and stick to that which is appealing; and, (g) follow the principles of *aṣṭāṅga yoga*.

We are made up of three natural qualities, which move like the potter's wheel. These are luminosity, vibrancy and inertia *(sattva, rajas* and *tamas)*. As each individual is caught with the qualities of nature, he has to understand them to subdue them. For this he has to get intellectual clarity and emotional stability and channel his energy with will-power. As he progresses in both of them, he realises that life and death are two sides of the same coin and he stops worrying about wants, dissatisfactions, non-fulfilment of desires, delusions, fear, fickleness, shakiness, uneasiness and depression.

In certain *āsana*, like in *Dvi Pāda Viparitā Daṇḍāsana* and *Setu Bandha Sarvāṅgāsana*, the mind is uplifted and fed with copious energy. There are also *āsana* like backward extensions where the mind is brought to get connected to the body with energy to think positively. For

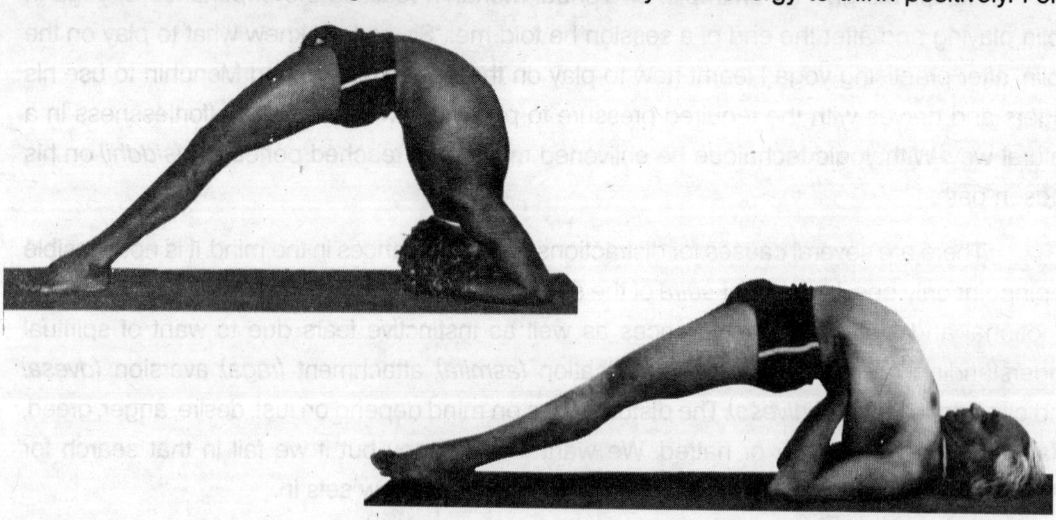

Plate n. 30 – *Dvi Pāda Viparitā Daṇḍāsana* and *Setu Bandha Sarvāṅgāsana*

instance, *Ūrdhva Dhanurāsana, Kapotāsana* or *Vṛśchikāsana* stimulate the front brain with energy to face emotional disturbances.

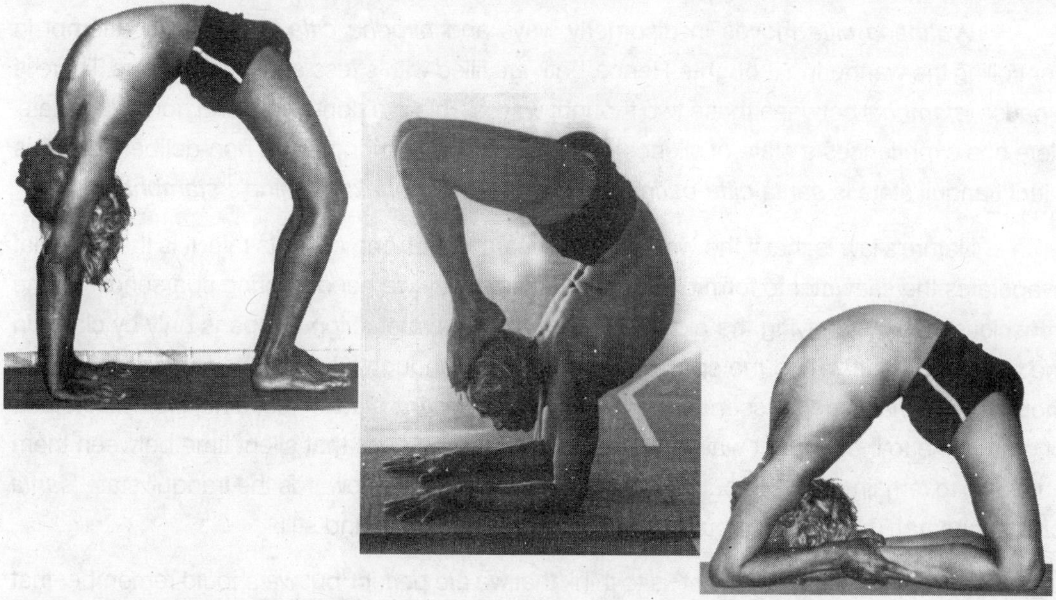

Plate n. 31 - *Ūrdhva Dhanurāsana, Kapotāsana* and *Vṛśchikāsana*

Ujjāyī prāṇāyāma also charges energy with short retentions after each inhalation. *Viloma prāṇāyāma,* where the breath is retained with interrupted inhalations, uplifts the mind with confidence and hope, and builds up stability and not allow the mind to get disturbed and distressed or diversified.

VII.4. - Do *āsana* and *prāṇāyāma* stop thought waves

Yoga is meant to stop mental modifications *(yogaścitta vṛtti nirodhaḥ).* In the third chapter Patañjali explains that *vyutthāna nirodha saṁskārayoḥ abhibhava prādurbhāvau nirodhakṣaṇa cittānvayaḥ nirodha pariṇāmaḥ* (*Y.S.,* III.9) - when the *sādhaka* loses attention, he has to return towards the restraint of consciousness *(nirodha pariṇāma).* When sharpness of attention diminishes and subliminal impressions surface emerging imprints rise *(vyutthāna saṁskāra).* Watching these and learning to check them is restraint.

Though Patañjali had spoken in the earlier chapter about the restraint on *citta,* he explains in the third chapter what *vyutthāna citta* is, and the ways to restrain it.

Vyutthāna citta moves in disorderly ways and *nirodha citta* is a forceful attempt in controlling the wandering thoughts. Hence, both are filled with stress and strain factors. There is a pause (*stambha*) between these two thought waves. This is a non-stress and non-strain state. Here one experiences a state of silence, which occurs unknowingly and non-deliberately. This silent tranquil state is *śanta citta pariṇāma.* It is *manō-kuṁbhaka* or mind's *stambha vṛtti.*

Nature's law is that if the weather is unbearably hot, one expects rain. It is the heat that evaporates the seawater to form clouds. In the same way we need to bring sparseness to the consciousness by rarefying the clouds of thoughts. This rarefaction happens only by clarity in the head and heart. When the sparseness comes in a thoughtful state, the force of emerging thoughts *(vyutthāna)* gets lessened. This effectively affects the state of restraint *(nirodha).* Instead of giving time to the thought waves to arise or restrain, increase that silent time between them and learn to remain quiet without waves. This is transformation towards the tranquil state *(śanta citta pariṇāma).* This is how thought waves are brought to a stand still.

It is but natural for many of us to think that we are perfect, but we should remember that we are born with defects. The defects are of three types: a) intellectual, b) emotional and c) instinctive. Patañjali calls them afflictions. These afflictions affect the body, mind, intelligence and consciousness.

If ignorance and ego are intellectual defects, pain and pleasure, happiness and sorrow, attachment and aversion are emotional defects. Whereas fear of death, planning life as if one is immortal is an instinctive defect. These defects bind us in the web of sorrow causing fickle-mindedness, indecision, tremor in the body and unrhythmic shallow breaths.

Patañjali gives a list of psychological, psychosomatic, neurological and psychiatric impediments, which have roots in sorrows and afflictions. In one way or the other we get afflicted and affected by them.

Any disease from a simple cold to cancer eclipses both body and mind. Physical and mental laziness, idleness, languor, slowness and dullness affect our physical and mental activities. Doubt, confusion, indecision, non-confidence, carelessness, forgetfulness or heedlessness retards our mental progress. On account of these, one loses self-confidence and quality of action and one suffers from this thinking power as the mind flickers and fluctuates. The dexterity and verbal intelligence is the cause behind such defects. These perplex any thinking person.

How did Arjuna get caught in the web of emotion *(viṣāda yoga)*? He saw his relatives, friends, teachers and elderly ones whom he adored. He was caught in attachments and refused to fight. Lord Krishna had to ignite and awaken Arjuna's intelligence *(buddhi)* by introducing the eternal Soul, the imperishable entity existing in him, to eradicate the emotions, which were hidden in him as instinctive defects. Lord Krishna engaged Arjuna in battle by removing these defects, advising what his duty was. For people like us, Patañjali gave *aṣṭāṅga yoga* as a remedial measure to understand these defects as well as showing ways to come out of them.

One has to give his head and heart to solve such problems and win the battle by practising *āsana* and *prāṇāyāma* as one cannot solve these perplexities by mere thinking. Lord Krishna explained this to Arjuna and finally made him act, and Arjuna had to agree saying, . . . *kariśye vacanam tava* (I shall act according to your word). Here, the *jñāna* led towards *karma*. Krishna advised him to do *jñāna pūrvaka karma* (action with matured intelligence), without thinking of the result by indirectly introducing *bhakti* in him.

When we have to do *āsana* and *prāṇāyāma,* the action has to coordinate with the thought wave and the thought wave has to understand the action so that there is understanding between the mind and the body. Through these two aspects of yoga the communication and communion between the body, mind and intelligence connect the outer body to the inner body and the outer mind to the inner mind and remove imbalances in thinking and acting. This type of act brings union between the factual intelligence of the body with the analytical intelligence of the head.

While practising *āsana* and *prāṇāyāma,* one has to keep in mind that if the root is firm the tree grows healthy and bears flowers and fruits. Practice of yoga should be in such a way that one derives perfect intellectual, emotional and instinctive health, which in turn brings an untainted bliss and makes one feel the sense of auspiciousness.

Body is the abode *(deśa)*. One has to tie a knot between the body and the mind while practising so that the *citta* presents itself *(prajñā śakti),* consistently and constantly in the entire body, feeling the energy *(prāṇa śakti)* spreading from the bottom of the soles to the crown of the head. Then defects in body and mind fade out.

VII.5. – Is it possible to live without ambition, pride or ego

Ambition, pride and ego are commonly understood as aims in life, yet we cannot survive in the world without ambition. They are the keys to activate life. Even children are not free from ambitions. The question is how does one creatively use ambitions without turning them into greed and selfishness into selflessness. The dividing lines between these are very thin, fine and subtle for the mind to distinguish between them. It needs deliberation whether to aspire for wisdom or be caught in ambitions.

Do we not motivate children to drink milk tempting them that it is good for strength? Also do we not motivate them with hopes about their future? In the English language 'ambition' is the only word for all aims. But in *Sanskrit* literature we have words like *āśā, abhilāṣā, ākānkṣā* and *mahatvākānkṣā. Āśā* means hopes; *abhilāṣā* means having the desire for noble aims. *Ākānkṣā* means a wish or desire and *mahatvākānkṣā* means noblest wish or desire. *Āśā* aims at the temporal level whereas *abhilāṣā* aims at a certain spiritual level. *Abhilāṣā* is pure hope. Is it possible to master any art, science or philosophy without *abhilāṣā?* The *mahatvākānkṣā* indicates the greatest and the noblest desire to reach the Self or the *ātman,* wherein the desires *(vāsanā)* are made to evaporate. Desires arise from the knowledge of memory of past perceptions. *Āśā* means a wish, a desire or an expectation. It is like a matchstick to ignite interest as a choice. *Āśā* as hope is pure at the beginning but later gets contaminated with lust and greed, and becomes *ākānkṣā.* When the *ākānkṣā* gets multiplied, desires increase. When the first hope is achieved, one becomes greedy and likes to expect more and more. He becomes selfish in his motives and develops unwanted conceited thoughts. What man needs is *mahatvākānkṣā* – the great, pure, untainted, crystal clear aspiration which leads him towards pure knowledge and wisdom.

Ambition no doubt motivates. Once that ambition or motivation is fulfilled, then my advice would be to proceed and keep the mind open to learn to receive and absorb what comes in presentation. Act without the taint of ambition. The absorption sets in and not ambition. Ambition makes us work within a restricted frame of mind looking for the benefits. If we are caught up in ambitions, they lead us in the long run towards pride and ego bringing sorrow and affliction.

Let us not build castles of ambitions. Let us convert ambition into aspiration towards constructive thoughts for earning new knowledge. Undoubtedly the achievement for us is towards *adhyātma darśana: nirvicāra vaiśāradye adhyātmaprasādaḥ* (*Y.S.,* I.47) – from proficiency in *nirvicāra samāpatti* comes purity. Luminosity *(sattva)* flows undisturbed, kindling the spiritual light of the self.

VII.6. – Intelligence of the brain and brawn

Brain has analytical intelligence, while brawn has factual intelligence.

Intelligence grows in two directions – horizontal or emotional and vertical or intellectual. Intellectual knowledge is essential in order to get success in vocation. This is the vertical growth of intelligence. In order to understand man-to-man, or to understand pleasures and pains, love and attachment, family happiness and contentment, emotional intelligence or horizontal growth of intelligence is essential. Brain works on intellectual intelligence and mind on emotional intelligence. The emotional problems cannot be solved intellectually, but with mature knowledge that comes from the heart, they are solved.

Science has made man's intelligence grow vertically, but without a broad base. See how rural people or villagers are warm, affectionate and embracing, whereas sophisticated city men think of themselves, their survival, their satisfaction, and are careless of their fellow beings. When one looks into the flower, he enjoys the flower and appreciates, from his heart, the Creator's creation, whereas an intellectual looks at the flower from his head and before appreciating it begins to dissect it to know its origin.

Practice of yoga needs both types of intelligence, where the brain is made to descend to the level of the brawn, while the mind is made to look within the brawn. The head gathers knowledge from action, whereas the heart gathers experiences and feelings.

Perceptive knowledge moves more easily outwards than inwards. As one loves to take the fragrance of a flower, has he ever thought of taking the fragrance of a breath or has he any day heard the inner sound or the inner voice of his existence? The feel of the external touch of joy is experienced easily, but to feel the touch of joy in the deeper layers of the being needs yogic practices.

When we are doing *āsana, prāṇāyāma* or *dhyāna,* we have to be aware of every portion of the outer and inner body. Then we are in contact with the self. If we live in a state of non-dual state, we bring the intellect of the head in unison with the intelligence of the heart. We make each cell or fibre of the body as intelligent as we are intelligent in the head and heart. Here the brain and brawn get wedded to each other.

VII.7. – What is a balanced brain

We do not know how the brain mysteriously imprints each experience moment to moment. The reason may be that we live mostly with the past or the future and do not observe the present. The moment we live in the present, the fluctuations of the past or the future do not rise. When we witness the present, there cannot be any other thought. Perhaps at this time it may be possible to know the functions of the brain. A moment is the minutest part of time. We have to learn to witness moments and from there it may be possible to watch the movements of moments to realise what moment is.

The brain is the seat of intellection, ignorance and arrogance. It is the seat of afflictions and fluctuations as well as of thoughts and actions. The brain is the main intellectual organ, which plays a great role in imprinting the experiences of worldly life and spiritual life.

The front of the brain is the conscious brain, which is ever active and aggressive. It thinks logically and projects the future. When it does not respond, it means that it is either clouded with pride or dominated by *avidyā*. When *vidya* rises to the brim, it subjugates the pride and leads one towards clarity and humility. That is why I insist, while teaching, to abandon one's thoughts and to receive the instructions without pre-conditions. Then one is sure to learn better.

In yogic practices, all the four hemispheres of the brain and the four chambers of the heart are brought to a balanced state. This state of development frees one from pleasure and pain. It does not allow past experiences to surface, nor to think of future plans. At this balanced state, what remains is only witnessing and experiencing. This state is known as *samāhita citta*.

I am not a layman to yoga. But being a genuine practitioner of yoga, I observe and witness whatever occurs in the *sādhanā*. Whatever I learn I impart to all.

Patañjali explains four types of *samādhi*, namely *vitarka, vicāra, ānanda* and *asmitā*. Here *asmitā* stands for matured intelligence taking one close to the self.

A balanced state is when the intensity of the afflictions is reduced, and oscillation of consciousness from the past to the future or from the future to the past is arrested, and the present state is witnessed. This is the balanced state of brain in man.

VII.8. – Empowering memory

Memory is an important faculty that stores information, remembers incidents and taps the consciousness for action or reaction. As we all know, the physical body is built upon food. So also, the mental body is structured on memory. Memory is the abode for all imprints to set in *(smṛti saṁskāra)*.

We all know that memory, being one of the modifications of the consciousness, it gets mixed up with other *vṛtti* and *kleśa* as well as desire, anger, greed, anxiety and worry. All these fuel the memory and ruffles it in creating confusion in the consciousness. Practice of yoga cleanses the memory and filters and purifies it to develop maturity. Patañjali uses the word *smṛti pariśuddhi* meaning total purification of memory (*Y.S.*, I.43). Perfect memory helps the consciousness in its journey towards one-pointedness *(ekāgratā)*. The raw memory disturbs the consciousness and doesn't allow it to remain steady and one-pointed.

One should know that it is a skill to improve memory. This is still a necessary tool to remember the words that were read or to express the experience in toto, without colouring it with emotional or intellectual dressing. Truthful practice of yoga transforms the nature of memory to be clear and clean. When memory is clean and pure *(smṛti pariśuddhi)*, mind remains clean and pure, says Patañjali.

Clear memory is dependent upon right perception tallying with the discriminative intelligence *(vivekakhyātiḥ)*. Work, experience and words have to coincide with scriptures as well as from the matured teachers in the chosen field. Pancaśikhācarya[1] says, *ekameva darśanam kyātireva darśanam* – there is only one knowledge; discriminative knowledge *(viveka-khyāti)* and that alone is the knowledge.[2] Forgetfulness or negligence grows weeds and impede the consciousness to acquire ripe memory.

Forgetfulness is the basic fault wherein one perceives and memorises only partially, creating room for confusion. On account of this, he forgets to remember what has to be remembered and stores unwanted thoughts, ideas and events as memory.

For memory, Patañjali says: *tajjapaḥ tadartha bhāvanam* (*Y.S.*, I.28). The reverential repetition of the sacred syllable *āuṁ (praṇava)* with contemplation on its meaning and feeling helps the *sādhaka* to develop right memory. It means that as a student, he has to learn to listen, read with respect and rethink on what he hears and reads so that he develops a right memory, for memory to get ripened.

---

[1] (1st century AD). A great authority on *sāṁkhya darśana* and the third on the lineage of the founders of *sāṁkhya* tradition, after sage Kapilā and Āsuri. Reputed as the author of *Ṣaṣṭhi-tantra,* he is often quoted by Vyāsa.

[2] Quoted in *Vyāsa-bhāṣya,* under I.4.

Parents force their children to study in schools or colleges expecting their children to grow as per their ideas. This acts as a hindrance on the child and the child loses natural interest and memory power. The parents have to lure children with attractive words and not their wishes, which retard the growth and memory. If they are rightly channelled on the studies of their interest, then they improve memory power on their own. Heavy stress on studies causes strain on the nerves, brain and mind, which affects their memory power.

Śīrṣāsana, Adho Mukha Vṛkṣāsana, Adho Mukha Śvānāsana, Ūrdhva Dhanurāsana, Viparīta Daṇḍāsana, Setu Bandha Sarvāṅgāsana, Sarvāṅgāsana, Halāsana and *Viparīta Karaṇī* recharge the battery of memory, and refresh the memory to get back its power. Repeated movements from *Halāsana* to *Paśchimottānāsana* bathes the brain with adequate oxygenated

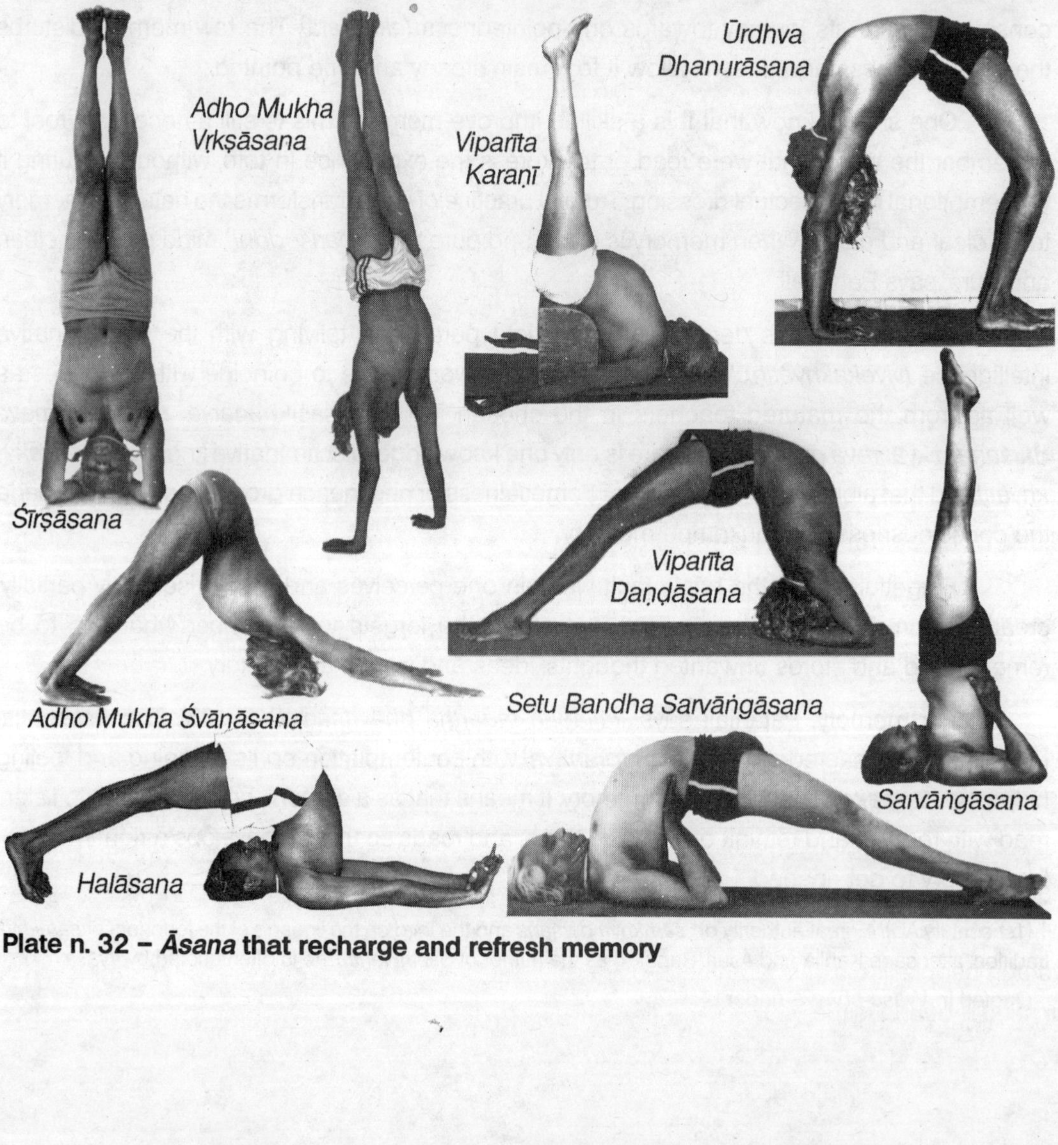

Plate n. 32 – *Āsana* that recharge and refresh memory

blood supply and sharpen the brain and mind to a considerable extent. *Prāṇāyāma* too helps in improving the memory, but when the body, brain and nerves are tired, then one should stick to *āsana* only. They refresh fast. When not tired, *prāṇāyāma* can be tried with short in-breath retentions *(Antara Kuṁbhaka)* for five to ten minutes and not more. It triggers freshness, helps to retain memory power and frees one from the stress factor.

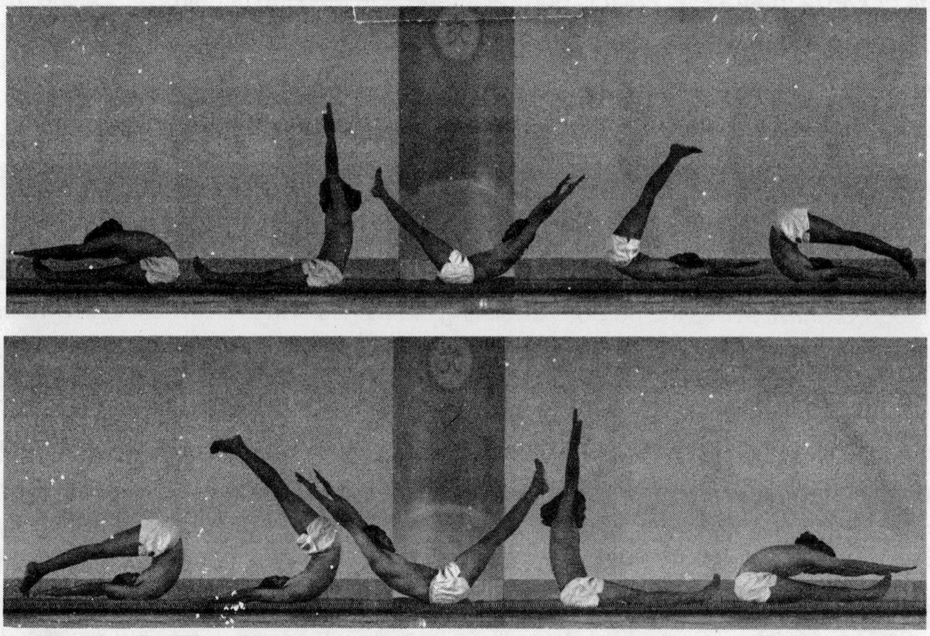

Plate n. 33 – *Paśchimottānāsana, Halāsana, Paśchimottānāsana* bathing the brain

VII.9. – Does culturing the body culture and civilise the mind

This Institute has an outer wall with *āsana* figures on it. Because of these figures, it is identified as the Yoga Institute.

Suppose one sees land without fences, it appears vacant as a vast space. The moment it is fenced, the space gets limited. In the same way, the mind has space. But, as it is fenced by the frame of a body it gets a place with the body as its walls.

If the mind moves, nerves trigger, breath throbs and brain acts as if these were in close relationship within the frame of the body. Often we feel the mind closer to the body than to the self. When the mind goes closer to the self, then that person turns to become a yogi or a saint. Average people like us are bonded in pains, pleasures, attachments and infatuations. As such our mind is bound to the body and body to the mind. When we get a stomach upset or headache, the message goes to the brain and we feel as if the world is falling on us. This means that our mind is suffering more than the stomach or the head. We don't separate our "mind pain" from the stomach upset or headache. The pain is in the stomach or somewhere and not in the mind. Instead of brooding on them, we have to tap the brain to find ways and means to eradicate these afflictions, so that both brain and brawn work in unison to face the facts and find alternative means to get rid of them. Does not this body awareness in the form of pain change the moods of the disturbed mind to act to get rid of pains?

Practice of *āsana* and *prāṇāyāma* makes one understand the factual intelligence of the body and makes the analytical intellect of the brain act rightly. This is *dharma-pariṇāma*. *Dharma-pariṇāma* is the transformation towards the good that is to be held (*Y.S.*, III.13). This is what our yogic practice does.

Fortunately the body, the temple of the self, has all the capacity to reach that state through yoga, so that it serves the purpose of fulfilling the wishes of the self. When such awareness comes, then the mind, moods and behaviour change for higher living and better thinking.

Though *āsana* and *prāṇāyāma* practices appear as a physical science, they definitely constitute a mental science. For example take *Dvi Pāda Viparīta Daṇḍāsana*. Here the brain and mind see inside the body. Is it not interesting to notice how the brain and mind recede inwards? See while in *Paśchimottānāsana* how the mind comes in to contact with the outer body. For melancholic people backbends are taught with eyes wide open so that they charge their energy to tickle the body and the mind. Similarly, hyper tense people find calmness and quietness in the forward bends. In these *āsana*, though the mind is in close contact with the body, they bring calmness in the nervous system.

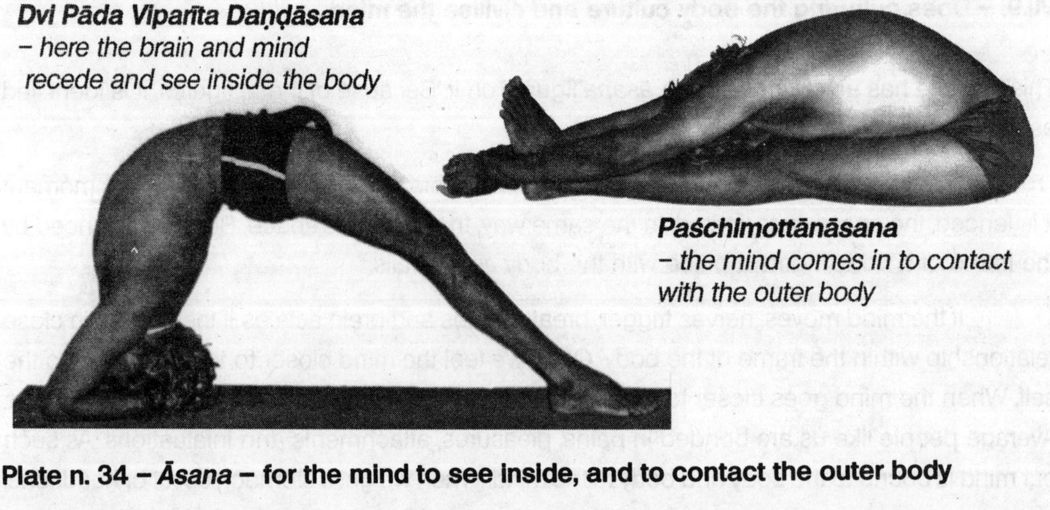

Plate n. 34 – *Āsana* – for the mind to see inside, and to contact the outer body

Supta Kūrmāsana

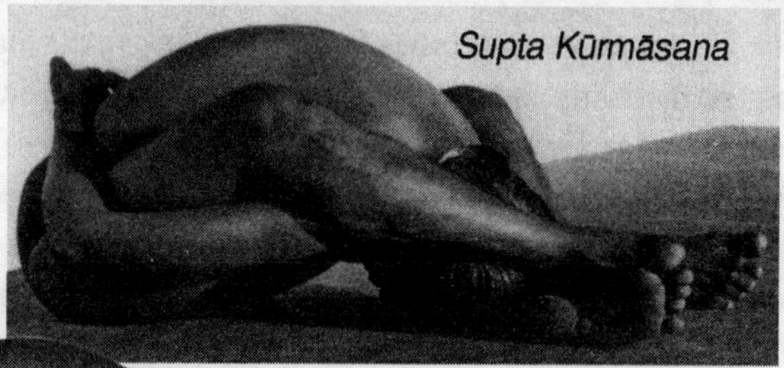

Paśchimottānāsana

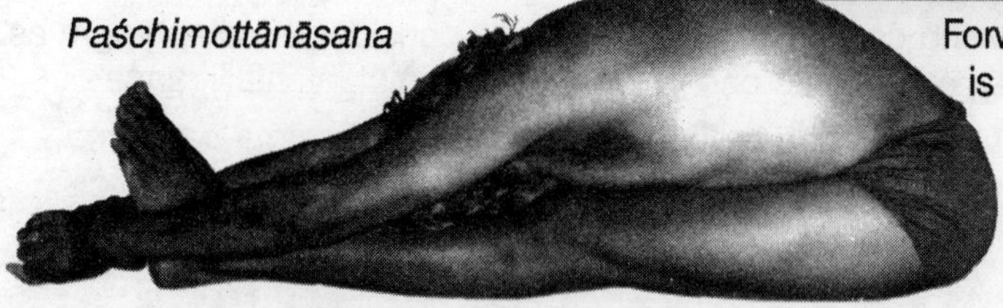

Forward bends – though the mind is in close contact with the body, they bring calmness in the nervous system

Plate n. 35 – Calmness and quietness in forward-bends

This way, if one studies the effects of different *āsana* on the mind, he realises how moods and behavioural patterns can be changed according to the sequential pattern of practices.

In the practise of *āsana* even the five elements *(bhūta)* – *pṛthvi, āp, tej, vāyu* and *ākāśa* – with their subtle counterparts *(tanmātrā)* – *śabda, sparśa, rūpa, rasa* and *gandha* – get affected on biological levels.

In this way if we study the varying states of mind in each *āsana* by penetrating further deep into the body, we realise the interconnection between the various layers of consciousness and learn how the culture of the body influences the mind for it to get cultured well.

VII.10. – The diaphragm is the medium between the body and the Self

No doubt the diaphragm is a muscle, but it has a great bearing on the mind. It is the only muscle that makes one draw in vital energy. When there is fear or sorrow, the diaphragmatic muscle sinks and shrinks making the breathing heavy and emotionally shaky.

Yoga makes one learn to develop elasticity in this muscle. Most of the *āsana* and *prāṇāyāma* help the diaphragmatic muscle to extend and expand, which assists the deep breath to take place.

In olden days people suffered from physical diseases; today we suffer from stress-related diseases. In both the cases the functioning of the diaphragm gets affected. Expressions like "I want to be like that", "I want to be competitive", "Come what may", cause tension in the diaphragm creating stress factors. Although the challenge is from the head, the stress is on the diaphragm. The more the stress one feels, the harder the diaphragm becomes causing cardiac problems, as the door of the mind gets jammed or squeezed. If the diaphragm spreads, it takes the physical, emotional and intellectual loads with comfort. If this muscle gets hardened, fear sets in, in place of confidence, inviting cardiac diseases. Hence, I consider the diaphragm as the medium between the body and the self.

VII.11. – What is the inner body

The inner body is that which covers the single non-oscillating mind, intelligence, consciousness, the 'I' and the self. The outer mind is that which dabbles with the organs of action and senses of perception.

The outer body is made of flesh, muscles, bones and skin. Many of us soon feel these parts of the body while doing *āsana* or *prāṇāyāma*. The peripheral mind being close to the outer body, gets stirred to awareness and awakens the body.

The inner body, which is not easily cognisable, is the lungs, heart, intestines, liver and so forth. The inner body being organic, practice of *āsana* and *prāṇāyāma* helps one feel and recognise the organs and their functioning.

Besides the organic body, this inner body also includes the stable mind, intelligence, consciousness and self. Mind is the bridge between the inner body and the outer body. While practising *āsana* and *prāṇāyāma*, the mind carries all the gathered information to the intelligence during its journey from the outer body towards the self and from the self towards the outer body. Mind being clever and cunning carries the sensitivity of pains to the intelligence but avoids transmitting when in pleasure. Only, it approaches the intelligence *(buddhi)*, for guidance when it is indecisive. Gradually practice makes the mind move closer towards the inner body. Here begins the inner journey for the mind to move closer and closer towards the intelligence for it to illuminate the consciousness for the Self to remain in its absolute state. This is the inner body.

VII.12. – How yoga improves the intelligence

Buddhi or intelligence is not an acquired discriminative knowledge, but experiential wisdom that comes from the filtered right skill of action.

Vyavasāyātmikā buddhirekeha kurunandana I
Bahuśākhā hyanantāśca buddhyao'vyavasāyinām II (B.G., II.41)

Arjuna, the filtered experiential wisdom is one. It does not oscillate, whereas the undecided intellect scatters in many directions, and remains endlessly diverse.

Before understanding this action-oriented intelligence *(buddhi)*, know that memory and mind assume a false identity as intelligence. When memory and mind are in doubt, they remain empty. Intelligence *(buddhi)* judges the information of memory and mind, discriminates by putting them into action again and transforms them into non-changeable experiential knowledge and understanding.

Concerning its development, we have to follow the example of a gardener who removes the weeds first, before sowing the seeds for good crops. We have to remove first the weeds that cloud our body and mind for judicious development of intelligence.

Yogis of lore never discriminated body from mind as they follow each other. They wanted a healthy balance between the brawn, the brain and the mind. Hence, they found out various *āsana* to keep all the sheaths of the body and mind healthy to live in a harmonious way.

VII.13. – Can we feel the effects by a minimum practice

One begins to feel the benefit of yoga even with minimum practice of thirty to forty minutes a day in two weeks' time. At our Institute, we conduct classes with intense attention at a stretch for two hours and the members who attend class once a week feel the effect of yoga for the whole week.

As one begins to practise, one feels elated in one's total well-being. Time bound practice has limitations. Only a beginning has to be made. If one adopts and practises with zeal as part and parcel of life, then the time factor has to be forgotten. Only intensity in *sādhanā* takes one beyond one's expectations.

Secondly, yoga is not meant to live within the frame of the mind but to cross over and go beyond the mind.

VII.14. – The relationship between relaxation and awareness

We have been provided with four hemispheres of the brain, which are biologically explained, Patañjali explains them on an intellectual level as: argumentative centre, synthesis centre, elation centre and conscious centre. Similarly he explains the four biological chambers of the heart at an emotional level as: friendliness, compassion, gladness and non-attachment.

The head cultivates attention while the heart cultivates awareness. Both attention and awareness are the key for good relationships. The practice of relaxation pacifies these chambers of head and heart when one takes to the active part of yoga. They blend these two intelligences to integrate, communicate and commune with each other. This brings pensivity in the heart, which automatically helps to develop attention without tension. This then leads one towards relaxation in attention and awareness, maintaining sharpness in his vocation. This is nothing but alert passivity: alertness in the heart and passivity in the head is the essence of yoga.

VII.15. – The seven states of consciousness and emotions

We have been endowed with seven states of consciousness and as such we should know that we also have such states of health and emotions. Go back to the earlier volumes where I have mentioned that the mind, intelligence and ego are all encased in the abode of consciousness – *citta*.

Suppose in a family, mild skirmishes take place and one gets upset and disturbed. Do we think such upsets are intellectual disturbances or emotional disturbances? Is it not purely emotional disturbance?

The head is the seat of the intellect and the heart is the seat of emotions. The mind expresses itself through the body and the body gets affected and expresses explicitly for the mind to get the feel of it. Here I am deliberately using the word 'mind' for consciousness as it is easy for many to grasp. The mind speaks through emotions and the body expresses them in its own inarticulate language, like the brain thinks and the organ of speech that expresses it.

Emotions like joy, anger, fear, grief, pity, affection and love are expressed through the language of the body. When one is emotionally disturbed, the chest caves in along with the sternum and the brain cells dip, creating mental dullness. This is how the inner emotions affect the body. See, when one is in joy, his chest lifts and expands like a fighting cock, filled with joy in his heart. Here, the mind expresses through the body by its reactions.

Take for example *Sarvāṅgāsana.* Many sink their chest, caving the sternum in. Naturally one has to recharge the back muscles and ribs to move in by lifting the shoulderblades in and shoulders back so that the chest opens and the sternum 'caves' out. This re-adjustment and re-positioning of the trunk in *Sarvāṅgāsana* brings quietness and suspends the emotional thoughts.

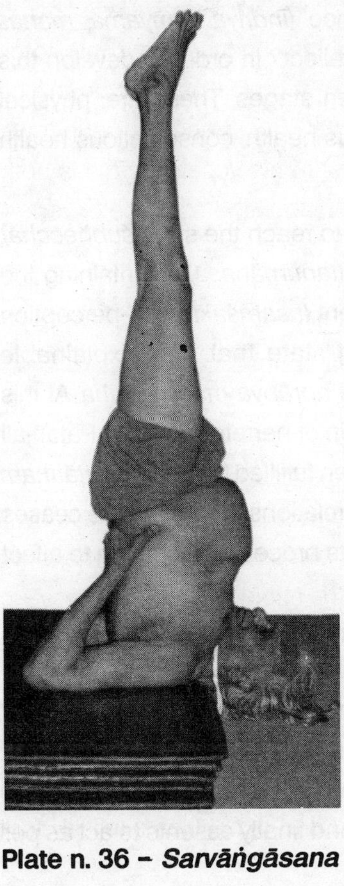

Plate n. 36 – *Sarvāṅgāsana*

Haṭhayoga Pradīpikā says that emotions have a bearing on the nerves and nerves on mind;

Indriyāṇāṁ manōnatho manōnāthastu mārutaḥ |
Mārutasya layo nāthaḥ so layo nādamāśritaḥ ||
(*H.Y.P.*, IV.29)

Mind is the master of senses, and life force (element of air) is the master of the mind. The vibration of life force is felt on the nerves and suspension of vibration (sound) controls and smoothes the nerves, which affects the mind. Hence the nerves are the masters of the mind. If the nerves are strong, mind remains calm and stable.

Tension in the face, dilation of the pupils, tremor of the body, tingling of the skin, increase in breath rate, sudden sweating, are signs of emotional as well as psychological imbalances and disturbances. In some, the blood pressure goes up or down, stomach contracts, mouth dries, which in turn disturbs the hormonal secretions adversely.

To come out from these disturbances, Patañjali explains the healing process through the *sūtra* I.33*: maitrī karuṇā muditā upekṣāṇām sukha duḥkha puṇya apuṇya viṣayāṇām bhāvanātaḥ cittaprasādanam.* Normally, when someone is happy about achievements, the others become jealous of him.

If someone seeks a pious and virtuous life, the others try to find defects in him even though they are negligible. When one has defects or vices, the other may become happy. This is the human mind.

Patañjali says that when someone is happy, share that happiness with friendliness. If someone is in sorrow, share it with compassionate action. If someone is virtuous, be glad and joyous. If someone has vice, do not criticise but guide him and be indifferent and aloof. Is it not a mental cure for emotional healing? (*Y.S.*, II.33).

Now, the place of emotions in *sapta prajña* – the seven states or seven-fold consciousness. The seven states of consciousness are: (a) raising consciousness *(vyutthāna citta),* (b) restrained consciousness *(nirodha citta),* (c) tranquil consciousness *(praśānta citta),* (d) attentive consciousness *(ekāgra citta),* (e) settled consciousness *(nirmāṇa citta),* (f) fissured consciousness *(chidra citta)* and lastly, (g) divine consciousness *(divya citta).*

Their awareness is awareness in the body, senses, energy, mind, intellect, consciousness and self. Does not awareness of senses, mind and intelligence *(indriya saṁyama, manas saṁyama* and *buddhi saṁyama),* control the emotions and intellect? In order to develop this awareness, we need sound health. This health is also in seven stages. These are: physical health, moral health, mental health, intellectual health, conscious health, conscientious health and divine health.

The *Yoga Vāsiṣṭha* explains the *sapta prajñā* as desire to reach the soul *(śubhecchā),* reflection to reach the soul *(vicāraṇa),* attenuation of the mind *(tanumānasā),* maintaining the intelligence with crystal clarity *(sattvāpatti),* state of non-attachment *(asamśakti),* non-perception of objects *(parārthabhāvanam),* and lastly the experiencing state that is unexplainable *(brahmavidvaiṣṭam).* As the *Upaniṣad* say, *tato vācaḥ nivartante aprāpya manasāsaha.* At this stage the organs of speech and mind retire as they cannot explain or narrate this state. Patañjali explains this state of the *sādhaka* as one whose purpose has been fulfilled (*kṛtārthan*); *kṛtārthaṁ prati naṣṭam api anaṣṭam tadanya sādhāraṇatvāt* (*Y.S.*, II.22) – the relationship with nature ceases for the emancipated beings because its purpose is fulfilled, but its processes continue to affect others.

These days, meditation has become a treatment for emotional disturbances, whereas meditation requires total physical fitness, emotional stability and intellectual clarity. An emotionally disturbed person is gloomy, dull, lonely and sorrowful. How can he meditate? In *Bhagavad Gītā* one comes across Arjuna, who had all these emotional disturbances. Lord Krishna took him in his hands and treated him in various styles of yoga to bring him back to normalcy. At the end, he thanks Lord Krishna for relieving him from delusion and grief and finally assents to act as per his duty (*B.G.*, XVIII.73). That is how the seven-fold consciousness, the seven states of awareness and the seven states of health have to be understood through the light of the eight petals of yoga.

VII.16. – Is there any state beyond yoga

Is there a state beyond yoga? Is it a fantasy or a poetic expression? Hard for me to comment! When we say that if our consciousness is extended like a bow, we have reached a state of bliss. In bliss, is there a room to think or speak? If a dagger is kept in the scabbard, it rusts. If one sharpens the sword each day, it maintains its sharpness and shines. In case we have experienced this bliss, are we able to keep that state steady? Who knows? By entering the world of pure dance we may lose what we got and enjoy remembering the past experiences. This bliss state is easy to describe but hard to maintain. If a dancer does not maintain his practice, can he dance? It is the same for all of us if we neglect *sādhanā* and stay in the past glory. Therefore let us sharpen attentively the sword of our intelligence, by taking it out from the scabbard of the consciousness and polish the scabbard – the body – so that we experience bliss and talk less about it.

Remember the words of Patañjali who advises us to continue and persist *sādhanā* even when we have experienced *samādhi.*

VII.17. – On death and dying

Birth and death are beyond man's control. They don't belong to our domain. Life departs when the time comes. According to our scriptures, death is a natural phenomenon of *prakṛti* (nature) while life is *vikṛti,*[1] as Kālidāsa puts beautifully in *Raghuvaṇśa.* Birth and death are not in our hand. But life in between birth and death needs to be shaped, baked and cultured. Lord Krishna

---

[1] Generally translated as 'evolute', it means formation or matter assuming a form. According to *sāṁkhya* philosophy, all forms of *vyakta* (manifested matter) are *vikṛti* (*Sāṁkhya Kārikā* of Īśvarakṛṣna, 3).

says that life is in unmanifested form before birth, it becomes manifest after birth and goes back to its unmanifest form in death (*B.G.*, II.28).

Death and dying are two different things. Death is a full stop to the present life, but dying is a process. By the word death one should not get frightened by the dying process. It is told that: "Every form of meditation is in essence a rehearsal of death." But I do not think so. For me meditation is a new life. It is a death from worldly pleasures and enlivenment towards spiritual light. A Zen adage says, "If you die before you die, then when you die, you won't die." This means that one has to live positively until death. This is what *abhiniveśa* means. We die due to the fear of death rather than actual death.

I am neither concerned about death nor dying. But I would say this much. If my body becomes fully non-functional though living, I would consider it as my death. So, I do not waste my time on thinking of death but do yoga to live holistically every moment. Face the fear of dying courageously; then death becomes glorious and majestic.

SECTION VIII

ADJUSTMENTS IN PRACTICE

SECTION VIII – ADJUSTMENTS IN PRACTICE

As a good number of students from all over the world were approaching me individually for right adjustments, I thought that this is the best place to touch this subject here so that it would benefit thousands of readers at the same time.

Hence, I have grouped the members' doubts according to the anatomy of the human structure, and touched on it for correct adjustments according to the needs.

VIII.1. – Why a background is needed for adjustment

Adjustment in practice is not just to acquire a "better *āsana*". It is the entire approach to practice that needs to be done judiciously with awareness so that a state of parallelity exists not just on the outer appearance of the presented *āsana*, but that parallelity has to resonate throughout all the sheaths of the self.

One has to begin and end in the adjustment of an *āsana* in such a way that the human anatomical structure is not disturbed or distorted.

Any distortion or wrong positioning in the *āsana* reverberates creating changes in the muscles, joints and fibres and clamour in the mind and intelligence of the practitioner, jarring all the sheaths of the self. During the practice of *prāṇāyāma* any gasped, sucked or pressured inhalation or exhalation is wrong.

There is much more than the alignment of the outer frame of the body to be attended to in the presentation of the *āsana*. As it is through their correct, even and measured placement (with ascension, extension and expansion), the senses of perception find their place of neutrality from where they change and begin their involvement with inner perception. Again it is with the sensitively determined position of the outer limbs that the mind has to act, like smooth pouring of oil from one vessel to the other. Thus, each one has to begin from the outer, to become absorbed and immersed into the inner dimensionless space. This way all the sheaths of the self occupy the entire being with intelligent awareness pervading the body throughout. Hence, all the sheaths have to be attended to co-ordinate while practising *āsana, prāṇāyāma* and *dhyāna*.

By this undistorted abiding of the vehicles of the self with the Self, there are no longer any divisions. This way the aim of yoga practice is established throughout practice.

VIII.2. – Stretching and strengthening of arms

Birds have two wings for flying higher and higher. For man, the shoulder blades are the wings to stretch higher and higher. Hence, stretching the arms over the head is important. The shoulders may be stiff due to negligence, or due to frozen shoulders and shoulderblades.

When one stretches the arms over the head, the upper arms do not stretch straight due to non-attention at the armpits, shoulder joints and shoulder blades. In order to stretch the arms above the head, one has to soften the skin on the outer side of the armpits and roll the shoulders backwards. Then, bringing the inner shoulder blades down, roll the shoulders in and stretch the arms up. It is better to move the upper arms behind the ears without bringing the head forward or down. Extend the arms from the side ribs without protruding the pelvis and thighs or the abdomen. Often I use a rod between the arms and the back of the head to get full extension of the arms. The following *āsana* help for stretching and strengthening the arms – Rope movements, *Paschimanamaskārāsana* (*Namaskāra* behind the back), *Baddha Hastāsana*, arm movements in *Tāḍāsana* as in *Gomukhāsana, Vātāyanāsana, Sālamba Sarvāṅgāsana* II and *Halāsana*.

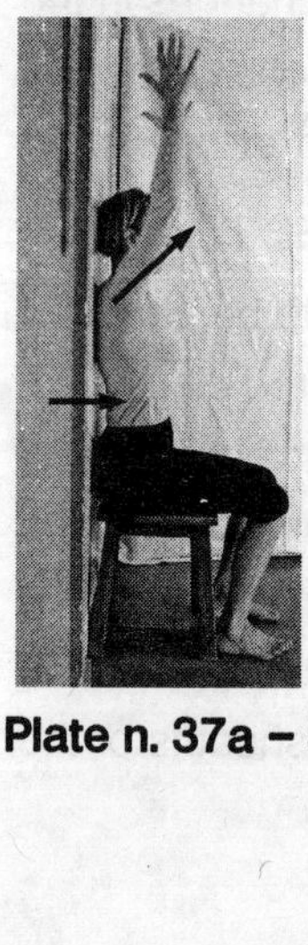
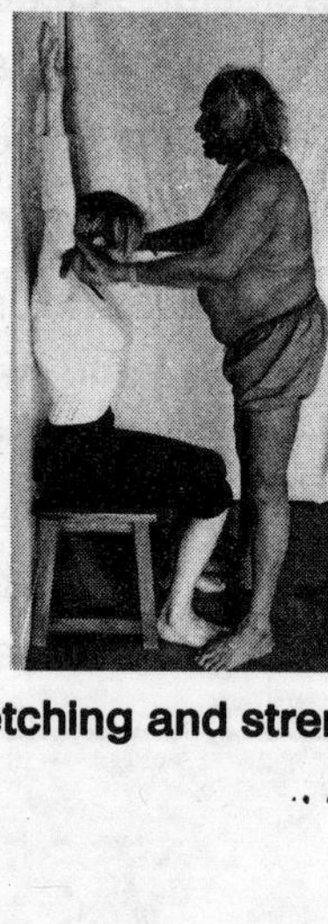
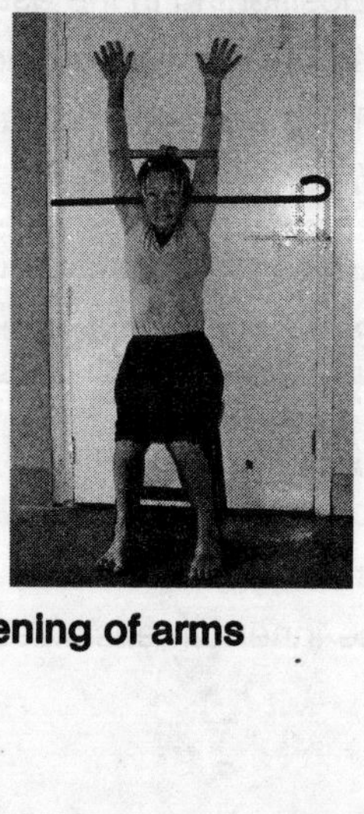

Placing a rod to get a full extension of the arms

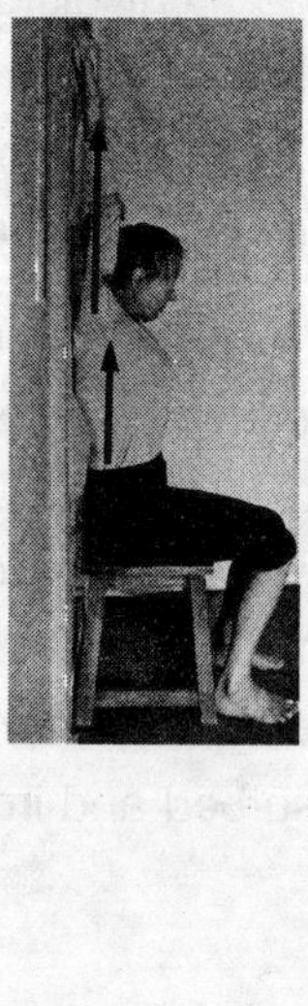

Plate n. 37a – Stretching and strengthening of arms

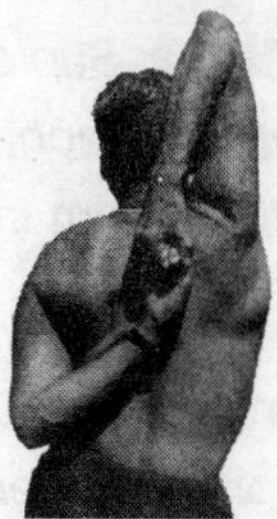

Gomukhāsana arms

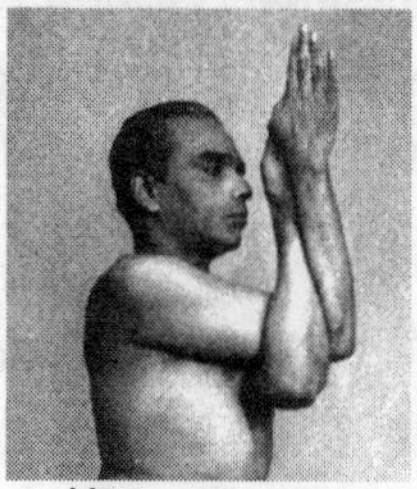

Vātāyanāsana arms

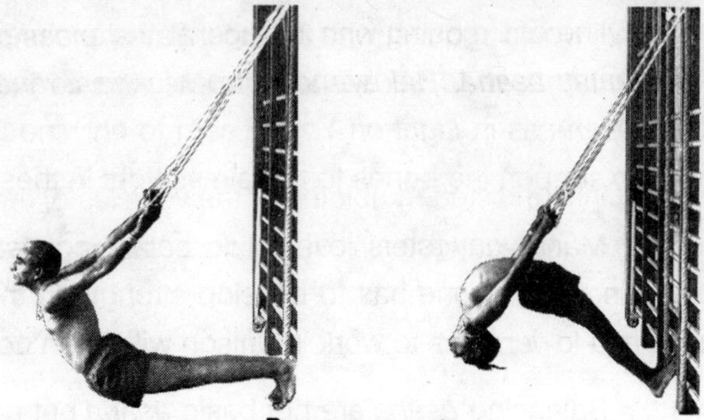

Rope movements

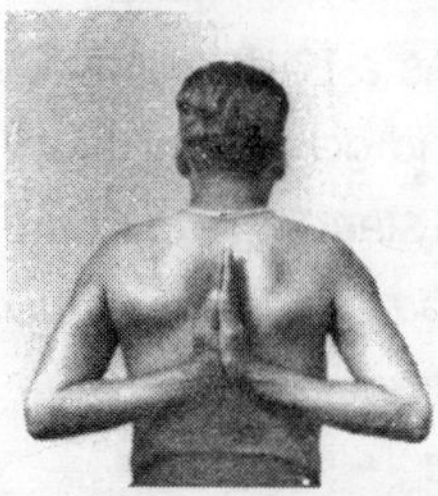

Paschimanamaskārāsana

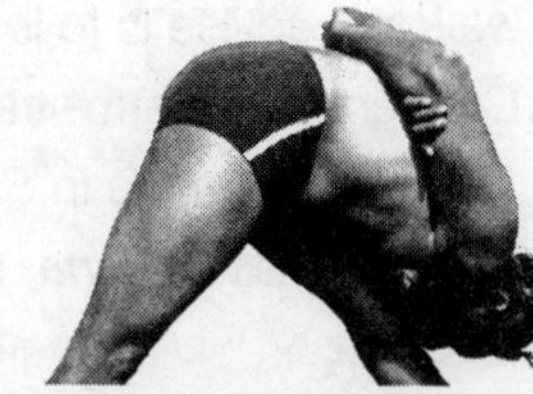

Baddha Hastāsana arms

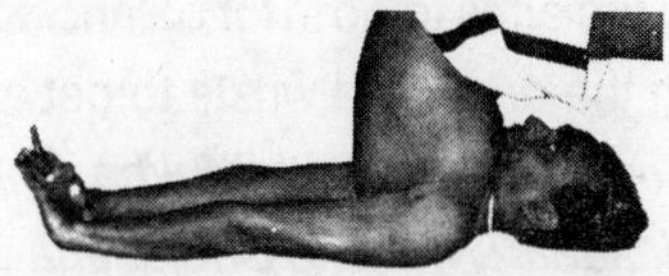

Halāsana or *Sarvāṅgāsana* II arm position

Plate n. 37b – Stretching and strengthening of arms

VIII.3. – On bow legs and elbow pain

It is most important to know that our knees bear most of our weight in all walks of life. Hence, they the main support and holder of all our labours in action. They bear the body weight at all times in all movements and functions. Therefore neglect or postponement of treatment to knee injury is not good. In order to work on the cartilages, tendons, ligaments of the knees, one has to begin from the head of the calves, the source and end of the thigh muscles, by creating space there to correct the injured or painful parts. It requires careful and correct adjustments with the concerned parts of the knees.

Regarding bow knees or knock knees, one has to use a soft brick to create space and a belt to bring-in the parts that need to come closer to each other and sit in *Daṇḍāsana* or lie down in *Śavāsana*.

In *Utthita Trikoṇāsana,* learn to stretch the leg to shift the weight from the outer side towards the inner side of the leg. To do this, do not rest the outer edge of the feet on the floor, but shift to the inner feet. In *Vīrāsana* also, rest the head of the metatarsals on the floor.

About the elbows, *āsana* with the help of the ropes improve. Perform *Sālamba Sarvāṅgāsana* using a stool for the elbows and the weights on the palms. For *Halāsana* use the stool to place the feet to stay longer.

I would request one to look at the pictures of *Vīrāsana, Baddha Koṇāsana, Supta Pādānguṣṭhāsana, Halāsana, Adho Mukha Śvānāsana, Adho Mukha Vṛkṣāsana, Pincha Mayūrāsana* as in *Light on Yoga*. Learn to entwine the forearm muscles and harden them in order to support the bones to remain straight in these *āsana*.

Many youngsters love to do balancing *āsana* on the arms. Before thinking of the balancing *āsana*, one has to develop strength in the elbow joints as they control the upper arms and lower arms to work in unison with even co-ordination.

Balancing *āsana* are not basic *āsana* but power building *āsana*. As a baby learns to stand, tries to walk and leaps after learning to walk, my advise is to learn and go step by step, preparing the arms to go in for balancing *āsana*. Concentrate on arm stretch in standing positions, entwining the arms and wrists to get accurate balancing of arms in *Sālamba Śīrṣāsana, Adho Mukha Vṛkṣāsana, Ūrdhva Mukha Śvānāsana, Pincha Mayurāsana, Chaturaṅga Daṇḍāsana, Bhujapīdāsana, Dvi Hasta Bhujāsana* and *Ṭiṭṭibhāsana*.

A new terminology has come into yoga now as power yoga. All these balancing *āsana* are nothing but power yoga in today's yoga.

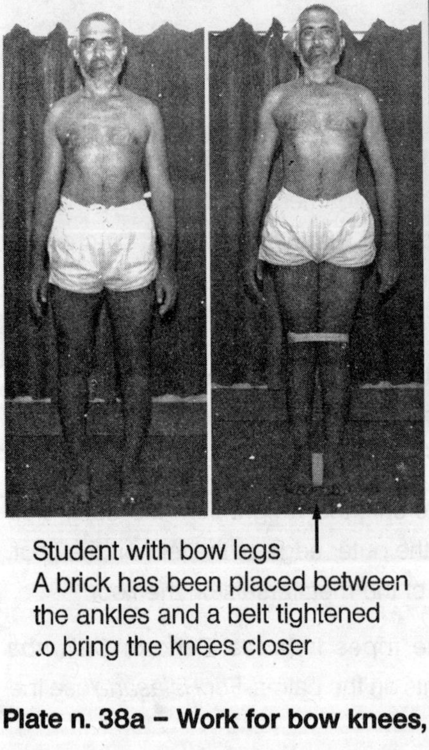

Student with bow legs
A brick has been placed between the ankles and a belt tightened to bring the knees closer

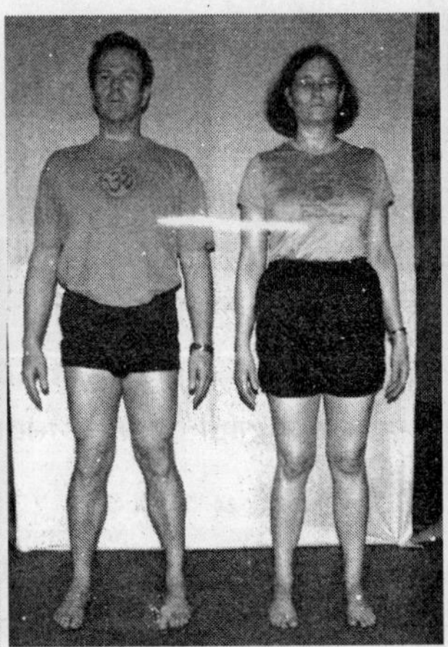

Both students have knock knees

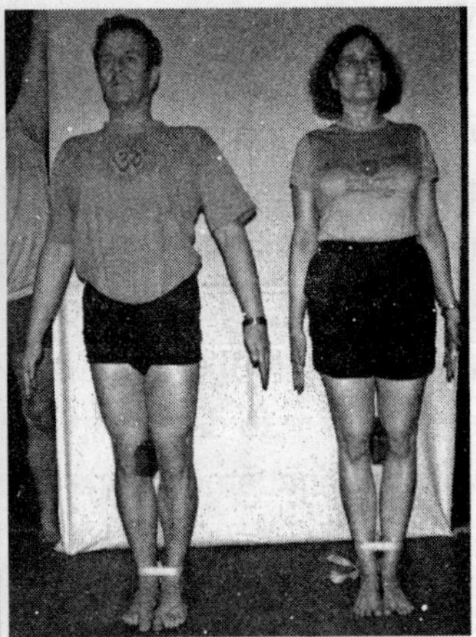

The brick is placed between the knees and the belt to the ankles

.. also in *Daṇḍāsana*

Plate n. 38a – Work for bow knees, knock knees and arms

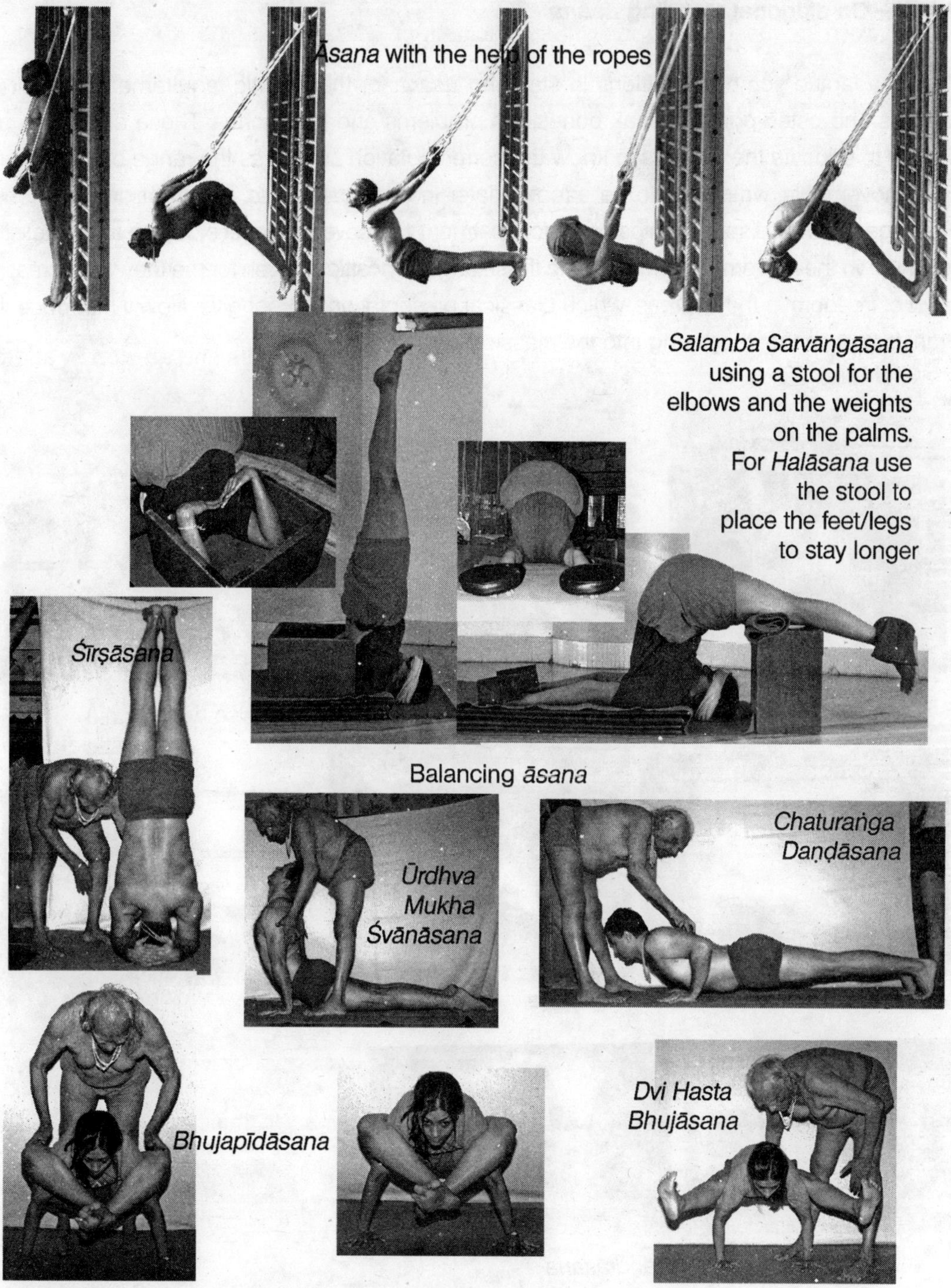
Āsana with the help of the ropes
Sālamba Sarvāṅgāsana using a stool for the elbows and the weights on the palms. For Halāsana use the stool to place the feet/legs to stay longer
Śīrṣāsana
Balancing āsana
Ūrdhva Mukha Śvānāsana
Chaturaṅga Daṇḍāsana
Bhujapīḍāsana
Dvi Hasta Bhujāsana

Plate n. 38b – Work for bow knees, knock knees and arms

VIII.4. – On diagonal standing *āsana*

I have adapted some innovations in standing *āsana* for therapeutic requirements for osteo-arthritis and osteo-porosis, weak bones, hip problems and backaches. These alterations are meant to educate the patients to know the correct rotation as well as the range of hip, leg and arm movements, which are to be adopted later in classical *āsana*. I thought of this in 1992 when people with displaced hips came for treatment. I discovered it after studying and practising on my own the movements that occur in these angular positions. Even for me they were creating a lot of freedom in these areas, which classical presentation did not give. Now, I introduce the transformation that they bring into the classical way of practising.

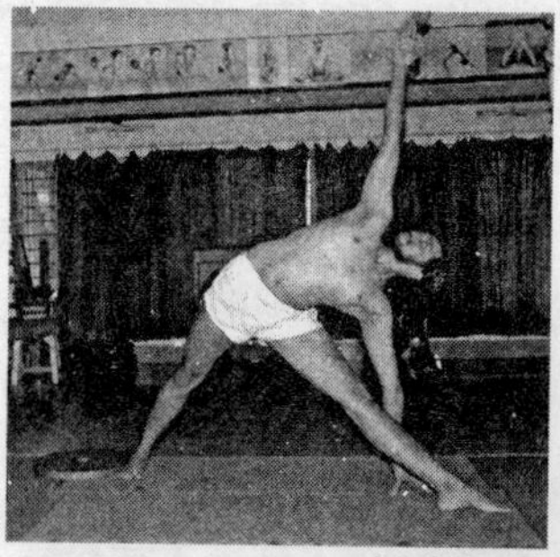
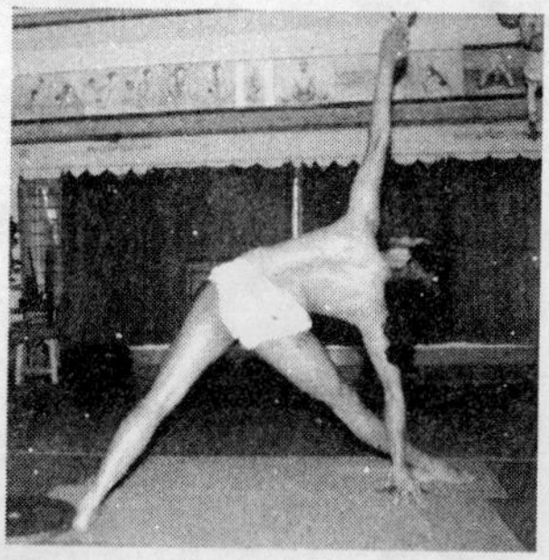

Utthita Trikoṇāsana

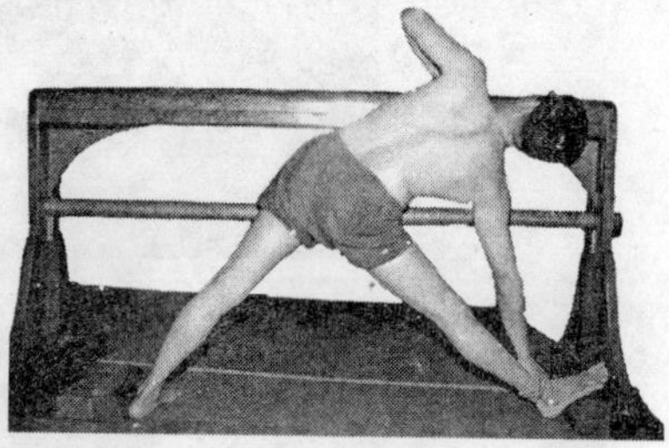

Also with the aid of a trestle

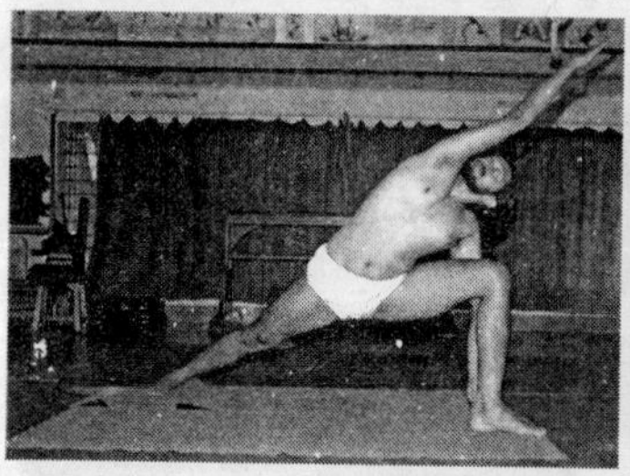
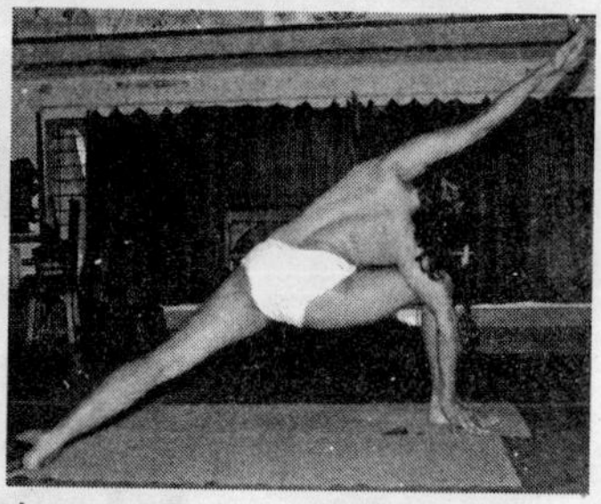
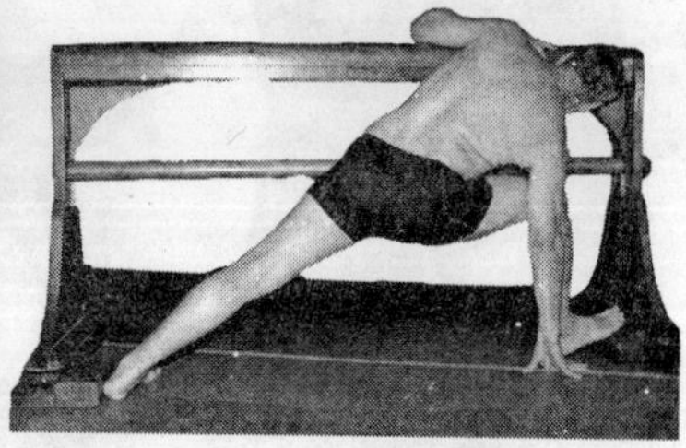

Utthita Parśvakoṇāsana

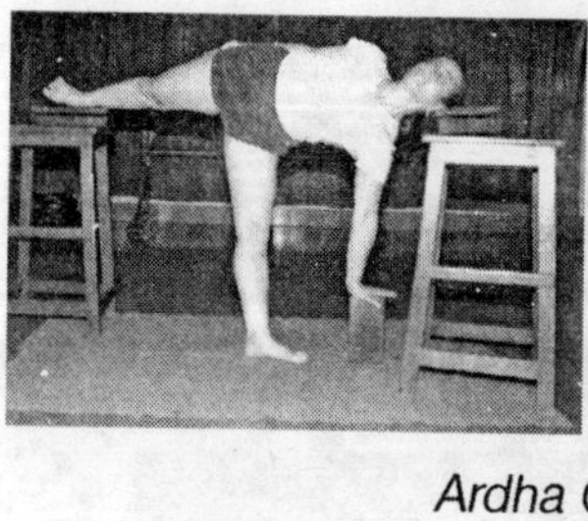
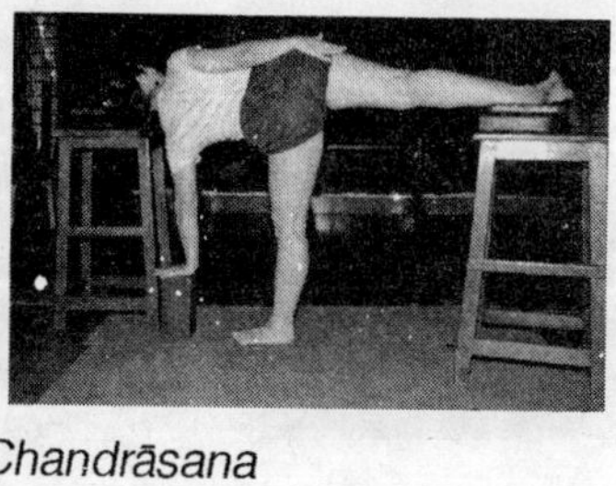
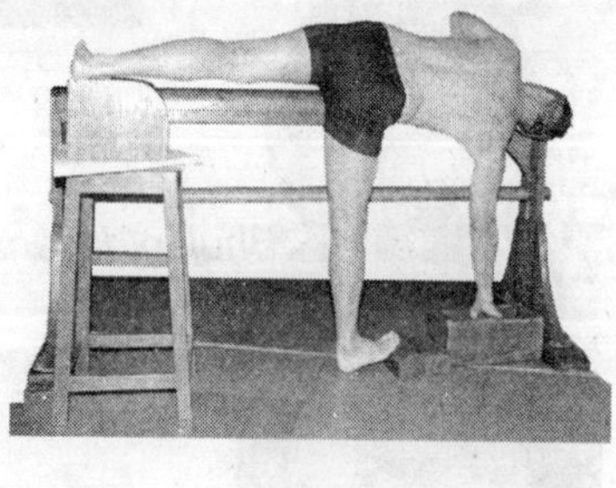

Ardha Chandrāsana

Plate n. 39 – Angular standing *āsana*

Often I find people are more familiar with their anterior body than with their posterior body. While the anterior body can be seen the posterior body cannot be seen. The angular standing *āsana* give the sense to feel the posterior body and to adjust to enhance the restricted movements in the lower spine, buttocks, hips and sacroiliac areas and arms. When a healthy body like mine began getting a better feel from the movements, then the ideas struck me to help and work on people to derive better and quicker benefits than what they were gaining by keeping the legs in line to each other. Here the rotator muscles of the hip joints and shoulder joints rotate to the maximum level where classical positions do not act, or move, so much.

People suffering from sciatica, pelvic lock, cracked or projecting tailbone, rheumatism and arthritis began experiencing relief as they could create space in these areas. In fact, when one does standing *āsana* with the anterior body facing the wall, he finds that he needs lot of correction as he can trace the lack of movements in his back.

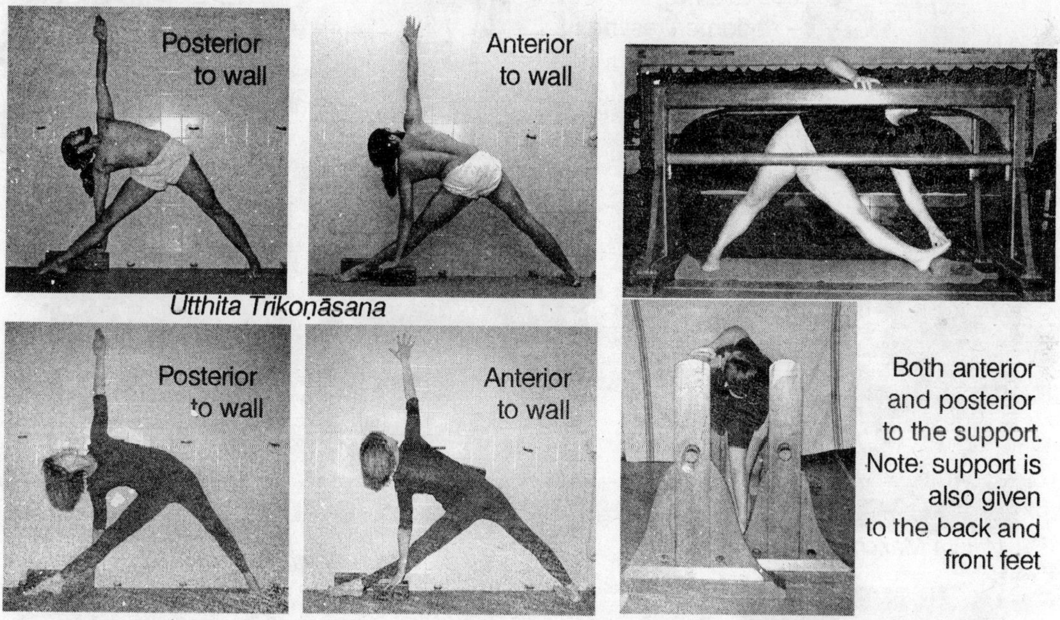
Posterior to wall
Anterior to wall
Utthita Trikoṇāsana
Posterior to wall
Anterior to wall
Both anterior and posterior to the support.
Note: support is also given to the back and front feet

Plate n. 40 – Support for standing *āsana* – anterior and posterior

VIII.5. – On lumbar pain in forward bends

Lumbar spondilitis and spondylosis give pain for some in backbends and for some in forwardbends. At the same time some feel relief through forwardbends, while others do so in backbends.

If the pain is felt in forward bends, then it is better to use a firmly rolled blanket between the thighs and abdomen in order to roll the lower torso over it to bend forwards. This relieves the pain immediately. If one is slim and tall or the spinal muscles narrow or the trunk may be broad but the spinal muscles narrow or for any previous injury, rest the abdomen on a high stool with pillows and do *Uttānāsana, Adho Mukha Śvānāsana* with wall ropes, *Prasārita Pādottānāsana*, chair *Bharadvājāsana*, standing *Marīchyāsana, Utthita Hasta Pādānguṣṭhāsana, Mālāsana* with folded blanket between the legs and abdomen and *Pavanamuktāsana* on a bench. These *āsana* relieve lower back pains.

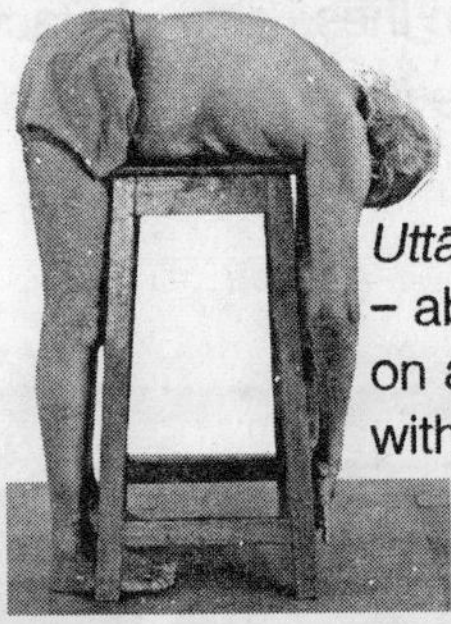

Uttānāsana – abdomen resting on a high stool with pillows

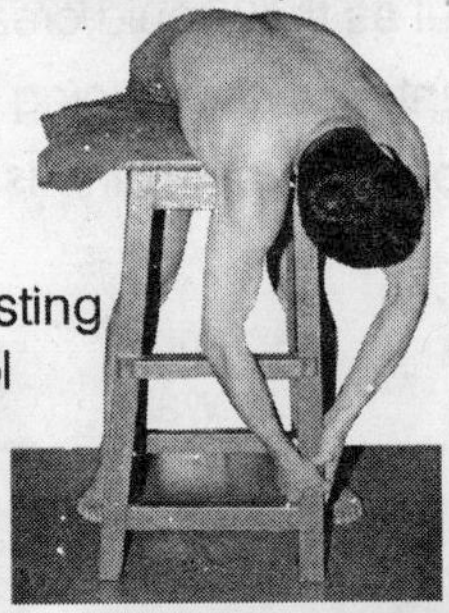

(Parśva Uttānāsana)

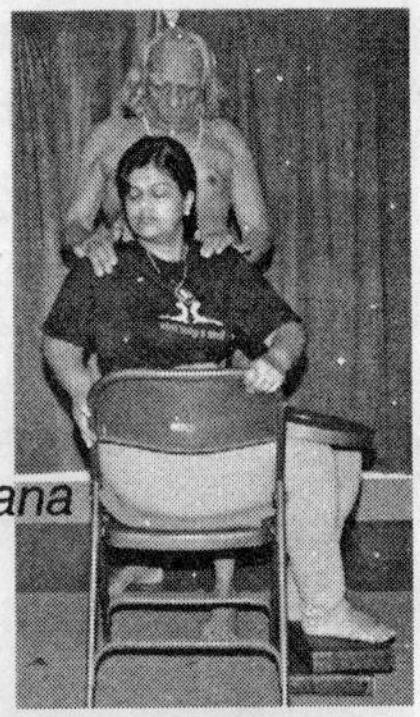

Bharadvājāsana – chair

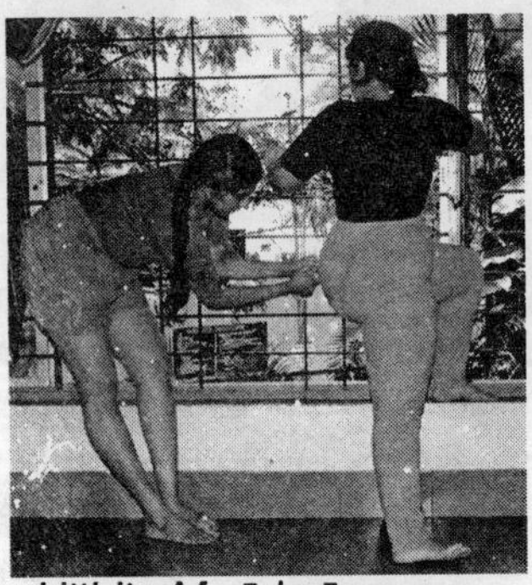

Utthita Marīchyāsana

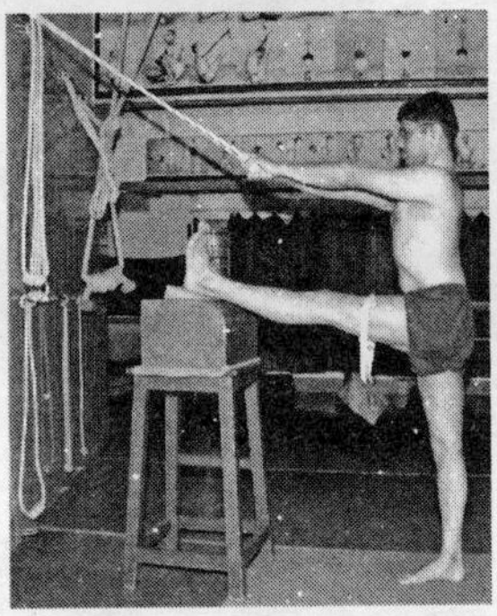

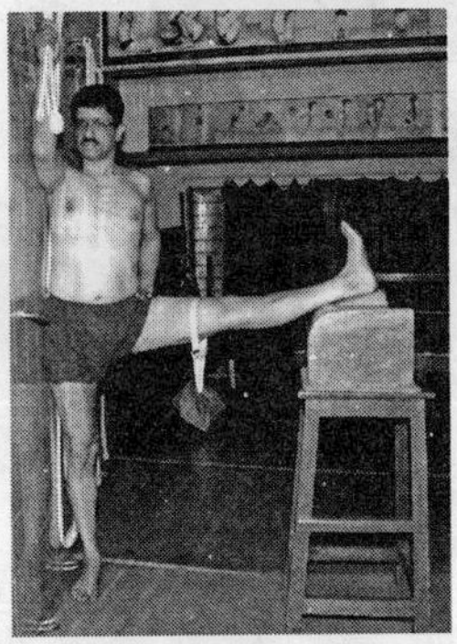

Utthita Hasta Pādānguṣṭhāsana 1 & 2

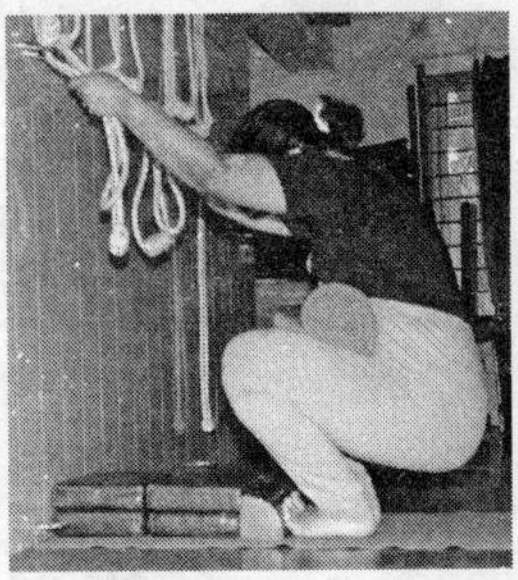

Mālāsana with folded blanket between the legs and abdomen

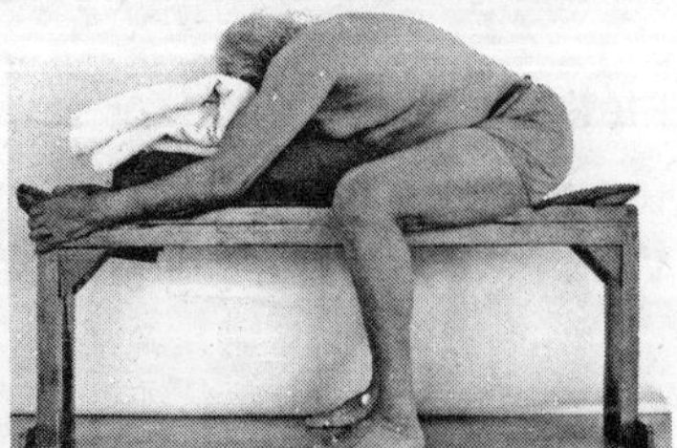

Pavanamuktāsana on a bench

Plate n. 41 – Examples of *āsana* that relieve lower back pain

Let me draw attention on lateral twists for lumber pain. The lateral movements are very good for lumber problems. Begin from simpler twistings without creating hardness in the abdominal muscles for the spinal muscles to extend, without the stress. Train the abdominal muscles and organs to remain passive while performing lateral twists because most people suffering from back aches use their abdominal muscles in their movements due to the fear of injuring the spine. Hence, at the time of practising *āsana*, it is advised to keep the abdominal muscles soft by rotating the torso instead of straining them. Keep the abdominal muscles passive and move them first so that you use the spine as a churning rod and see that the lateral part of the spine rotates freely with the torso. Follow the *āsana* like a) *Pārśva Daṇḍāsana*, b) *Pārśva Vīrāsana*, c) *Pārśva Baddhakoṇāsana*, d) *Pārśva Upaviṣṭakoṇāsana*, e) *Pārśva Pādmāsana*. They relieve the soreness of the spinal muscles, lessening the pain in the affected parts.

One has to observe carefully and adjust the spinal muscles to run parallel to each other. Then toning takes place and they respond well and remove fear complexes. When the above *āsana* come well, it is easier for one to understand the complex advanced twists such as *Marichyāsana* III, *Ardha Matsyendrāsana* and *Paśāsana*. They all act as boons for lumbar problems. If the lumbar and sacral parts are sore, then my advice would be to do *Śavāsana* covering the space between the floor and the lower back area with a soft thin silk pillow or cloth to cover the vacant space that occurs between the floor and the back. Then place two pillows or a bolster on the lower abdomen and thighs and place weights that are used for weight lifting on them. There, these weights soften the spinal nerves and make the spinal muscles loose. This is actually *Śavāsana* to the lumbar and sacral areas. Then one can use yogic traction as shown here.

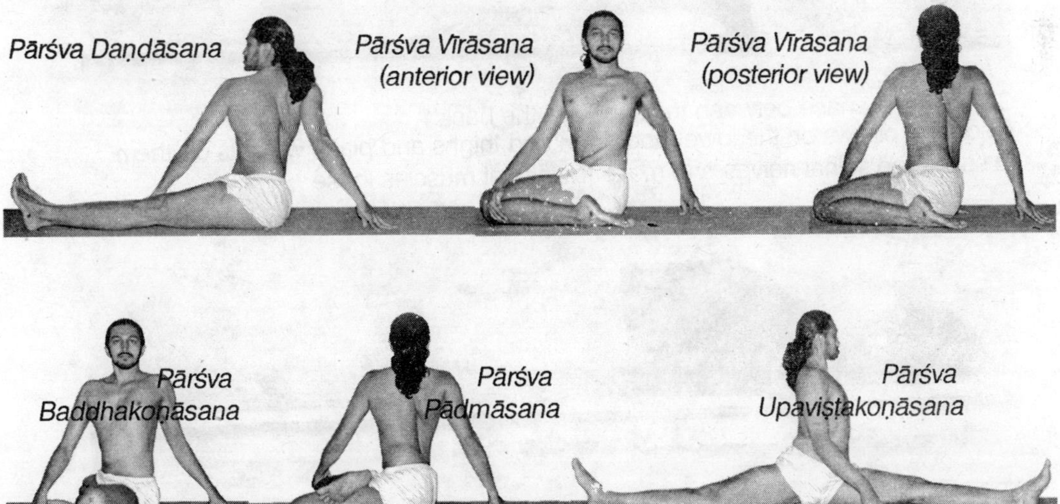

Plate n. 42 – The Lateral Twists

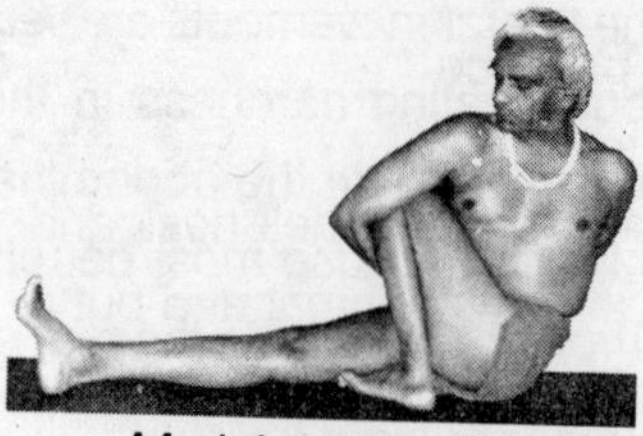

Marichyāsana III

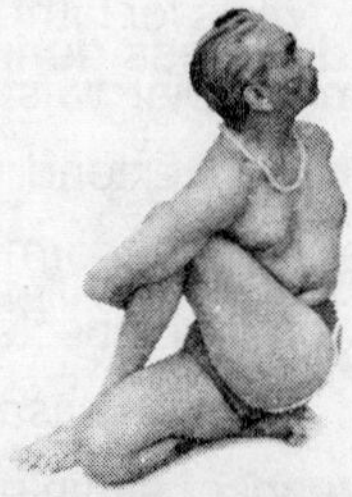

Ardha Matsyendrāsana

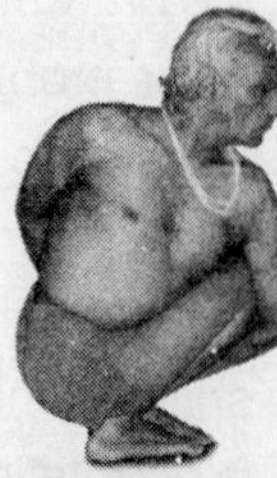

Paśāsana

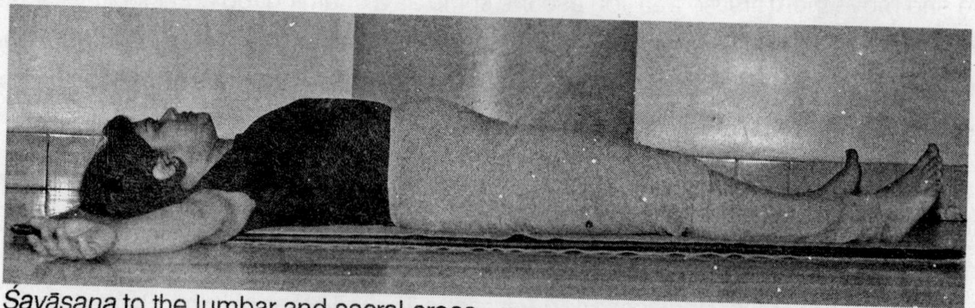

Śavāsana to the lumbar and sacral areas

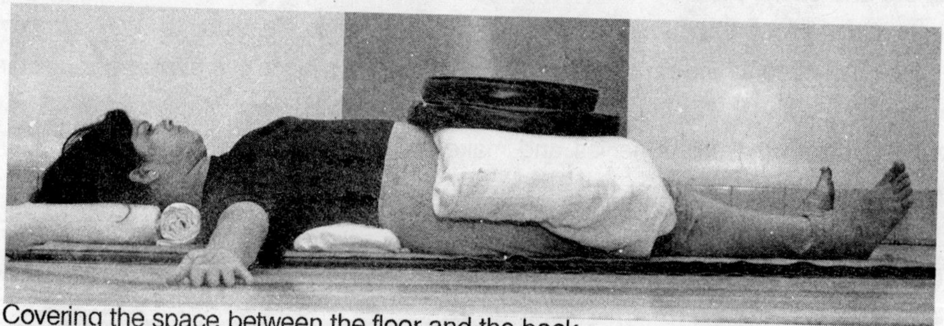

Covering the space between the floor and the back
Place two pillows on the lower abdomen and thighs and place weights on them to soften the spinal nerves and make the spinal muscles loose

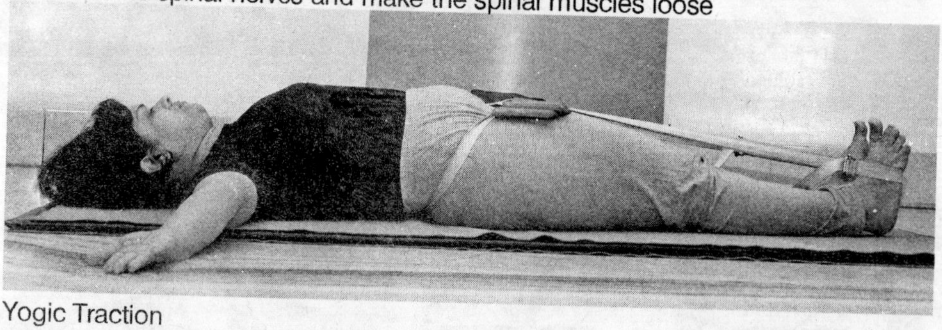

Yogic Traction

Plate n. 43 – Understanding the classic *āsana* and lumbar, sacral *Śavāsana*

VIII.6. – Feel of dryness, sickness and dizziness during *āsana* practice

People who are slim, weak and tall feel this dryness in practice. They protrude their neck and throat in *āsana* and *prāṇāyāma.* Even in the daily walk of life they stress the throat and put a strain on it without paying any attention to these parts.

As they use their neck to do the *asana,* first they have to learn not to over extend their neck and throat in backward extensions. They compress the back but extend their neck and throat. They should learn to do *Ūrdhva Dhanurāsana* with head lifted up towards the ceiling as far as possible. Their throat gets relaxed and soft and the strain disappears by this way of presentation. So keep the head looking up at the ceiling in backbends.

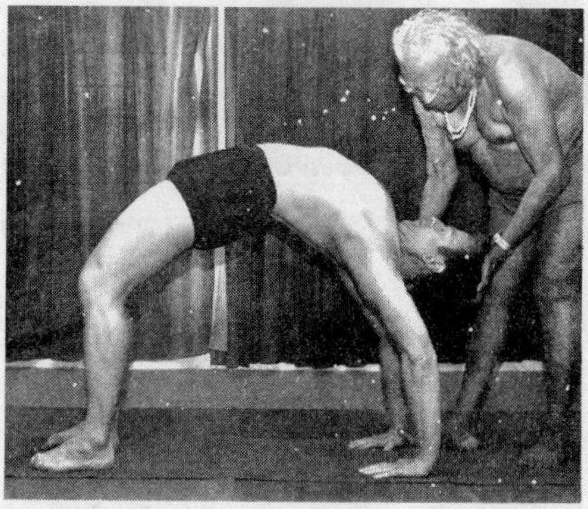

Plate n. 44 – *Ūrdhva Dhanurāsana* with the head raised

In such people, their sternum caves in more than normal. They suck the tongue towards the throat in their practise and block the throat. This makes their breathing heavy and hard, which in turn strains the brain. Blocking the throat by the tongue creates tightness in the brain and makes the skull rigid. This makes them believe that their practices are intense.

Read carefully "Hints and Cautions" in *Light on Yoga,* where I have mentioned not to harden the brain cells. If the tongue is sucked in, the brain cannot watch or observe or catch the mistakes that the body is doing. So better watch the tongue and keep it in a natural condition as in sleep, then no signs of exhaustion and dehydration are felt. Often laboured breathing, holding the breath unknowingly and clinching the teeth, causes dryness. Deliberately avoid all these happenings.

Dizziness comes on account of obstruction in respiration, or due to poor digestion, weaknesses, thyroidism, spondylosis, over exertion, and hyper elasticity in the body.

One feels dizzy or blacks-out mostly in the standing *āsana.* The moment one feels this at once do *Uttanāsana,* resting the head on a bed or stool, *Adho Mukha Śvānāsana* or *Adho*

Mukha Vīrāsana in between two standing *āsana*. This relieves both dizziness and blackout. Dull functioning of the liver, unknowingly holding the breath, practising *āsana* after a short interval of meals and low blood pressure cause dizziness and blackout.

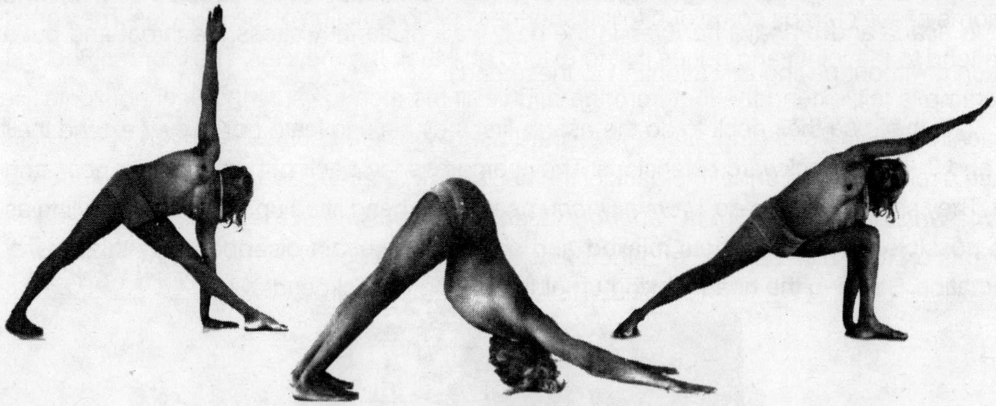

Plate n. 45 – *Adho Mukha Śvānāsana* in-between two standing *āsana*

For such students, it is better to start practice with forward bends and then the standing *āsana*, or do *Utthita Trikoṇāsana – Uttānāsana, Utthita Pārśvakoṇāsana – Uttānāsana*. This is called a *viloma* sequence. Do *Setu Bandha Sarvāṅgāsana* on a bench and half *Halāsana* with legs on a stool. Then one will not feel dizzy. This method is good for people with low blood pressure.

People with liver problems, indigestion, constipation, low metabolism and diabetes feel sick and dizzy. They have to start with simple non-irritating but stimulative *āsana* for some months before going for twists and difficult *āsana*. One has to judge one's capacity before attempting complicated *āsana*. Find out which *āsana* are congenial and help to relieve such conditions.

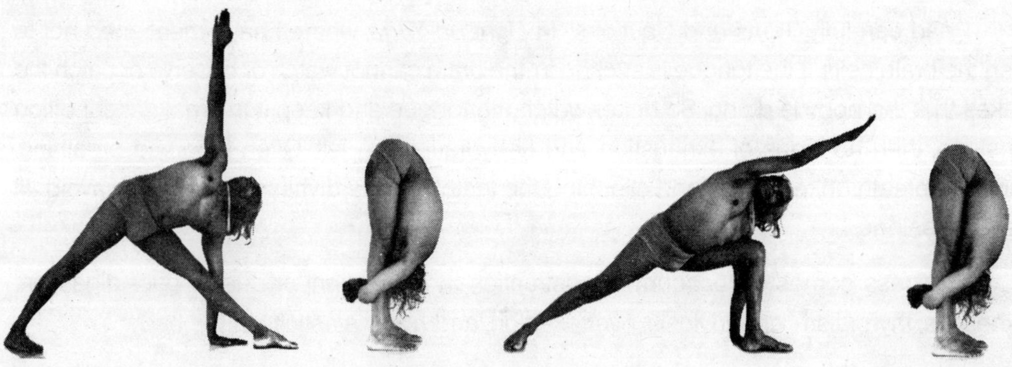

Plate n. 46 – *Viloma* sequence in *āsana* practice

VIII.7. - On cramps

Cramps come if the joints and the bones are not activated with co-ordination of the muscles, or in some cases cramps come due to the shortness or constriction of the muscles. Then one has to attend to the joints and bones first to extend and then the muscles. The moment the feeling of cramp is felt, extend the foot from the middle of the arch towards the heel horizontally and vertically in all the standing *āsana.* In forward bendings; keep some weight on the thighs and place a rolled blanket under the back of the heels. Do *Vīrāsana, Baddhakoṇāsana, Adhomukha Śvānāsana, Daṇḍāsana, Supta Pādāṅguṣṭāsana* and *Halāsana* with legs on the stool and place weights on the calves and extend the heels towards the floor.

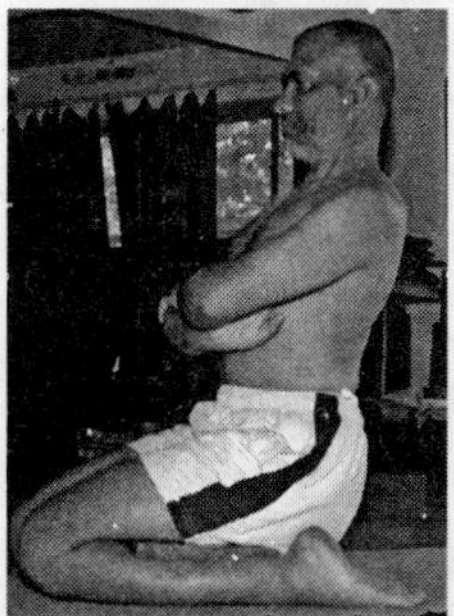

Vīrāsana

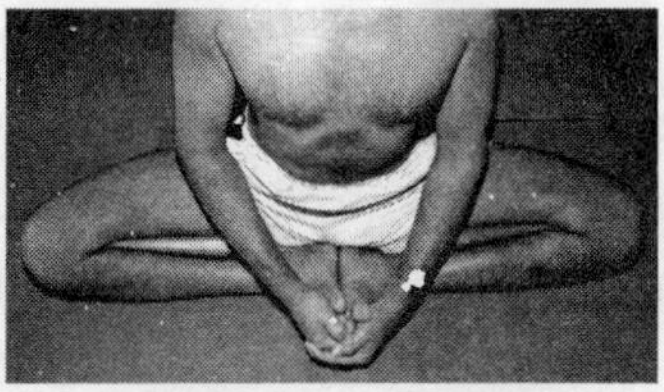

Baddhakoṇāsana

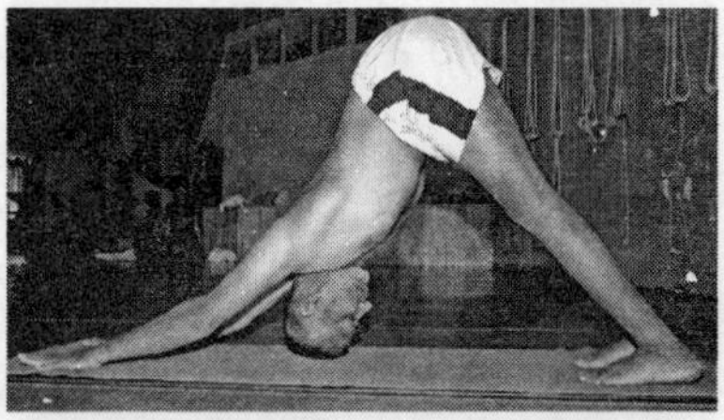

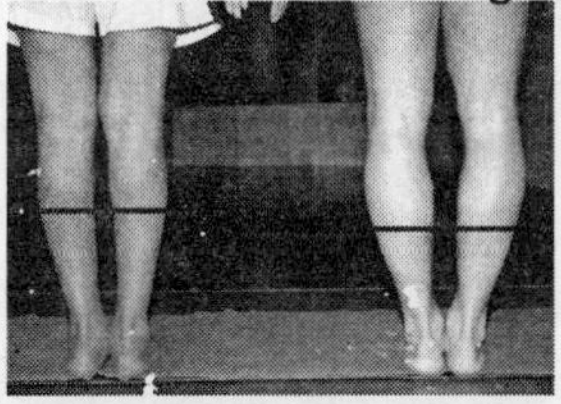

Short and long calf muscle length

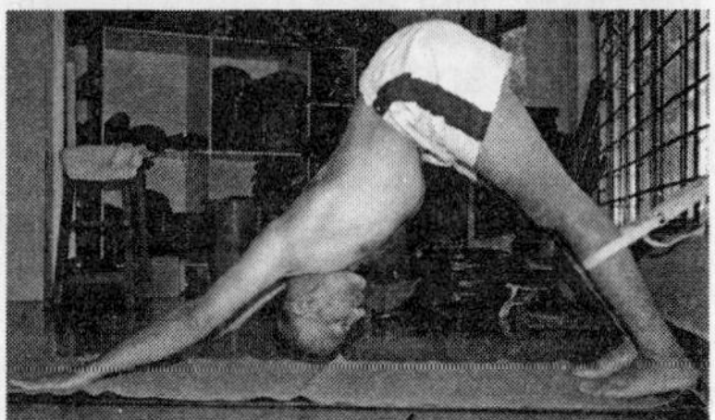

Adhomukha Śvānāsana with a belt to open calves

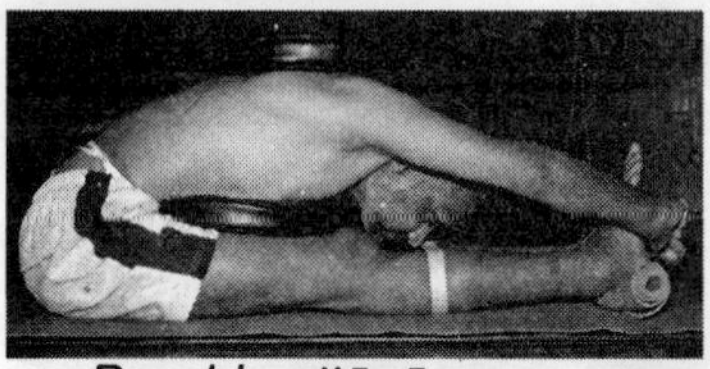

Paschimottānāsana with a roll under the heels and a weight on the thighs

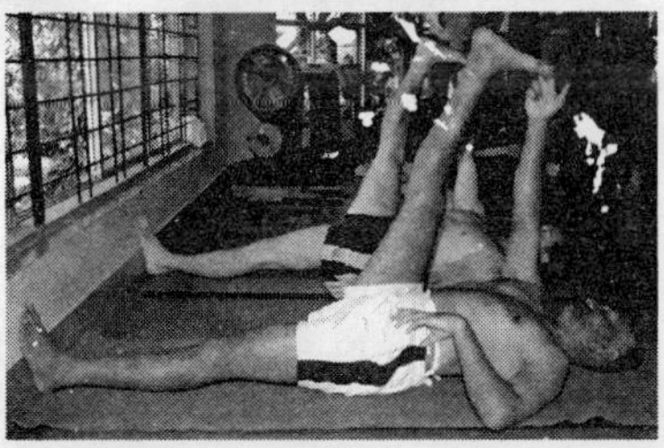

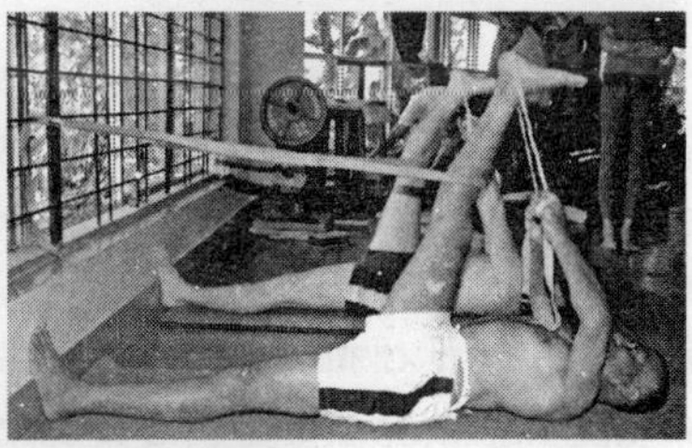

Supta Pādāṅguṣṭāsana and using belts

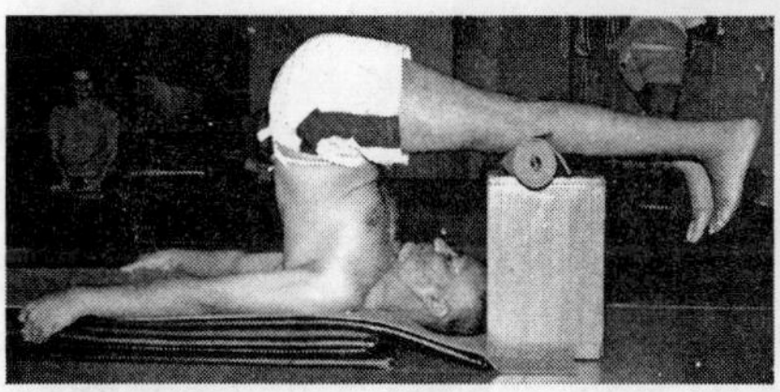

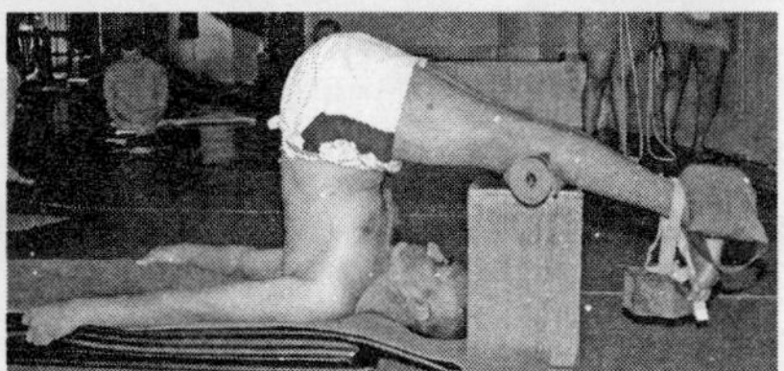

Halāsana with a weight to extend the legs

Plate n. 47 - Cramps

VIII.8. – If forward bends are easy why are backbends difficult

Those who do forwardbends with ease, should know that the spinal muscles of their bodies are toned and tuned only to move in that direction. For them backbends appear hard. Similarly, those who do backbends with ease find forwardbends difficult. This is on account of imbalance of the fluid in the system. Those who are good in forward bends do not show interest in backbends, and those who are good in backbends do not show interest in forward bends. As harmony and balance in body and mind have to build up in all parts of the body evenly, one has to culture the body by performing forward, backward or lateral movements as well as sitting and standing *āsana* sequentially. This way of adjustment in *āsana* transforms the restricted movements into a wholesome growth.

In forwardbends the posterior muscles of the spinal column extend and create space; in backbends anterior muscles of the spinal column extend and create space, whereas in twists creating space activates the lateral muscles of the spine and body. If one trains the spinal muscles only in one direction, then it is not a right practice or a right toning and tuning of the body. Just as a musician tunes his musical instrument to get the tone, one has to tune the physical and physiological systems of the body and strike a balance in forward bends, backbends and lateral movements of the spinal muscles with proper balance and concord. This is toning of the spinal muscles for a better all-round rhythmic growth.

VIII.9. – On physical and mental fatigue

Mental fatigue is experienced when the brain and the nerves get tired. Over-exertion, shock or fear and mental disturbances cause this fatigue. It is also associated with languor, dullness, oversleeping, uneasiness and unhappiness. Mental fatigue is first felt at the base of the back of the neck.

Physical fatigue is mainly felt in the structural body. When the system dries up and the limbs and the nerves fail to respond due to want of strength, indigestion or constipation, physical fatigue results

Both mental and physical fatigue can be lessened by practising the *āsana* that rest and rejuvenate body, brain and mind. Wrapping the eyes in *āsana* like *Adho Mukha Vṛkṣāsana,* rope *Śīrṣāsana*, forward bends, backbends with support of a chair or back bender, *Sarvāṅgāsana* with the help of a chair, half *Halāsana* and *Śavāsana* with elevated chest and weights on the legs are very effective in removing both types of fatigue.[1] It has to be practised for at least two weeks increasing the time of stay in each *āsana*.

Find the reason behind the fatigue, and adjust *āsana* and *prāṇāyāma* accordingly.

We are psychosomatic beings. It is difficult to demarcate between the psycho and the soma. I often say, where the body awareness ends, there the mind awareness begins. It is the same with physical and mental fatigue. If fatigue in the body is explicit, the mind gets implicitly involved and vice-versa.

VIII.10. – How to begin practice after sickness or injury

We teach children to learn the ABC's and gradually make them learn all the letters of the alphabet before they are made to read. In the same way, if something happens to me and I miss the practice for a month, I will not jump foolishly to start where I stopped a month ago. I have to start as a beginner with simple *āsana* and gradually tone the body, and then add a few difficult ones to re-educate my cells and fibres to get back the rhythm. When I know that my body is ready to shift into a strong practise, I go back to my original standard of practice.

When the body gets trained, toned and tuned, then anyone can go to the optimum level of practice. If the body refuses to respond, one should not use force. If a child is 'haughty' or 'naughty' and the parents are strict, does the child heed their advice? They cool down and try to sober the child. Similarly, our body is our child. We have to behave skilfully and adjust according to conditions and needs with both admonishment and cajolement. This way we can come back soon to our original standard of practice. As the mother follows the baby, let the mother, the mind, go with its child, the body, and later see that the body (child) follows the dictates of the mind (mother). This means the body is tuned to do complicated *āsana*.

[1] See Plate n. 66, p. 315 for examples of eye wrapping

A sculptor sculpts the stone carefully to bring out the figure. A woodcutter carefully cuts the wood and carves artistic designs. We as practitioners of *āsana* or *prāṇāyāma* have to follow the same way to learn the subtleties of the subject. We have to sculpt the mind and carve the body for response and challenge. When one wants to learn dance or music, or any form of art, is it possible to perform perfectly the moment the master begins to guide? It requires gradual practice with patience.

If body is not prepared and he forces his practice, then he suffers pain and aches and loses interest, so think, listen to the sound or vibrations of the body and practice. Then interest sets in and one will not skip or escape from practice on one pretext or another.

As back bends are difficult to do at once I restart the backbends carefully and judiciously and build them up gradually without pain or lack of interest. I shall observe the same attitudes for forward bends, and in course of time intensify all. But I will not oscillate my thoughts.

Therefore judicious balance in thinking and acting is needed to practise when a gap or hindrance comes in any *sādhanā*.

If this happens to me, I start from the simple *āsana* and judge the progress I make, and then extend my mind to proceed towards the complex *āsana* like backbends, twists and forward bends, or I begin with forward bends, twists and backbends, or start with twists, backbends, then do *Adho Mukha Vṛkṣāsana, Pincha Mayūrāsana, Adho Mukha Śvānāsana* and then forward bends, ending up with *Śavāsana* to clear my doubts on practice after injury or sickness.

VIII.11. – Difference between a healthy and an un-healthy pain in *āsana*

Sitting on a chair for a long time creates discomfort for many and so they move forward or turn to the sides. Often one puts an effort while doing an *āsana,* if the felt pain is soothing, then that pain is healthy. If the same pain persists and irritates even after the practice, that pain is unhealthy and wrong pain. We have to learn and find means to transform this wrong unhealthy pain into a right healthy pain. One has to wait in the *āsana* and trace how the pain occurred. Then, analyse the painful part with the non-painful part of the same areas. Then he realises that the non-painful part has more space and freedom than the painful part, which felt compression, or disturbance. A little tolerance to stay in the *āsana* is required to study the pain. Unfortunately, if pain occurs we give up the *āsana* instead of studying it. Let us bear that pain. In order to bear the pain, one has to relax the temples on both sides. This releases the tension of the brain cells and the unbearable pain becomes a bearable pain. When it becomes bearable then analysis is possible. Start analysing the corresponding part and learn to adjust the muscles to find the means of healing by studying the functions of those muscles in the counter parts. Then the unbearable pain transforms into a good pain, which can be transformed into a soothing healthy pain by right adjustment.

VIII.12. – Need of subtle adjustments for progression in *āsana*

If one has to progressively proceed in learning, then attention is needed to catch the missing points for subtle adjustments in each *āsana.* it can happen if one develops the way of watching attentively so that he can judge by trial and error and decide to reach a right approach for decision making.

In the beginning, confidence is needed to gain stability. One can reach stability through adjustments in action and pursue that action to learn to reach a perfect *āsana.*

There are various stages to undergo training. Commencement to learn *(ārambhāvasthā)* is the first one. Then comes intent and endeavour *(ghaṭāvasthā).* From here one has to be intimate with the practice to gain knowledge *(paricayāvasthā)* by acquainting both the intellect *(vidyā)* and intelligence *(buddhi)* to reach the final stage namely consummation *(niṣpattyāvasthā).* The practitioner (doer), the instrument *(buddhi)* and the object (*āsana*) has to become one in the *sādhanā.* Then that *sādhanā* is pure *sādhanā.*

One has to aim to reach this level. One has to begin to learn from the gross skeletal body. By this the body gets toned, understanding sets in and intelligence starts to vibrate for adjustments and readjustments till the final goal of the *āsana* is reached.

Here, I would like to tell you a story from a *Purāṇa.* Once a very dull and insensitive pupil was brought to a *guru* by his mother. The *guru* knew about his dullness and he entrusted him with a simple job of taking the cows to graze daily and made him eat food with neem leaves, which taste bitter. The pupil went on eating his food for months with neem leaves without complaining of its bitterness. One day, he came to his *guru* and asked him, "Why is the food so bitter today Sir?" For this the *guru* became immensely happy, and said, "From today on, you are not going to get this food as you are fit to learn now". Then the *guru* commenced teaching him, as he recognised the sensitive development in his pupil's body and grey matter of the intellect in his head.

For the practitioners of yoga the four stages that were explained earlier act as a handy reference to make progress in practice. *Āsana* bakes the body for it to take proper shapes in positioning so that it begins to communicate with the mind. This is *ghaṭāvasthā*. The mind brings the intelligence to help further in learning. This is *paricayāvasthā*. As one introduces a new person and then become friends on their own, intelligence begins to cooperate while practising *āsana (saṁvedanā)*. Here the body gets yoked to the mind and the mind to the intelligence and finally the intelligence to the Self *(saṁyoga)*.

Finally the intelligence leads the practitioner to feel the presence of the self in each area of the body. Through this feel of self witnessing each area suggestions arise for new adjustments to do *āsana* in a better way as well as in the right way. This is the last stage of learning *(niṣpatty'avasthā)*. In this state, one earns judiciously the rhythm, balance, accuracy and precision in action, and by this he makes the Self to witness the *āsana*. Often yogis and saints call their actions as actions from the inner voice of the self or intuitive knowledge.

VIII.13. – Is there an *āsana* to make one happy

I am happy in any *āsana;* I do not demarcate. If I demarcate I am neither an artist nor a yogi. A *sādhaka* should have a choiceless and non-conditional mind in his *sādhanā*.

If an artists or musicians have choices, then they cannot be considered as true artists. It is the same for a yogi. If he has a choice, then he is not what he claims to be.

For me, any *āsana* whether it is simple or complex, I enjoy and feel the joy of practising and staying. If one asks for seeking happiness, as per his conditional mind, I may give a sequence here, but know that one should not do for the sake of pleasure to satisfy the organs of action senses of perception and mind. The *sādhanā* is to experience non-pollutable and non-alloyed bliss.

1) *Uttānāsana* (resting head on a small stool).

2) *Adho Mukha Śvānāsana* (fingers touching the wall and head on a bolster),

3) *Śīrṣāsana* with props. As there is no load on the neck, it soothes the brain. Independent *Śīrṣāsana* may strain the neck as many cannot stay in this *āsana* with ease and comfort.
4) *Dvi Pāda Viparīta Daṇḍāsana* on a cot with head on floor.
5) *Sarvāṅgāsana* with support of the chair.
6) *Halāsana* with legs resting on stool.
7) *Setu Bandha Sarvāṅgāsana* on a long bench of one foot wide, but neck on floor, with a pillow or bolster to rest the head.
8) *Bharadvājāsana* and *Utthita Marichyāsana*
8) *Śavāsana.*

All these *āsana* calm and satisfy the mind. These may take about forty-five minutes.

Know that these sequences are for health and happiness, but yoga *sādhanā* is meant to go beyond the frame of just health and happiness.

Practising beyond the frame of one's thoughts and mind leads him to the spiritual bliss and those who do within the frame of the mind end up in sensual happiness.

VIII.14. – About *Sālamba Śīrṣāsana*

Śīrṣāsana means balancing on the head by placing the top most part of the head on the floor which may vary between four to five centimetres. Watch *Tāḍāsana* and study the position of the head and space between the ears, neck and shoulders. Do *Sālamba Śīrṣāsana,* retaining the space between the shoulders and the ears as in *Tāḍāsana* and adjust the inner and outer banks of the deltoids to remain parallel to the ground as well as with each other. In *Sālamba Śīrṣāsana* observe the line from the centre point of the crown of the head to the middle of the arches of the feet. Attend to the lateral side of the body and ascend them to be in par with the centre of the body as in *Tāḍāsana.* To know whether the crown of the head is on the floor or not in *Śīrṣāsana,* watch the tip of the nose which has to run parallel from the inner end of the tip to the outer end of it and shoulders and shoulder blades at even level.

Do not droop the upper arms, allowing them to rest on the lower arms. Keep the energy of the lower arms holding the floor and upper arms ascending towards the trunk. This adjustment distributes the body weight evenly between the head and forearms. Suck in the spine in that upright position by holding the back of the thoracic dorsal skin close to the sternum. Refer to

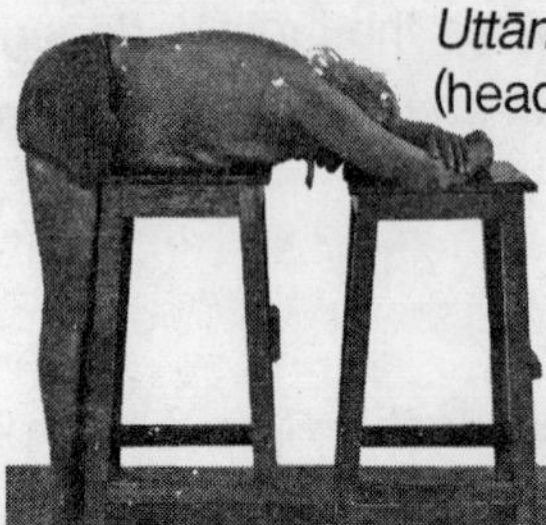

Uttānāsana
(head resting head on a stool)

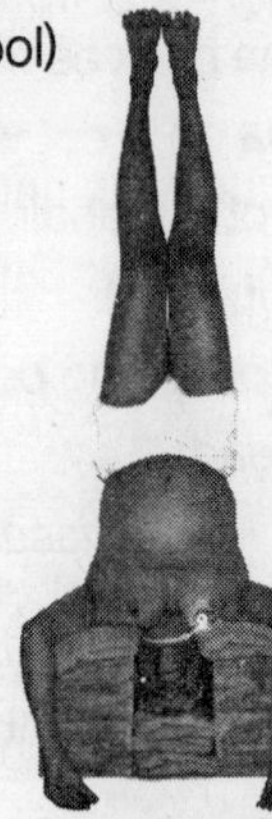

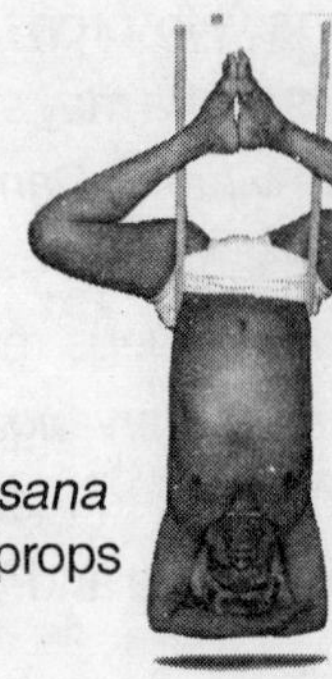

Śīrṣāsana
with props

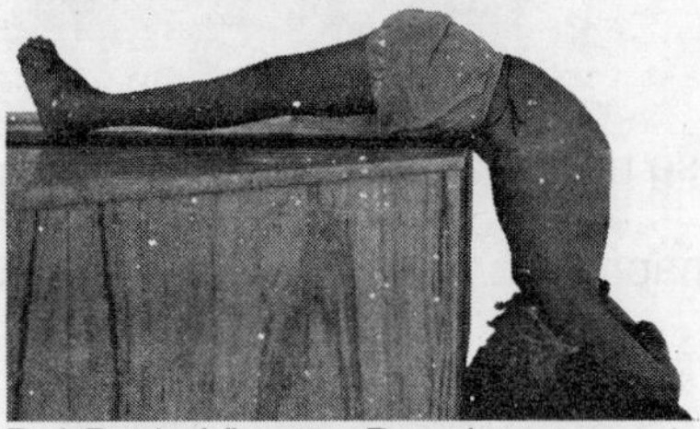

Dvi Pāda Viparīta Daṇḍāsana
on a cot with head on floor

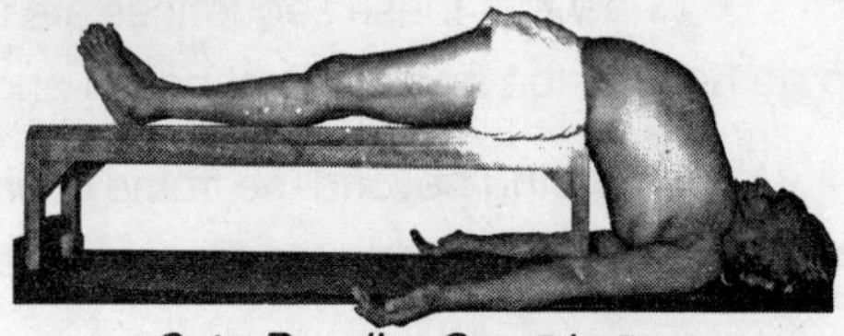

Setu Bandha Sarvāṅgāsana
on a long bench

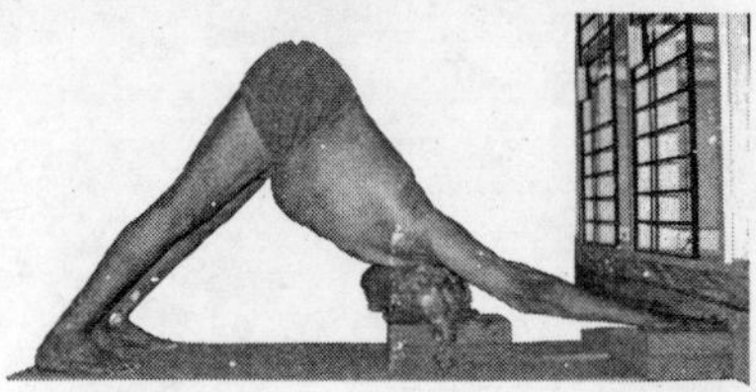

Adho Mukha Śvānāsana

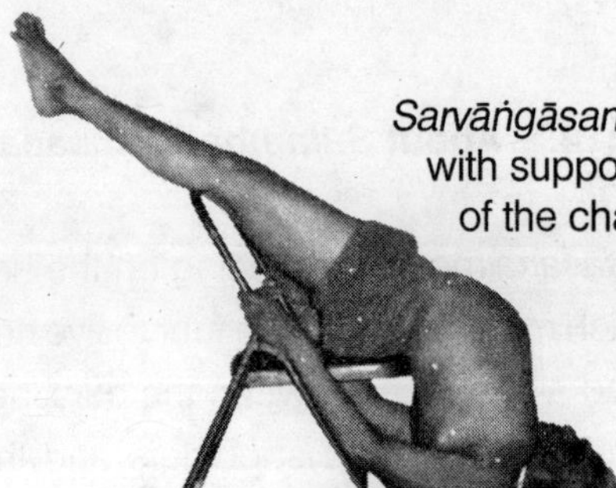

Sarvāṅgāsana
with support
of the chair

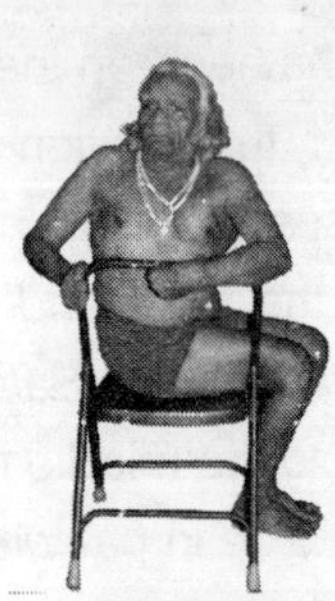

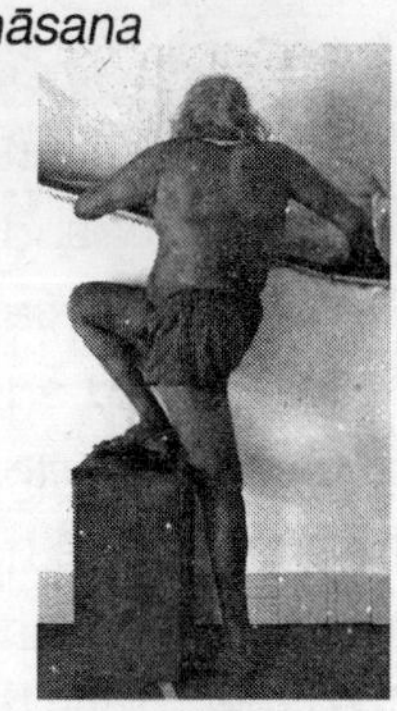

Bharadvājāsana and
Utthita Marichyāsana

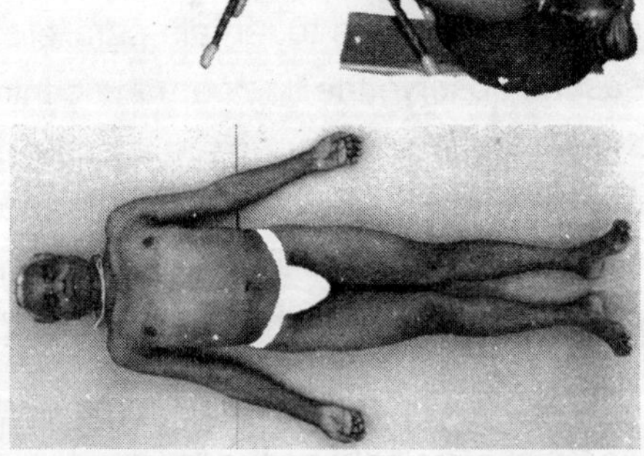

Śavāsana

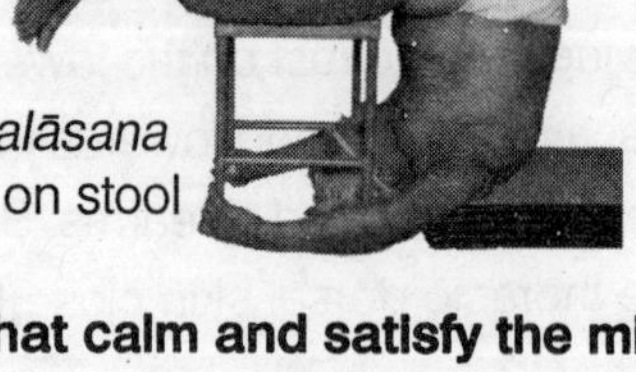

Halāsana
with legs resting on stool

Plate n. 48 – *Āsana* that calm and satisfy the mind

Light on Yoga and study the position to learn well. If one is a beginner, it is better to learn from a trained teacher.

In *Sālamba Śīrṣāsana,* though the fingers are interlocked, the moment one takes the head down the lower arms shorten. Therefore press the elbows and extend the lower arms dividing between the wrists and elbows and form a tripod. This helps to extend the arms in maintaining their stretch and length. In the presentation of the *asana,* the movement of the skin and flesh should not vary. The sense of touch on the inside as well as outside of the arms must be even. Ascend the arms and adjust the sides of the body to be at par with the centre body. This helps the spine to gain better balance. Awareness should be equal on all parts of the body. The nail corners of the big toes should stretch evenly and remain alert and active. Remember to rest the elbows in line with the outer width of the shoulders. Then weightlessness in *Śīrṣāsana* is experienced.

Also watch the imprint of the head, which gets marked on the blanket or a mat. One can see that dent imprinted on one side and on the other side the imprint on the blanket or the mat does not show that . This means that right at the start the centre of the head and the circumference around the centre of the head were not placed properly. The imprint of the circle of the head should be evenly printed and circularly visible.

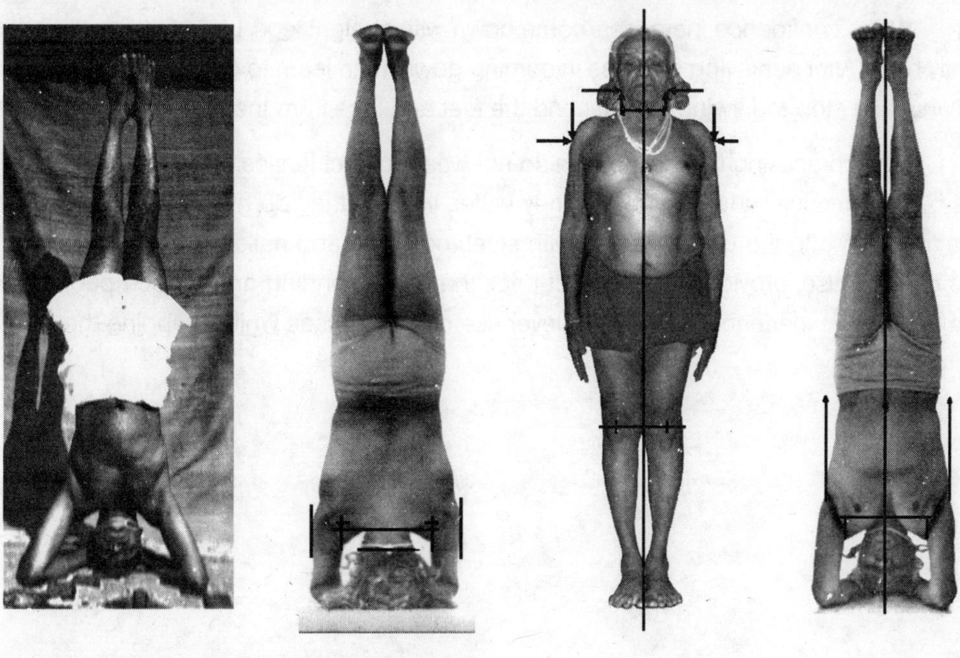

Plate n. 49 – About the balance of *Śīrṣāsana*

In case one wishes to balance *Sālamba Śīrṣāsana* on his own, he can use the corners of the wall so that the side walls protect and guide for the right position. For this he can ask someone at home to lift his legs. When the balance is acquired with confidence, then learn the art of going up or coming down. First learn to come down as the legs move with the current. Flex the knees, bend them towards the abdomen and lower the legs to the floor. Only remember not to bang the knees on the floor but to unlock the knees and bring the foot down to touch the floor. When confidence is gained to come down, then learn to go up placing the head six inches away from the wall. (Wall is to gain confidence.) In case you are not sure, learn from the teacher. Going up is against gravity. That is why one needs a teacher's help. Sometimes, if you feel you are losing the balance, do not struggle to hold the *āsana* but lower the legs one by one and let the bottom feet touch the floor. Then the knees will not get injured.

I suggest to not come down with straight legs at first. One way of learning to go up and down is to go close to the wall and take one leg after the other. The other way is to bend at the knees and swing the legs to go up. While reaching half way, keep the spine erect, tuck in the buttocks and ascend the bent knees. When the bent knees face the ceiling, stretch, extend and straighten the legs to be perpendicular to the floor. Similarly, come down with bent knees, tucking back the buttocks and rolling the spine, lower the knees towards the abdomen and bring the feet to the floor. This is the way to learn going up and down in *Sālamba Śīrṣāsana.*

When confidence increases, come down with straight legs, by first taking the buttocks slightly back. After achieving success in coming down, then learn to go up with a swing on the legs and later stop the swing and ascend the feet and legs from the ground without jerks.

While practising inverted *asana* do not wear contact lenses. Some feel irritation in the eyes by the pressure and sometimes they water. In case they do not bother the eyes, then I leave the choice to the users. People with steel rods, wire and nails in legs, spine, chest and arms can practise, provided they do not prick the corresponding areas. Such people should learn from well-experienced teachers. Never use contact lenses while wrapping the eyes with a bandage.

1st: Learning close to the wall taking one leg after the other

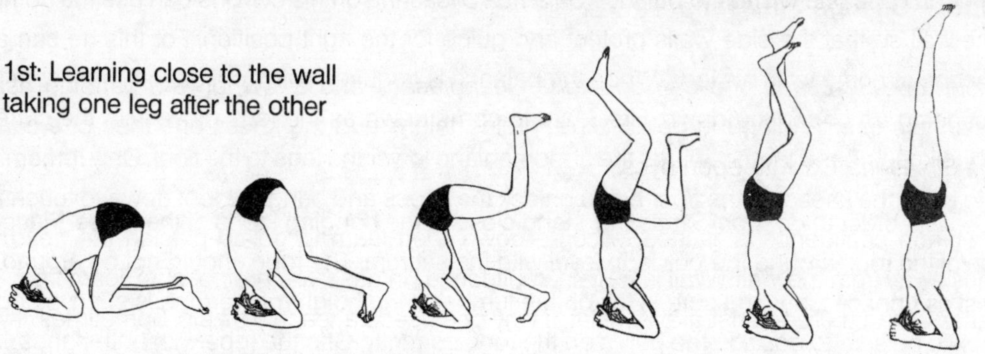

Next: Learn to go up away from the wall keeping both legs together but bent

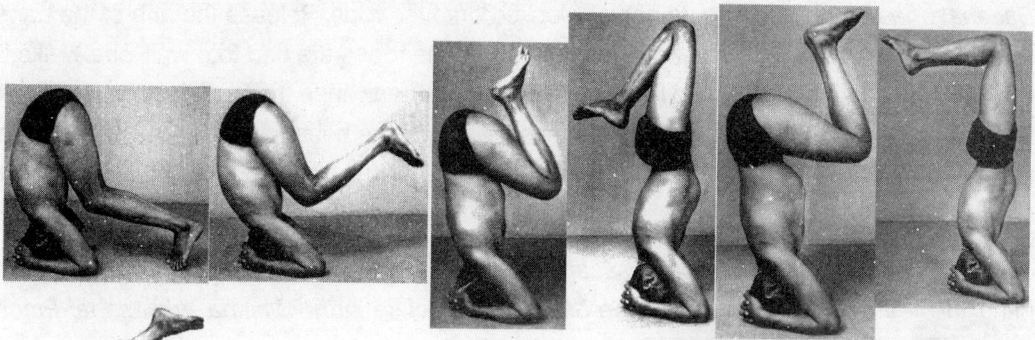

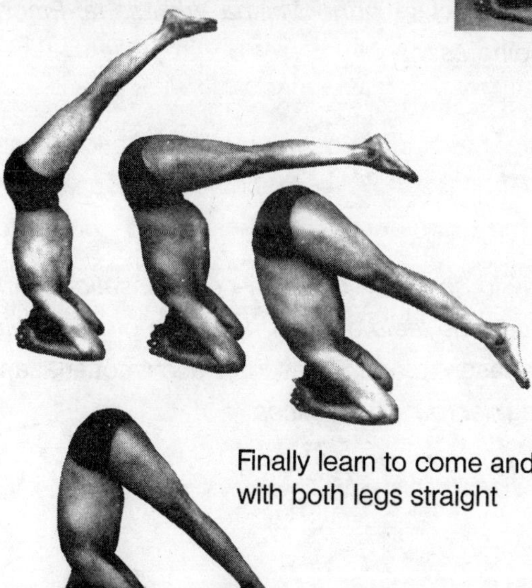

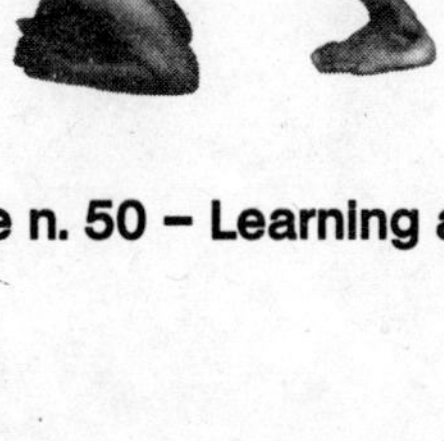

Finally learn to come and go with both legs straight

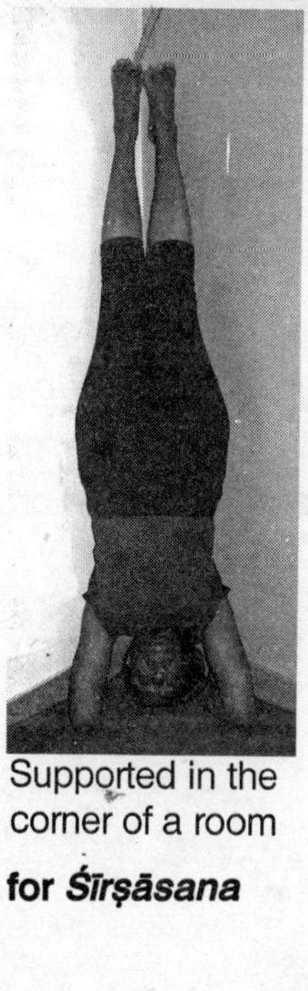

Supported in the corner of a room

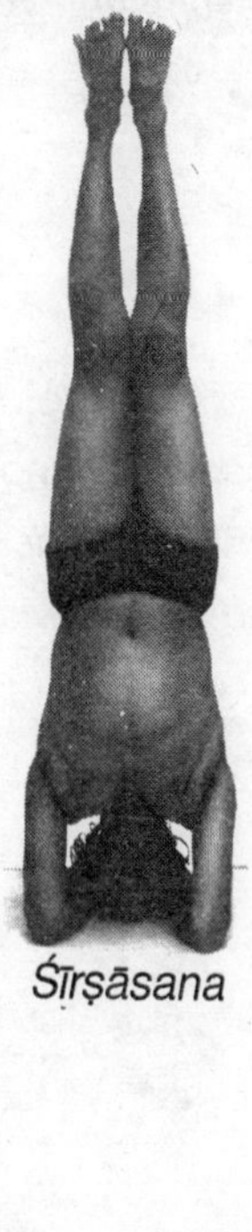

Śīrṣāsana

Plate n. 50 – Learning and increasing confidence for *Śīrṣāsana*

VIII.15. – On rope-*Śīrṣāsana*

Before rope-*Śīrṣāsana* one can do *Ardha Chandrāsana* and a few forward bending *āsana*. These help in extending the pelvic joints, groins, thighs and the knees and then one can do rope-*Śīrṣāsana*. Do with open eyes.

In order to do rope-*Śīrṣāsana*, stand close to the hanging loops of the ropes. Place the loop of the rope around the pelvis, in level with the sacrum. The rope should not be around the waist as unnecessary pressure is felt on the lumbar. If the height of the rope is short, stand on a box to be sure to position the pelvis on the rope correctly. Grip the rope with both hands, lean backwards and swing both legs up, spreading them apart wider than the ropes. Then entwine the legs around the rope, like *Baddhakoṇāsana* position. By circling the rope with the legs in *Baddhakoṇāsana*, the body gets actually locked onto the rope. Release the grip of the hands and extend the arms overhead (towards the floor). If the ropes are tied to a wall, one walks up the wall rather than swinging the legs up, and one either entwines the feet around the ropes or keeps the legs straight. On account of the suspension of the head in space, one may develop fear. In such case use two or three bolsters for the head to rest on them, then the fear goes and confidence comes to stay in the *āsana*.

To come back from *rope-Śīrṣāsana*, grip the rope with the hands, unwrap the legs and bring the feet to the floor. After *rope-Śīrṣāsana* practise *Adho Mukha Vṛkṣāsana, Pincha Mayūrāsana, Adho Mukha Śvānāsana* and standing *āsana*.

Note: *In rope-*Śīrṣāsana, *some are likely to get dizzy, or an icy-cold sensation in the head. Do* Adho Mukha Vīrāsana, *at once, whether one feels dizzy or not. Then proceed with forward bends like* Uttānāsana, Adhomukha Śvānāsana, Jānu Śīrṣāsana, Paśchimottānāsana *and lateral twists. Afterwards, switch on to the regular routine practices.*

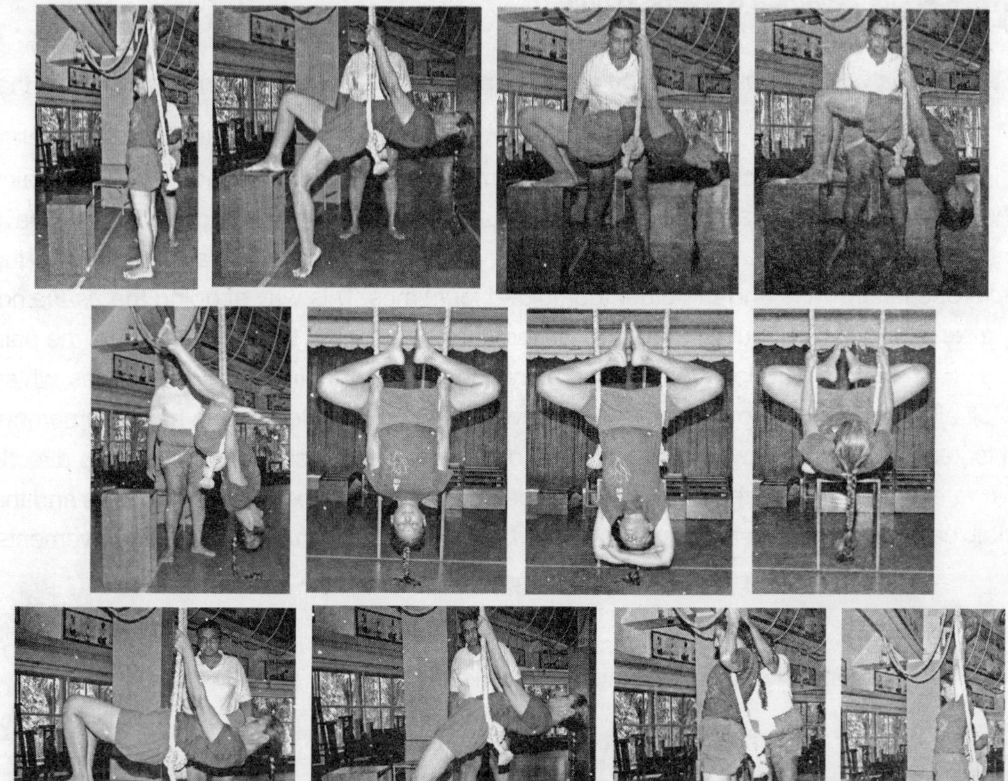

Plate n. 51 – Comming and going to Rope *Śīrṣāsana*

VIII.16. – About *Sālamba Sarvāṅgāsana*

In *Sālamba Sarvāṅgāsana,* many may get neck pains as the cervical spine cannot take that curvature needed for learning this *āsana.*

In my years of practice and teaching I came across numbers of people who got pains in their necks. I devised ways of performing this *āsana* without pain. I made those who have short necks, or cervical pain to do *Sālamba Sarvāṅgāsana,* using five blankets, placing the bottom one length-wise and the other four folded four times. This way of doing the *āsana* not only extended their neck but also gave relief from their neck pains. Even then in some the pain persisted. I prepared wooden wedges and placed them under their trapezium muscles, which took off all pains. This is the way has to learn even with neck problems. One has to remember well to keep the outer elbows in line with the outer shoulders. Pressurise the elbows directly downwards to manipulate the back ribs. Feel the sense of rhythm between the elbows and the back. In case of doubt, look at the plates of *Light on Yoga* and carefully observe all movements.

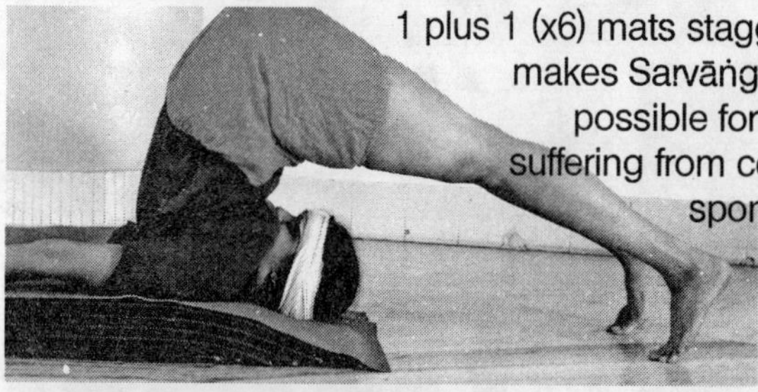

1 plus 1 (x6) mats staggered makes Sarvāṅgāsana possible for those suffering from cervical spondylitis

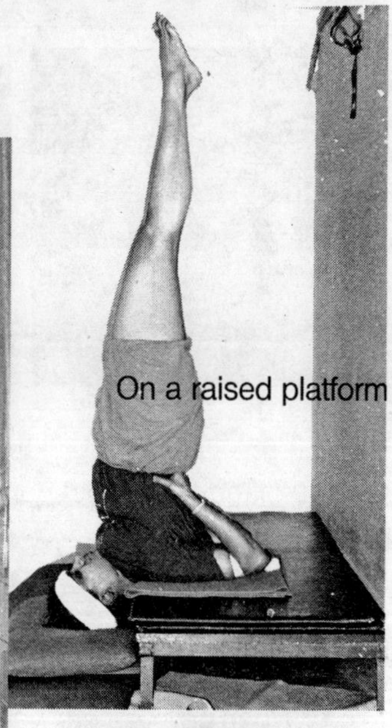

On a raised platform

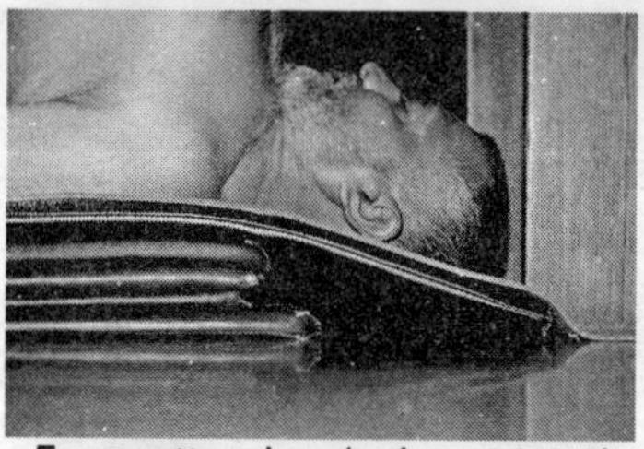

5 x matts plus 1 elongates the neck

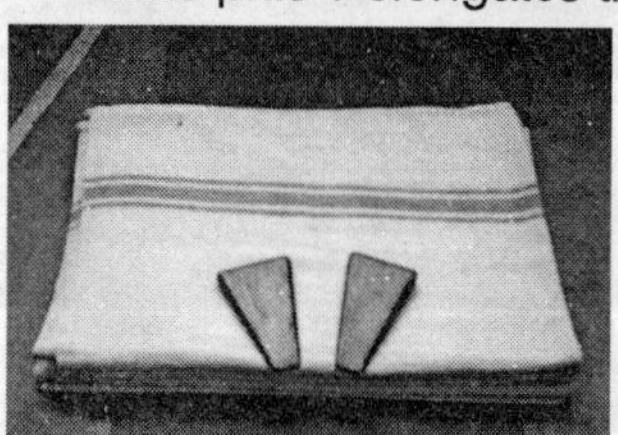

Wooden wedges under the trapeziums

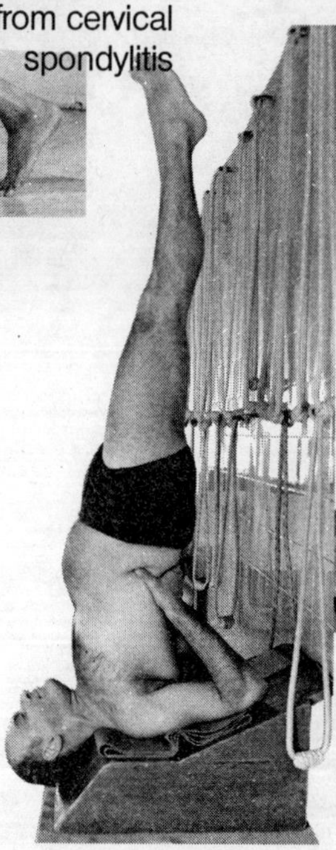

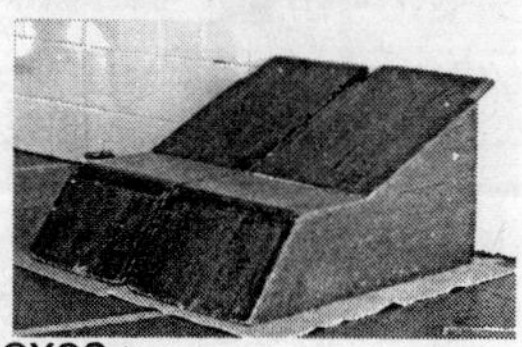

On 2 x *Simhāsana* boxes

Plate n. 52 – Preparations for relief of neck pain in *Sālamba Sarvāṅgāsana*

The famous *purāṇic* hermit Dattātreya had sixty-four teachers. He learnt from everyone, including the lowest of the low creatures. I took his clue and learnt the right action in *āsana* by looking at the movements of men and animals. Similarly, I advise you to look at your colleagues who unknowingly place their limbs in the right order. Catch their hairline adjustments and work by imitating their adjustments on the body. This acts as an eye opener to become a better practitioner and perform with self-awareness.

VIII.17. – Use of props

Many yoga practitioners are under the impression that the props I use are a central theme in my practice and teaching. It is not true. See my book *Light on Yoga* where I have presented all *āsana* without props except in *Sālamba Sarvāṅgāsana* where I showed use of a prop for those who were unable to practise properly.

Realising that genuine teachers are going to be rare, I evolved various props to make practitioners learn without teachers and at the same time not commit mistakes in their practices. Secondly, as many cannot reach that accurate precision in the *āsana*, I thought of alternative ways of not only protecting them from injuries but also of perfecting *āsana* by the use of pillows, blankets, blocks, belts, trestle and back bending planks. Finally, know that these act as a self-guide, self help in self-practice.

Basically, a practitioner without props does not have the sense of direction or he is unaware of the tilts that occur in *āsana*. Props correct such mistakes without the waste of time and energy.

In one's normal walk of life, he sits, stands, walks or drives and has the sense of direction. But on the giant wheel or a merry-go-round, he loses the sense of direction.

When newcomers want to learn *āsana*, they have no sense of direction. Take for example, *Parivṛtta Trikoṇāsana*. It takes a long time to understand the correct positioning of the left leg with the left arm, left abdomen with right arm, front and back of the torso on account of its revolving action.

Suppose one is doing *Śīrṣāsana*, the head is on the floor and legs are in the air. One does not know whether his feet are in the middle or swayed, to the right or left, or forward or backward. He may be using the stronger side for balance and not thinking of the weaker side and how it needs to be attended. When he does it on the ropes, he is not likely to go forward or backward or sideways. Similarly, when he does it against the corner of the wall, he remains parallel to the corner of the wall. Here the wall acts as a guide or a *guru* for him to know which way the body is tilting. In this *āsana,* one does not know whether the back has moved forward or the legs tilted or straight, but with the help of props not only the vestibular balance, but also the sense of direction for stability, the inner contact, connections and interrelations surface. Students who go for meditation are asked to close their eyes. Many become nervous and feel as if they are lost. *Āsana* practice done with the help of props gives a sense of direction creating courage to face the space.

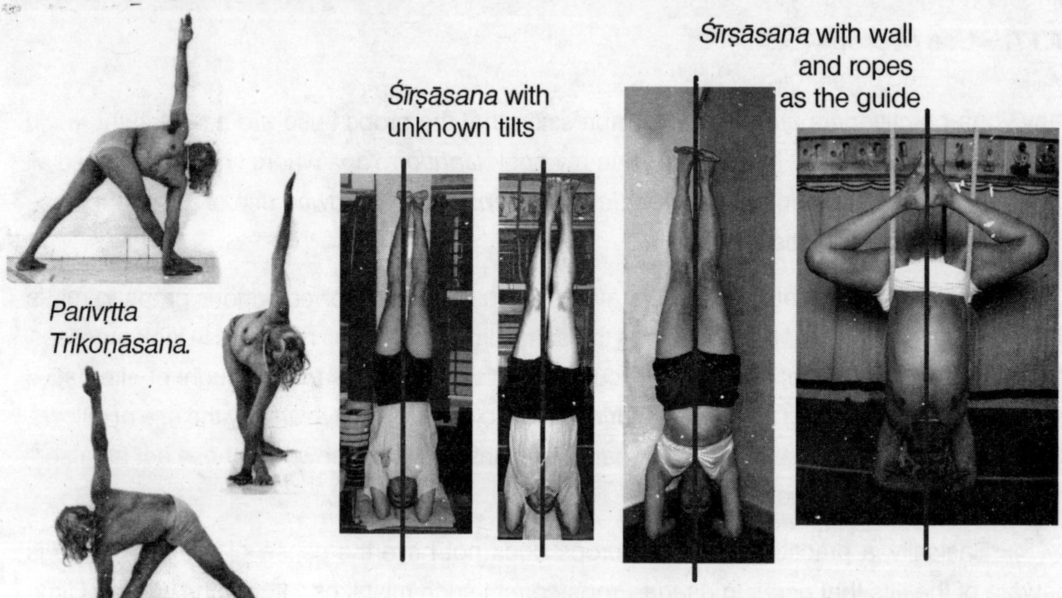
Parivṛtta
Trikoṇāsana.
Śīrṣāsana with
unknown tilts
Śīrṣāsana with wall
and ropes
as the guide

Note: The student in the wall-corner has a scoliosis, here the corner helps her to keep the teet, navel, throat and eyebrow in one straight line

Plate n. 53 – Props to give a sense of direction and create courage

So, props can be used by the practitioners for building up confidence and gaining control over the body, as well as a sense of direction. The moment these things are acquired, then my advice for them is to do independently and give up the props. Sometimes use the props and the wall as a threshold playing between dependency and independency. Practice with support for sometime and later try to be slightly away from the support, builds up courage to do independently one day. One must use the props to get the right sense of direction, alignment and understanding the *āsana.* When accurate presentation sets in, do independently simulating the feelings that come with the support of props.

Props act as a better *guru* when there is lack of movement, stiffness or instability in the body or in the adjustments of muscles, bones and joints. The props help in increasing the range of extensions, contractions, retractions, protractions, suctions and circumductions and help in reflecting on all these to learn the *āsana* in a shorter time saving one's energy. They initiate actions that are considered to be beyond one's imagination. Compare the movements of extension, expansion and circular action with props to those of the movemehts done independently. Then the importance of the props and their utilities are realised. Unless each one experiences himself, he does not know the value of these props.

Practitioners, who come with physical or mental disabilities, cannot perform independently, but they benefit from props. As in hospitals there are ICU wards, these props monitor the body of the practitioners by not allowing them to go wrong, but make them to experience the sense of well-being, comfort and confidence.

The aged or diseased people with negative mind, benefit by using the props on a permanent basis for their *āsana*. A cardiac patient can do *Setu Bandha Sarvāṅgāsana* on a bench, *Sarvāṅgāsana* with the help of a chair and *Śarapañjarāsana* on a platform to activate the ventricles. Polio patients need a trestle for standing *āsana* or back bends. They even help to learn *Paschimottānāsana*. People who do not dare to do independently can accomplish *āsana* with ease and comfort. Cardiac patients can conveniently do *Sarvāṅgāsana* on the trestle using their legs rather than arms. The person suffering with scoliosis needs to use the belts like a bracelet around the affected areas so that the muscles do not get pushed in wrong directions.

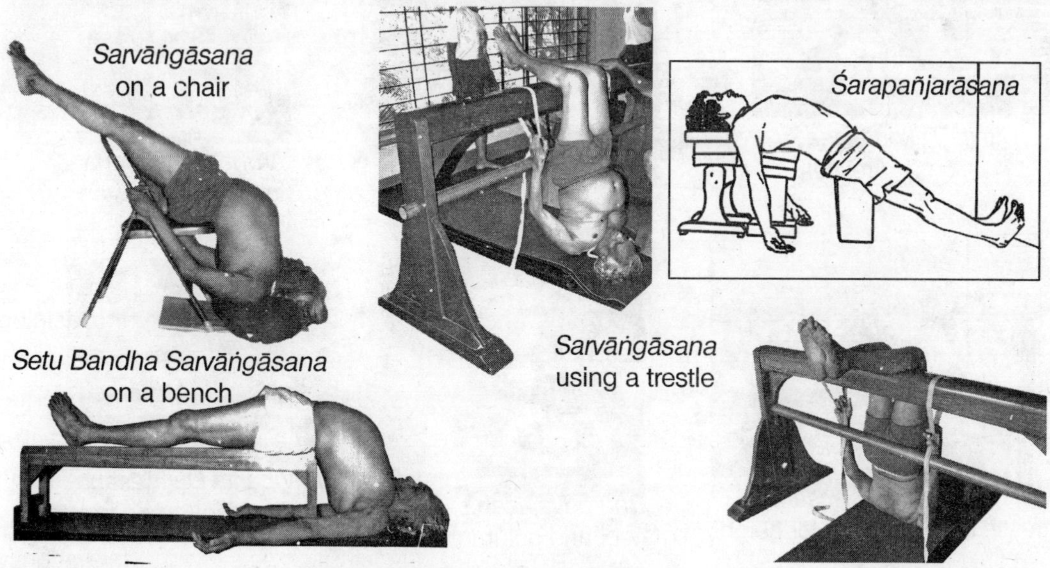

Plate n. 54 – Props as monitors for correct practice

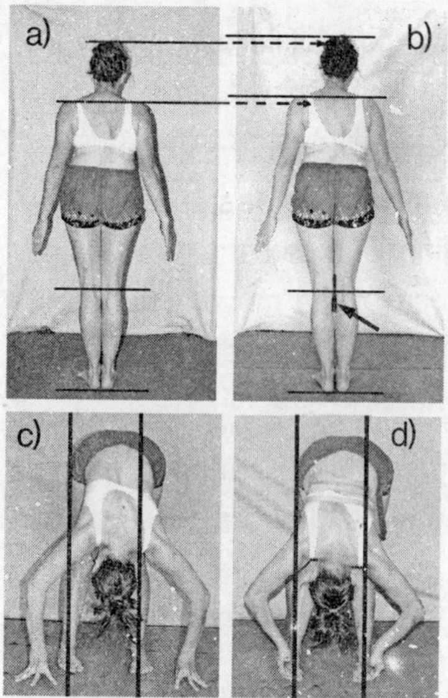

Both a & b are standing with heels on the same line. In fig-b a pad is placed between the inner knees, the result of this inner knee support is a lift of the spine. Note the level of the shoulders and the crown of the head that has increased its height

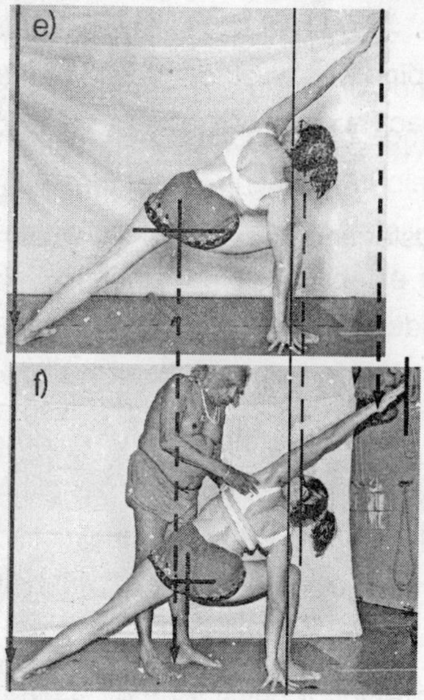

In e & f the belts are again used. See the extension to the whole spine from the tailbone, to the centre of the ear and to the tips of the fingers of the extended left arm. Notice how the spinal muscles work through-out its entire length.

In c & d a line has been drawn through the centre of the feet. d has the belts around the torso. Observe how that restraint bringing the outer body in centralises the spine.

Plate n. 55 – Use of belts for people with scoliosis

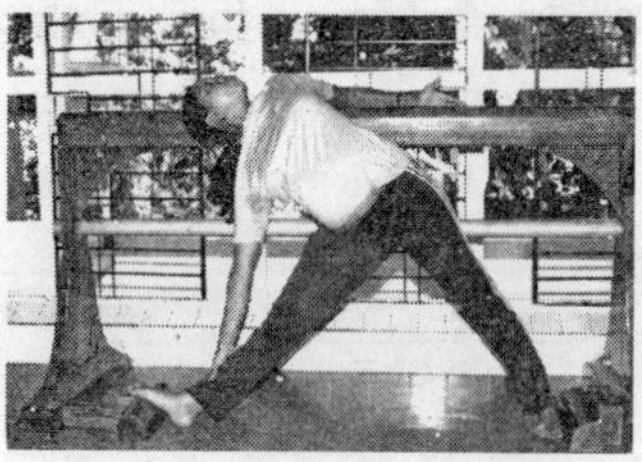

Utthita Trikoṇāsana (trestle)

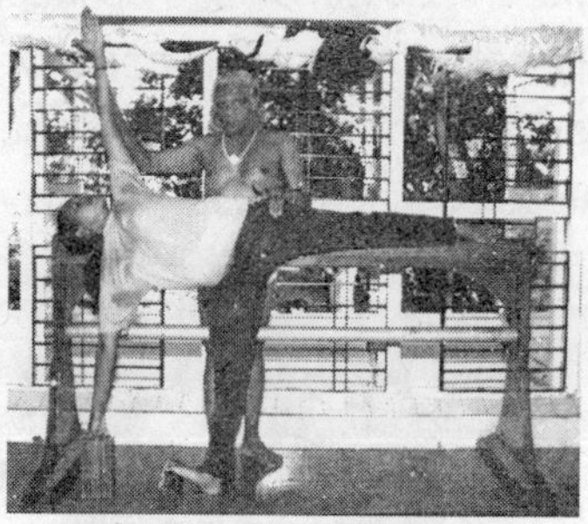

Ardha Chandrāsana (trestle & hand support)

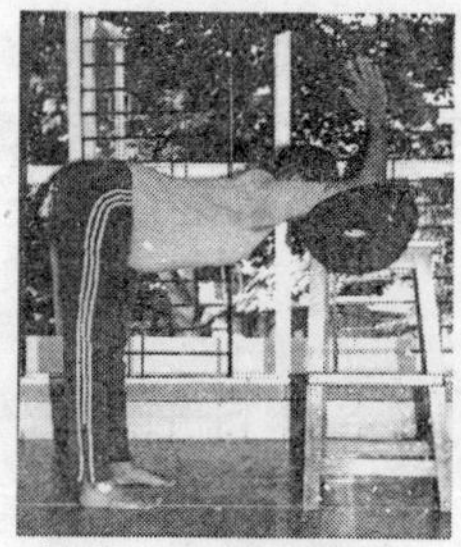

Ardha Uttānāsana (tall stool & bolster)

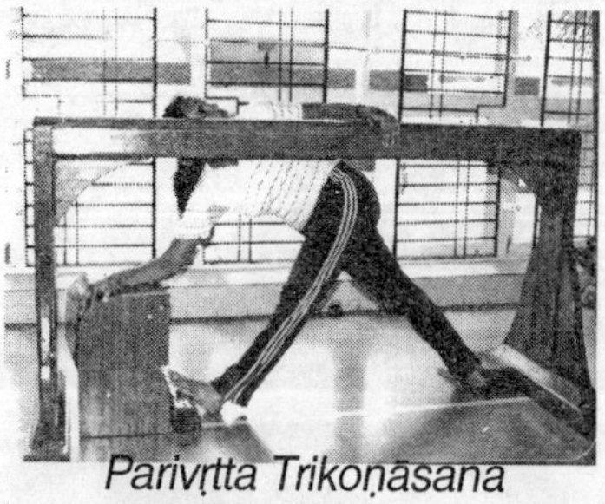

Parivṛtta Trikoṇāsana (trestle and 2 xboxes for height)

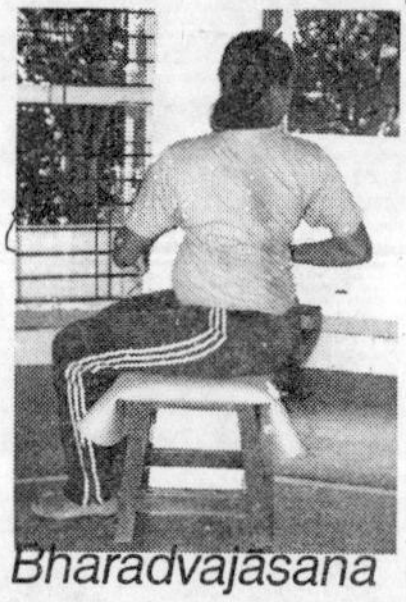

Bharadvajāsana (stool and column)

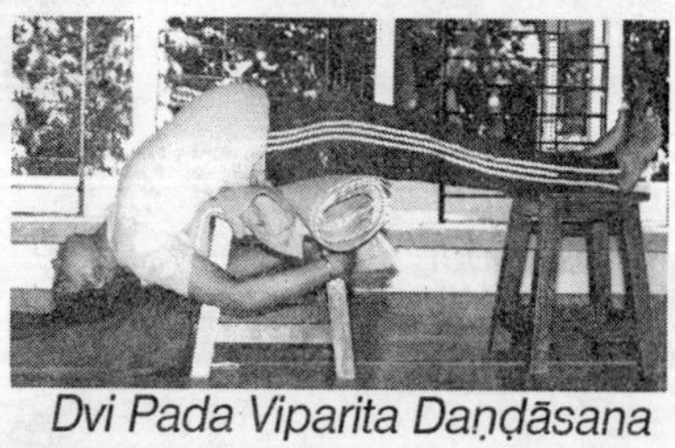

Dvi Pada Viparita Daṇḍāsana (2xstools, head supported on bolster)

Plate n. 56 – Use of props for practice during pregnancy

I had two severe scooter accidents. My shoulders and shoulder joints lost mobility. My spine was twisted. I was forced to take the help of props to get back the correct position of the back and flexibility for practising to the optimum level, which I could not have done independently.

Props help fast recovery from physical or mental fatigue. Afflicted persons recover faster and gain strength and energy.

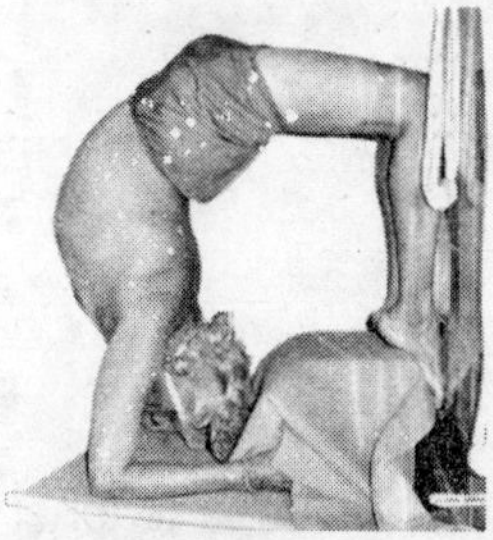

Vṛschikāsana using a box

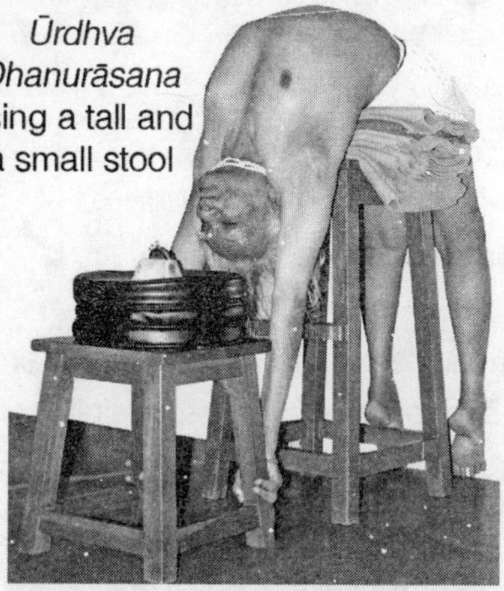

Ūrdhva Dhanurāsana using a tall and a small stool

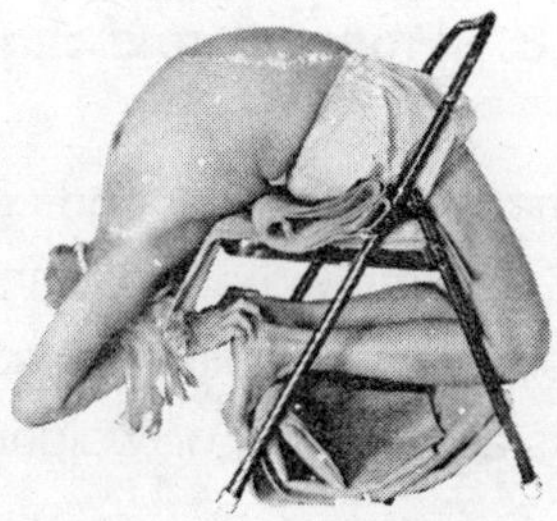

Kapotāsana using a chair

Plate n. 57 – Props for perfecting the challenging *āsana*

Though props are a boon to all, they have a great value especially for women, when they are pregnant or menstruating, or for any type of disorder. Women at the time of pregnancy can use the props to practise *āsana* safely.

The complicating and challenging *āsana* such as *Vṛschikāsana, Kapotāsana, Eka Pāda Rāja Kapotāsana* can be learnt to perfection through props without the sense of strain or stress or fear of injury.

I do not like anyone to depend on them but, use them for educating the body and mind. I continue even now, to think and develop new props. I have not yet lost my creative thinking.

I am now ninety years young, and I happily use the props to retain and sustain my practices rather than escaping them on the pretext of my age. Even at this age my body is strong, my mind is agile and my intelligence is steady and clear.

a) – The importance of props

The most interesting observation of the usage of props is that they allow ninety per cent of the practitioners to stick to their practices. At the Institute, those who perform independently come hours before the class and practice on props and ropes. This shows that props inspire them more towards yoga. Even for *prāṇāyāma* proper support guides one to align the body.

Props not only ignite zeal but also lead one towards a harmless practice without stress and strain. They simultaneously make one to enjoy extension, relaxation and rejuvenation as well as better understanding and right judgment in each *āsana*.

VIII.18. - From where did the usage of props originate

I started yoga in 1934 and circumstances made me become a professional yoga teacher in 1937. Being raw, both in practice and teaching, the responsibility of helping as a teacher was uppermost in my mind. I was searching and trying various means. By using heavy stones and bricks as 'supports' or 'weight bearers' to improve and perfect my own practice.

Often pieces from the stone and bricks used to graze and peel off my skin, yet I was using them to build up tolerance in the body and confidence in the mind to stay in *āsana*. Many of the *āsana* were painful but the weights were minimising the pains. I realised that it is possible to learn many *āsana* by these means, and the word 'prop' came in to vogue later. Sometimes I used walls, windowsills or doorsteps and corners of the walls for *Sālamba Śīrṣāsana:* I created

Storage container wooden planks and grinding stones

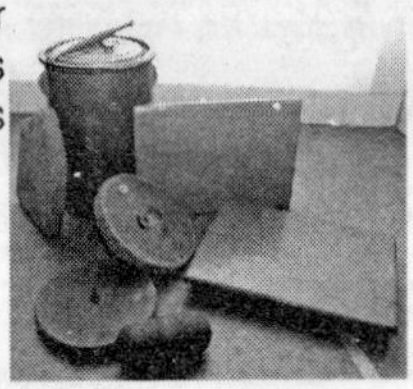

Water storage container for *Viparīta Daṇḍāsana*

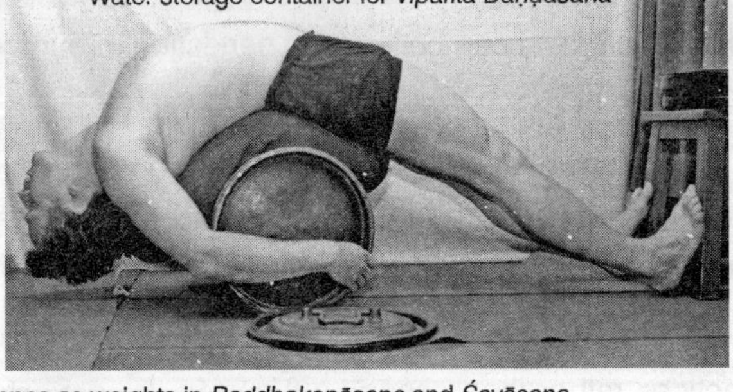

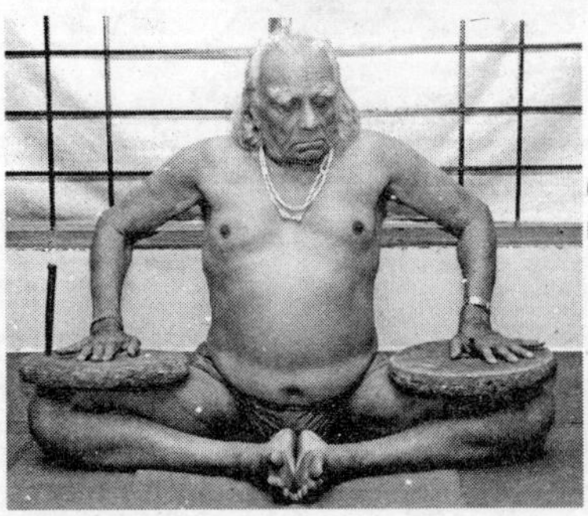

Grinding stones as weights in *Baddhakoṇāsana* and *Śavāsana* rasised wooden plank for chest elevation

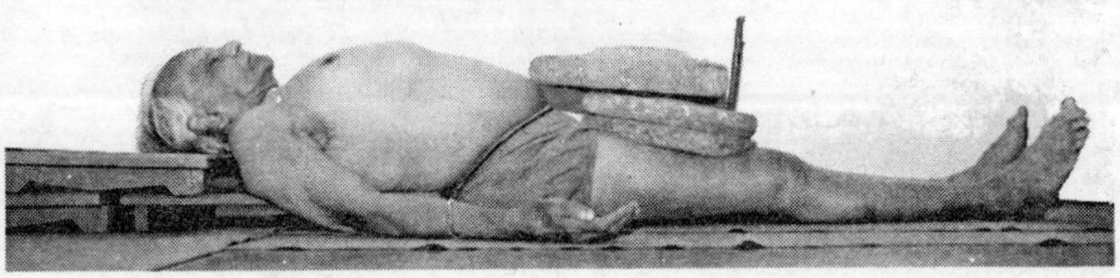

Plate n. 58 - Use of household equipment for practice

space between a door and a cupboard, used rolled mattresses for half *Halāsana*, windowsills for *Utthita* or *Parivṛtta Trikoṇāsana*, doorsteps and upturning a bucket to do *Ūrdhva Dhanurāsana* and so forth; later I used almost all household things, which were handy like chairs, boxes, cots, cupboards, wooden pieces, rollers, grinding stones, hard cover books and pillows. Even I used round drums or a chair to learn *Dvi Pāda Viparīta Daṇḍāsana, Eka Pāda Viparīta Daṇḍāsana, Chakra Bandhāsana* and *Kapotāsana*. Planks were cutting into my back (while trying backbends), but I persevered by changing the position of the plank, the brick or whatever.

After my marriage in 1943, I took a lot of help from my wife. I was asking her to sit or stand on my back explaining how to use a right pressure in forward bends, backbends and twists by showing the use of the arms and feet. Being my wife, she was shy to stand on my back, but I made her stand and I used her arms or feet as 'props', to see how much I could improve the forward bends, twists and backbends in my range. My wife did not know anything about *yogāsana* and, as such, she did not know how and where to help or give exact pressures on which muscle and so forth. It was like a zigzag puzzle for her. Through my assistance and guidance she learnt and continued helping me whenever I needed help. Those pressures helped me think of designs for the good of yogic posterity.

In fact, when I was guiding her to help me, I, at the same time, learnt how to help and grip different bodies; where to support without making them lose their balance. This pressure and help built confidence in me as the students were finding it easy to perform and be free from fear. These things initiated me to think of preparing the correct form or shape of the instruments, which materialised only after the opening of the Institute in 1975. As more and more people began approaching with multiple problems, I felt the necessity of props. In the early days students were benefiting with my personal help. At the Institute people began coming on a mass scale, hence I thought of providing instruments so that all could do at the same time. When the Institute was opened, I was the only teacher attending the morning and evening classes for years. I had only two options left. One was to help using my body as a prop for them to learn, which had its own limitations. The other was to create props for the members to practise on without the feel of pain or tiredness. Props made them to stay longer and longer with comfort. This made me think of various designs of instruments, to evolve ways and means for different *āsana*. At the same time in preparing the props, I had in my mind how to guide the suffering humanity in remedial treatments. All these were weighing in my mind to provide them the light of hope from despair.

I designed shapes for various *āsana* according to the anatomical curvatures and stretches that form in the body. Then I engaged a carpenter and I would test them by performing the *āsana* on the rough unfinished samples, advising him to chop a bit here or to add a bit there for performing rightly. I made him to re-shape each prop several times, until the required final shape was built for the correct presentation of the *āsana*.

The props are highly sophisticated and refined compared to the crude materials I was using at the time of learning myself.

The idea of rope *Śīrṣāsana* was the inspiration of ancient yogis who are said to have performed *Śīrṣāsana* hanging down from the branches of trees. My *guru* was tying ropes on two rings fixed to the wall, which restricted the movements of the body, where one could not stay more than a minute or two. For the full range of action in certain *āsana* through hanging ropes in the middle of the room was my idea. All the props used now like chairs, slanting planks, stools, stumps, bricks, foot rests, ropes, belts, are my innovations.

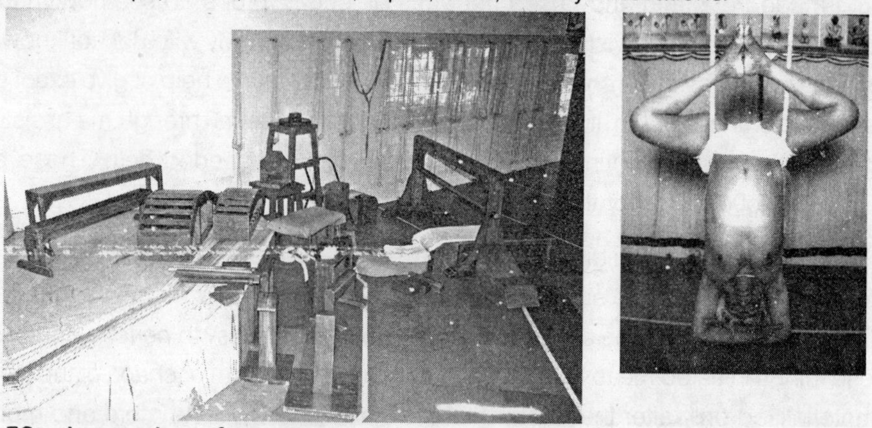

Plate n. 59 – Innovation of props

My *guru* had a hand written book on yoga titled *Yoga Kuranṭa*. *Kuranṭi* means a puppet or a wooden doll. Puppet shows are well known all over the world. *Yoga kuranṭa* is a method wherein one learns to manipulate one's own body in various *yogāsana* by means of a suspended rope, as if he were a puppet. Here the puppeteer and puppet are one, performing their own puppet show.

Bhīṣma, who was hit by arrows in the battle of the *Mahābhārata*, could not move to the side or sit. These symptoms made me think of cardiac attacks. Bhīṣma asked Arjuna to prepare a bed of arrows for him to rest. After studying the position, it struck me that the arrows were supporting the heart cavity, allowing a good circulation of blood through the coronaries, which prolonged his life. Bhīṣma inspired me to make and try its effects on patients of angina and other cardiac problems. I arranged bricks like arrows, which could support the thoracic dorsal spinal vertebrae and the heart muscles of the back protecting the cardiac nerves. I named this *āsana Śarapanjarāsana* or *Bhīṣmācharyāsana*. This became a boon for patients. *Viparīta*

Daṇḍāsana and *Kapotāsana* are the most difficult backbends. For those, I found means so that even the raw beginners can do with ease, without injury or harm. The stump is semicircular at top, the base has a stand and the stem fixed firmly on it for back protection. Here one can keep the legs taut and the feet touching and resting on a wall or a foothold.

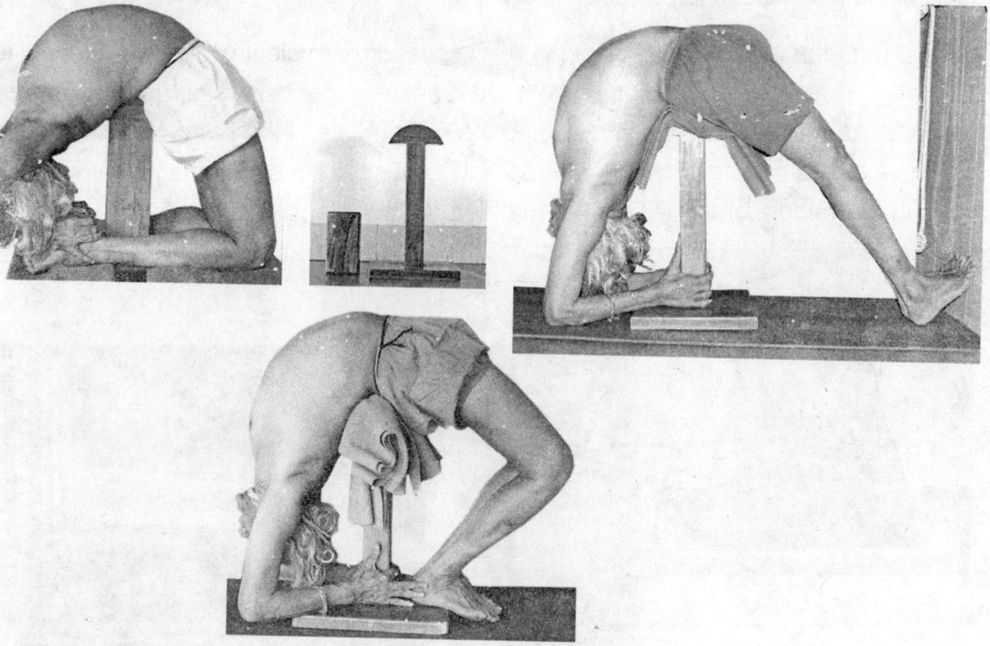

Plate n. 60 – Difficult backbends with the use of the stump

Reading the commentary on the sixth chapter of *Bhagavad Gītā* by Ramanujacharya, I came across the word *sāpāśraya,*[1] meaning hanging on, leaning against, depending upon support. This chapter is on meditation and Ramanujacharya in his commentary mentions to take support to sit for *dhyāna*. This was a moral support for my inventions. I felt that when he permits one to take support for meditation *(dhyāna),* one of the limbs of *aṣṭāṅga yoga,* then why not take the support for *āsana,* another limb of yoga? In fact, his suggestion of support is for the *āsana* in *dhyāna*. One should know that without sitting properly one cannot meditate.

Lord Narasiṁha, the incarnation of Lord Vishnu, is shown in temples as Yogā Narasiṁha with a cloth wrapped around his waist with bent knees and crossed legs. This gave me idea of wrapping the different parts of the body with belts or bandages.

---

[1] Ramanujācharya, while commenting on VI.3 *śloka* of *Bhagavad Gītā,* says, *Kāyaśirogrīvaṁ samaṁ acalaṁ sāpāśrayatayā sthiraṁ dhārayan...* Hold the body, head and neck upright and immovable (steady) taking a slight support.

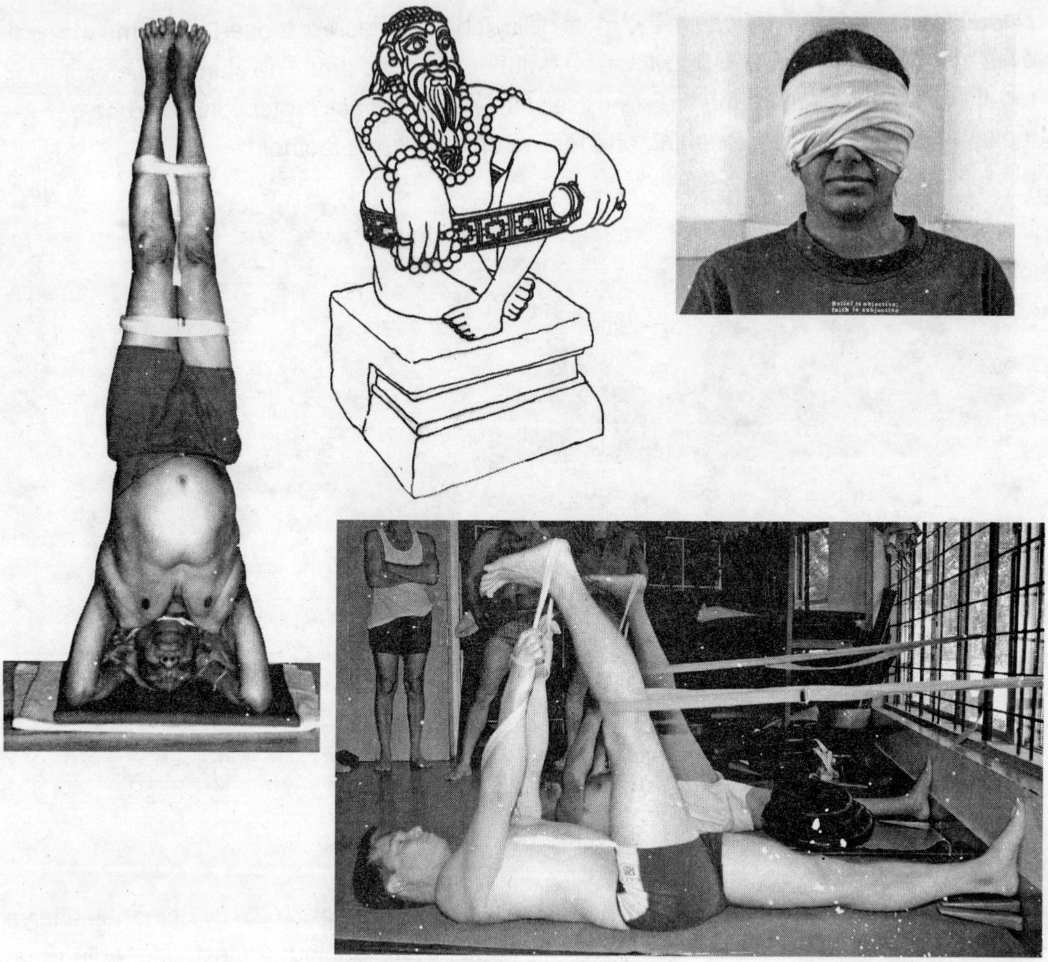

Plate n. 61 – Inspiration from Lord Narasiṁha

J. Krishnamurti used to talk a lot about the idea of alert passivity, saying that great sensitivity is necessary to create that state. As I had this experience in *Ṣaṇmukhī mudrā,* I wrapped his eyes with a necktie creating the same feeling in him. Thinking of Ramakrishna Paramahansa's story with the two *haṭhayogis* who prided before him that they could walk on water, for which the saint (jokingly or seriously) said to them that if a few paisa were given to a boat-man, he could have carried you across, so why waste time on *tapas* just to walk on water. This story came to my mind and instead of struggling to do *Ṣaṇmukhi mudrā,* which brings this alert passivity in the brain, a handkerchief, which may cost a rupee or two, was giving the same condition. Remembering this story, I told *Śrī* Krishnamurthi, "Sir, why use that great sensitivity to reach a state which one can realise it with a handkerchief?" He laughed at me.

Now, talking of the pros and cons of using props, one of the criticisms against me is that one becomes habituated to them and lacks the will to attempt doing independently. Is it the fault of the props? Never have I said to use the props on a permanent basis. I have said to use props as a guide to stop wrong practices. They do not allow one to go wrong and make one live in the correct *āsana*.

I am happy that those who were criticising these innovations are now using and writing articles on how to use, for deriving full benefit, has given me the satisfaction of seeing the usefulness of the props.

VIII.19. – Can one teach without props

In the early 1930s there were never general classes as there are now. I had general classes from 1936 for healthy people as well as in schools and colleges. I was giving private classes for people with physical and physiological problems. The real test of my knowledge began when the disabled, old and diseased started coming to general classes.

Whenever I was teaching privately, I was personally touching and attending to them, using my own body as props. I was getting feedback from their reactions by my support and the benefits for them were enormous. I was supporting them to perform as if I was performing that *āsana*. I never allowed them to go wrong. I was a teacher, patient and an examiner, and I was my own *guru*. I was cross-examining while I was assisting and teaching. I was adjusting my body properly for their needs. I was shaping their bodies as if I were doing the *āsana* for them. I was treating their problems as my own. No doubt, it was energy conserving for them and energy consuming for me. I gained knowledge on these practical experimentations on living anatomical bodies, and it helped me to know the man well. If one can work like me feeling each one individually, I am sure that many may go for other vocations, which are easy and soft.

I could help only limited patients before the Institute came into existence. When the Institute came, it was impossible to reach each and everyone in this manner. I had taught using my body as a support. It helped me to create the best of props for mass usage.

To run big classes at the Institute, I began using chairs, bricks, wooden planks and adjusted those props to fit exactly to each individual's needs. Pupils began performing fearlessly even the most difficult *āsana* like *Ūrdhva Dhanurāsana, Kapotāsana, Vṛśchikāsana* and so forth.

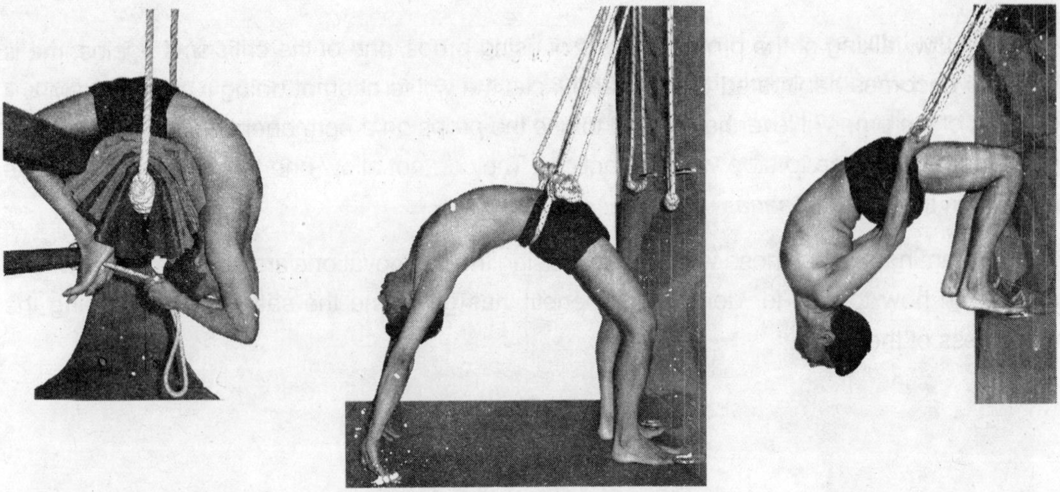

Plate n. 62 – props for fearless performance of difficult *āsana*

What I developed in helping students individually are the insights and the sensitivity in the fingers, arms, legs and toes became a magic touch that heals and exhilarates suffering patients without pain.

The difference between using my body as an instrument and the inert props is like comparing the handling a sentient being with that of a non-sentient object. Now I do guide how to make non-sentient object a sentient being while using props. I used my body with compassionate feeling towards the patients to give them maximum benefits. Only for a short period of time, I used to encourage them to try independently. In this process of teaching, I had to bear considerable pains within myself, as I was in awkward positions, supporting them to get the right positions. Besides pains and aches in my body and fatigue in the brain in teaching, I was cycling 20 miles a day, going place to place. I used to ask my wife to press her foot on my forehead due to this physical and mental fatigue and restlessness in the nerves. I learned through those pressures how to use weights for headache and brain fatigue. I made persons do *Setu Bandha Sarvāṅgāsana* or *Viparīta Daṇḍāsana* using my knees, twisting my feet and arms. I have even used the crown of my head, poking into their backs in backbends.

I have served thousands and thousands of people with my arms, legs and head. Even now when I know that direct help is much more effective than the props, I avoid props in certain cases and I use my body as a prop. I could handle each individual making the whole class of 30 or 40 people to do *āsana* like *Ūrdhva Dhanurāsana, Kapotāsana, Vṛschikāsana,* without injuring anyone. The group was never homogenous, some young, some old, some with physical or mental problems, some strong and some weak, some thin and some fat, yet I made them do these *āsana* adapting my strength and adjusting force according to the needs of each student.

As my present day students haven't seen that, they do not know what capacity and skill I had in those days. It was not only in backbends that I used to help in big classes, but I also helped them personally in balancing, forward bends, twistings and *āsana* like *Yoganidrāsana, Eka Pada Śīrṣāsana* and so forth.

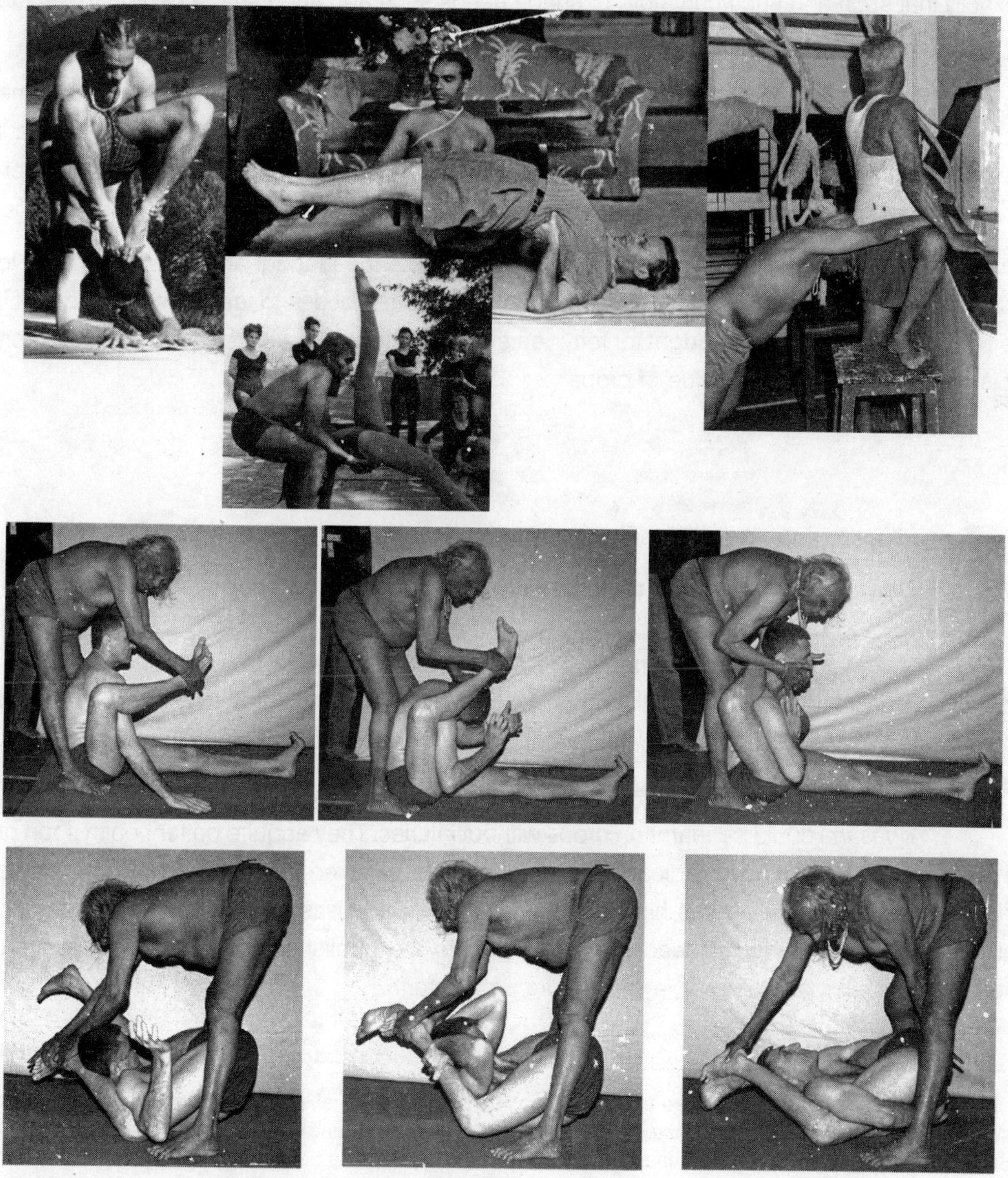

Plate n. 63 – Using my body as an instrument

They used to enjoy my help but my body used to ache for hours. People cannot imagine my aches and pains. With all these agonies of teaching, I built up yoga, which has been accepted now by the public though it took time. If I say that I am responsible for making yoga to reach the common people, it is not an exaggeration or a pride. Having taken such loads, I could say exactly that such and such curvature or shape needs such and such shape of prop to get the maximum benefit.

This is how I developed props evolving new ideas every now and then. As ideas came to me, proper adjustments for each individual on props gave them better benefits of yoga. I learnt even the art of spreading and using the blankets, where to fold, how much to fold, when to roll and where exact support is needed to derive maximum benefits within a minimum time.

So, to teach without props is not so easy. In yoga the teacher and the taught have to come closer to each other. It needs a tremendous thinking process to teach without props. If it is possible one can teach. I taught for forty years without props! Please keep this in mind. Then it is possible to realise the value of props.

VIII.20. – Does a demonstration of yoga with props attract audience

The demonstration on props will induce the audience to learn. As a stage artist, I have given lots of demonstrations with and without props to show how simple it is to do even the most complicated *asana.*[1] This made many introduce yoga with the use of props in health centres, gyms and other places.

Yogāsana could be learnt on props without injuries. They acquire better health soon or through props. Now, many medical research centres have taken interest in studying patients with cardiac problems, diabetes, high blood pressure, slipped discs, asthma and other common ailments with my method of teaching. Many papers are published on depression, asthma, scoliosis, metacarpal problems, eye pressure and so forth.

---

[1] In 1984-85 the author demonstrated *āsana* on props during Pune-festival, staying in *āsana* for long duration, which was appreciated by the audience. He did in Mumbai as well as in Pune showing the *āsana* independently and with props for aged, and also at the International Cardiac Conference held in Pune some years later, both with props and without props on cardiac patients, besides personal demonstrations.

I remember that whenever I gave demonstrations, I presented yoga as a pure art, with balance and poise, creating curiosity and igniting interest in yoga. As a science, I made it informative and educative. Yoga with props as a rehabilitation system has now been introduced in several medical centres. The most important benefit of the usage of props is that they make the *sādhaka* a lifelong student of yoga.

VIII.21. – The use of bandages

In yoga, we have *āsana, mudrā* and *bandha*. The practice of all these is meant to arrest, control, increase and divert this vital energy, wherever required. The bandage is *paṭṭā bandha*. It is used in three ways. Wrapping around the forehead is *śiropaṭṭa bandha,* around the eyes, *netrapaṭṭa bandha,* and around both, *śironetra paṭṭa bandha*.

This wrapping of a bandage is identical to *Ṣaṇmukhi mudrā*. As the students had difficulty to practise this *mudrā* even for five minutes, I found this method to get the effect of *Ṣaṇmukhi mudrā*. The effect of *Ṣaṇmukhi mudrā* is to make the senses to withdraw from the external world to the inner world within the body.

The senses of perception, eyes and ears are closer to the brain and mind and any disturbances in them distract the brain and mind of a person. If the eyes are the windows of the brain, ears are the windows of the mind or consciousness. The eyes puff out quickly when the brain is active. In sleep too, movements in the eyes occur if there is disturbance.

Sound disturbs the mind and the brain feels the stress. A mild vibration of sound reacts on the ears faster than an electronic machine, affecting both the mind and the brain. Though the ears do not show physical movement but hardness to hear is felt. The eyes react fast and become hard and tense.

Ṣaṇmukha means six-faced. According to Indian mythology, the six-faced Kārtikeya (son of Lord Shiva) is the leader of the divine army. *Mudrā* means a seal or a stamp. Kārtikeya is considered to be a great warrior filled with valour. In man, the eyes, nose, tongue, skin, ears and mind are the six faces.

In *Ṣaṇmukhi mudrā,* the palms and fingers are placed and adjusted on the eyes, ears, nostrils and on the upper lips to keep the brain passive and mind alert, and then to draw them inward to feel the presence of the soul.

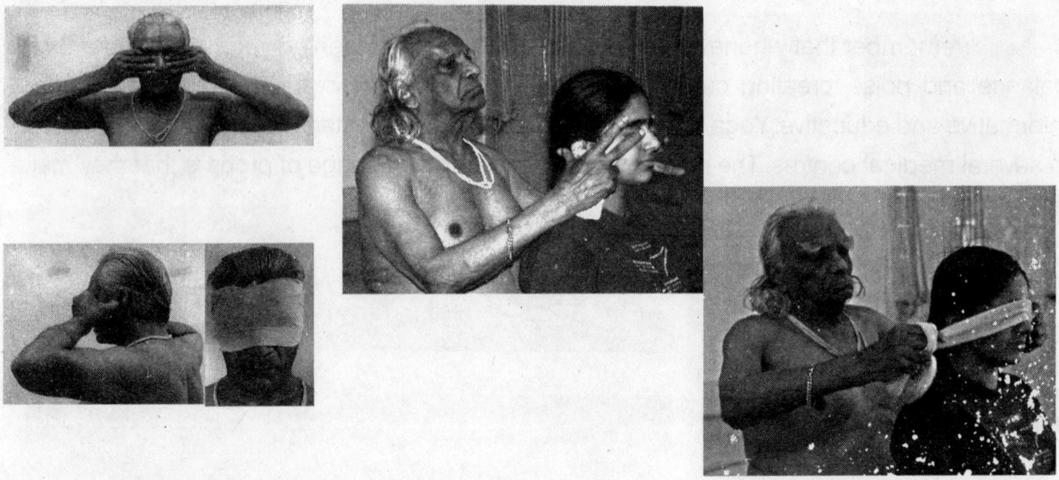

Plate n. 64 – Bandage for *Ṣaṇmukhī mudrā*

In the early days I used to take *Ṣaṇmukhi mudrā* personally attending to each and every one, either in *Śavāsana* or in sitting position. Even now, many see me in classes taking a few who are really suffering with emotional problems, nervousness, blood pressure or eye and ear problems. A few students in the 1950s came for treatment for glaucoma, myopia, ear pain, headache and migraine. As it was hard to handle all at one time in *Ṣaṇmukhi mudrā,* I wrapped the bandage around their eyes. I put it around the eyes from the front to the back by moving the nerves of the temples towards the ears, as if one is in *Ṣaṇmukhi mudrā.* I used to keep a small round plate, of three inches in diameter on the forehead, to quieten the eyes and disconnect the eyes form the floor of the brain. This was giving great relief in stress on the eyes. That was the beginning to find an alternative means of getting the effect of *Ṣaṇmukhi mudrā* without straining one's arms and fingers.

Due to the gentle pressure of the bandage the muscles and nerves on the floor of the brain get softened. As the eyes and ears recede towards the self, the vibrations in the senses of perception and throbbing in the brain and tossing of the mind come to a stand still. This wrapping the eyes arrests fluctuations soon and brings the brain and mind to a state of alert passivity experiencing both *manōlaya* and *citta nirodha* (passive mind and restraint in the consciousness).

Wrapping the bandage brings the blood pressure to normalcy in *Sālamba Śīrṣāsana, Sālamba Sarvāṅgāsana, Halāsana, Setu Bandha Sarvāṅgāsana* and *Viparīta Karaṇi.*

It is used as it helps the student to know the quality of quietness *(manōlaya).* After experiencing this quiet state of mind and brain I was advising them to learn to simulate *manōlaya* without a wrap.

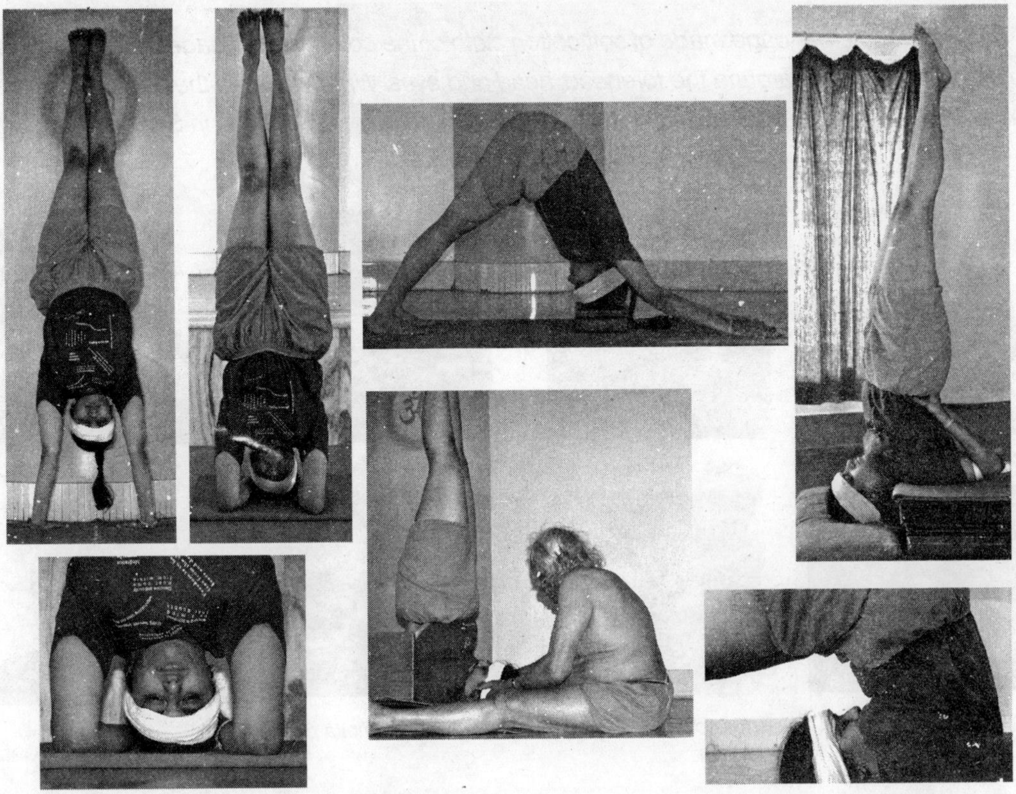

Plate n. 65 – *Āsana* with a bandage to know the quality of quietness *(manōlaya)*

In the case of headaches, eye burn, glaucoma and displaced retina, the use of bandage is not only compulsory but should be used as a ritual as precaution and treatment. In case of hypertension, glaucoma and displaced retina, wrap *(śiropaṭṭa bandha)* the clóth on the eyebrows or on floor of the brain and bring the eyelids down by using the fingers instead of the muscles of the eyes. When one has eye-infection or some serious problems, then the eyes are covered with folded bandage.

When irritation, tension and strain on the brain, loss of temper, dizziness, blurred vision or burning of the eyes surface, use a bandage in all *āsana*. However, in *Śavāsana* cover both the eyes and forehead *(śironetra paṭṭa bandha)*. Do *āsana* with eyes open when one is lazy, dull or dejected.

In my early years of teaching, I invented small bags filled with smooth cereals to enhance the effects of *Ṣaṇmukhi mudrā*. Later, many people began using sandbags. I suggest bags filled with semolina as it is better than sand. Who knows the dust of sand may reach the eyes and infect them.

*(**Note**: the bandage made of soft cotton cloth or the common bandage utilised in clinics be used as a wrapper around the forehead, head and eyes. When one ties the bandage around the head, the eyes feel cool, ears soft and brain and mind quiet as if one is in Ṣaṇmukhi mudrā.)*

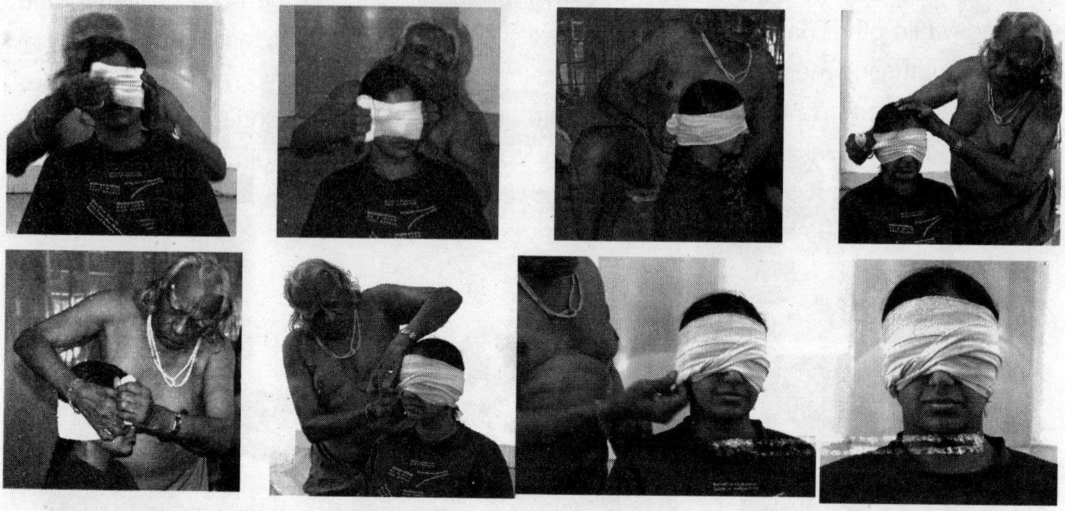

For *Śavāsana cover both the eyes and forehead (śironetra paṭṭa bandha)*

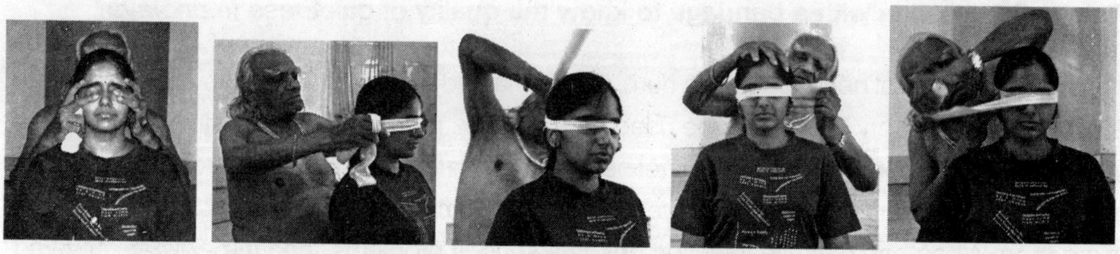

Hypertension, glaucoma and displaced retina, wrap (*śiropaṭṭa bandha*)
the cloth on the eyebrows or on floor of the brain
and bring the eyelids down by using the fingers instead of the muscles of the eyes

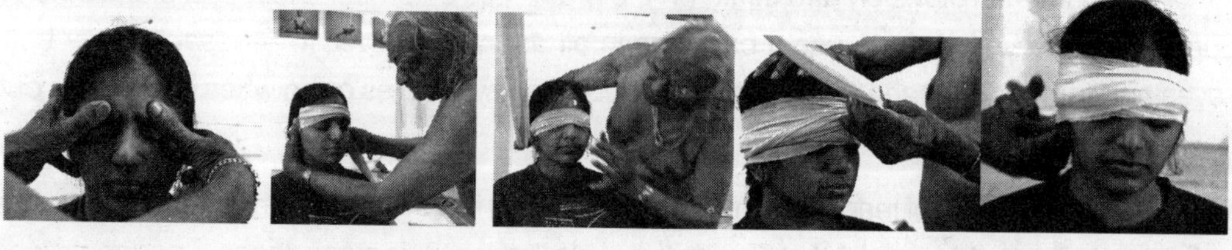

Plate n. 66 – Eye wraps

VIII.21 – Why in *Śavāsana,* does the body tilt, shake and take a long time to calm the mind

Often, when we do intellectual work, we think that we use only our brain, but it is not so. While the mental activities go on, the body gets involved. Some parts of the body get tense and hardened, while other parts remain loose, relaxed and lop-sided. Also, there is an emotional factor and fluctuating mental states, which affect the body and its physiology. The body shrinks, the muscles become taut, rigid, the diaphragm tenses and mind becomes restless. At this stage tilts and shakes take place. These bring undue fatigue and nervous debility. If one practises *āsana* with the support of props for some days, then restlessness turns into restfulness, the nerves are rejuvenated and regain the power and strength to restart *āsana* independently.

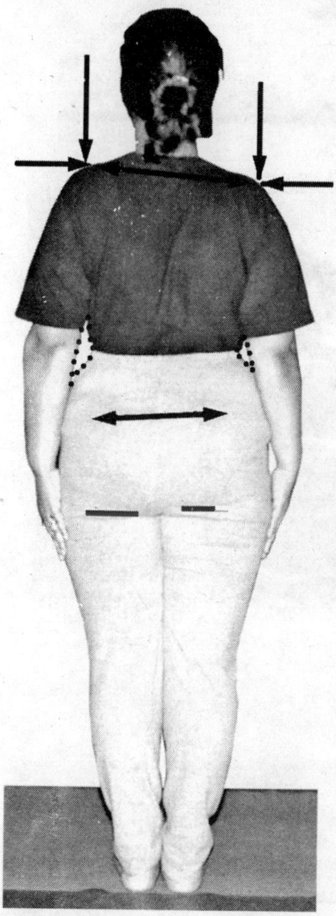

The level of the shoulders, buttock crease, sacram and the different space between the body and the inner arms indicate the tilts in the students body

Plate n. 67 – Tilts in the hips, shoulders and shoulder blades

In *Śavāsana,* tilts in the hips and wrong placement of shoulders, shoulder blades and arms have to be corrected and aligned by placing round plate weights.

People with suppressed or depressed mind, or feeble-minded with fear complexes, hypoglycaemia, low blood pressure, cardiac or asthmatic problems, can do *Śavāsana* with their chest raised by using pillows, bolsters, bricks or slanting plank. This kind of support brings freedom to the lungs and heart and helps easy breathing.

Śavāsana requires the training of the mind. If the body cannot relax, then the brain and the mind cannot relax, and vice-versa. Placing weights on the thighs releases the restlessness in the body. Similarly use a rolled towel on the upper back of the head and place a small weight on the forehead. This soothes the nerves and brain bringing pensiveness in the mind and body.

Besides keeping weights on the thighs and palms and wrapping the bandage around the eyes and forehead *(śīronetra paṭṭa bandha),* one can keep an appropriate weight on the forehead to relax the brain. Then *Śavāsana* happens effortlessly. After conditioning this way for a month or so, try *Śavāsana* independently. When you feel uncomfortable to do *Śavāsana* independently, then use the weights. I am sure a time will come when all will do *Śavāsana* effortlessly.

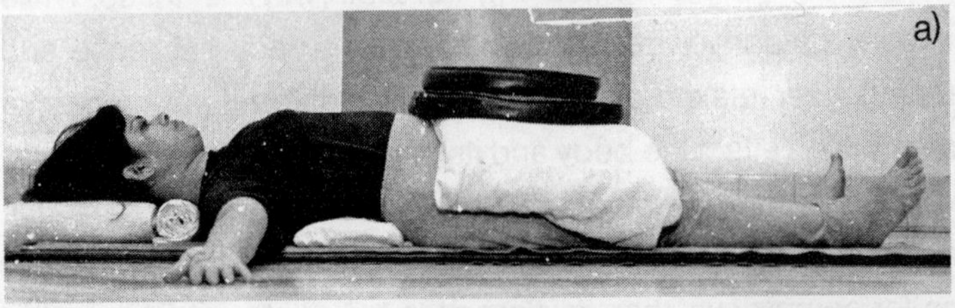

a) After adjusting the shoulders and hips a small folded cloth is placed between the lumbar and the floor. A pillow and 2x weights are placed on the thighs (a).

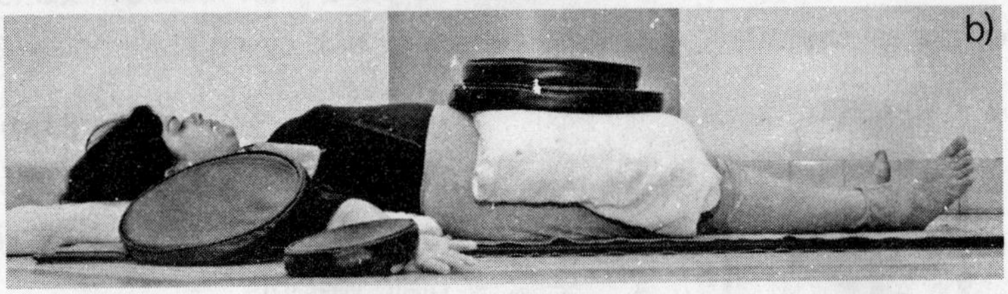

b) Next, weights are placed on the shoulders and palms (b).

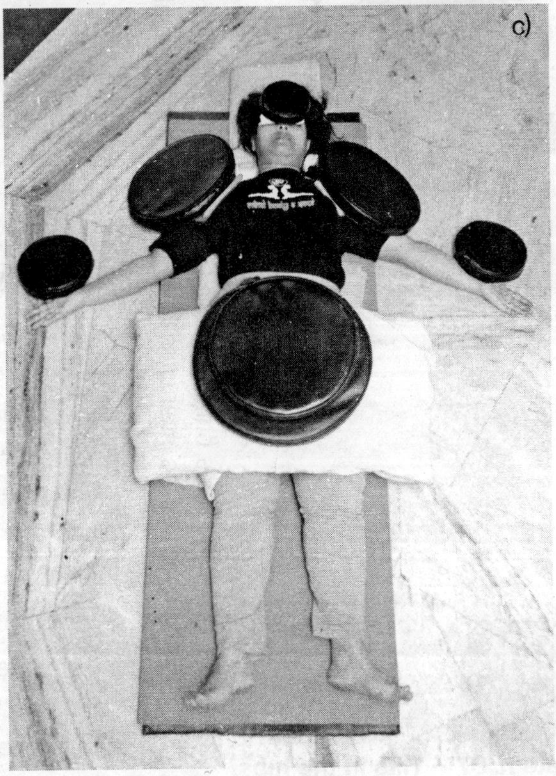

c) One can keep an appropriate weight on the forehead to relax the brain. Then *Śavāsana* happens effortlessly (c)

Plate n. 68 – Weights for *Śavāsana* to happen effortlessly

SECTION IX

ON PRACTICE – THEORY

SECTION IX – ON PRACTICE – THEORY

IX.1. – On personal practice

One has to know one's own standard of practice, mental condition and will-power and accordingly plan one's personal regular practice. In *Light on Yoga* I have given a 300 week course. As a mature teacher, now my advice is to divide those courses into 600 or 900 weeks according to one's intense, devotional and vigorous approach; which I did not realise when I wrote the book. It never struck me that all would practise ten hours a day like me. This was a blunder that I made in giving a 300 week course thinking that the whole world would practise like me.

Those who have that book can divide it into 600 or 900 weeks, following the sequences as explained on weekly basis to a two or three weekly basis. Then I assure you all of reaching the destination with ease and comfort.

When one drives a car he starts with the first gear, and then changes into neutral gear every time as he changes the gears. Similarly, to make sequences one has to think in what gear one is. One has to make the sequences in such a way that the movement of the spine and the movements of the muscles are extended advertently to the optimum level from the starting point, and return advertently in the same order by toning and tuning the body and mind. He has to see how far the body, nerves, muscles and joints co-operate and co-ordinate in order to enhance the range of movement in each *āsana.* Always end the practices doing the *āsana* that cool and quieten the body and mind. For example, if one ends the practice by doing *Kapotāsana,* then he is going to end up with pain and backaches. Perform *āsana* like *Bharadvājāsana, Adho Mukha Śvānāsana,* resting the head on a stool in *Uttānāsana* and *Paschimottānāsana* on bolsters. They cool the body and mind and the feeling would be as if he has not done *Kapotāsana.*

When we have to eat food, we heat it but we cannot take it if it is too hot. One needs to wait until the hot food becomes warm. Sequencing is of two types. Sequencing of *āsana* is one thing; the other sequencing is the way to begin, continue and how it should end up. In the former, one has to study the anatomical range in the body as well as the *āsana,* and accordingly introduce *āsana* wherever it fits in for each one's physical and mental capacities. But the sequencing of *āsana* at the end must be in a way that he comes back to the natural condition of coolness and quietness as if the strain of practice is not felt at all.

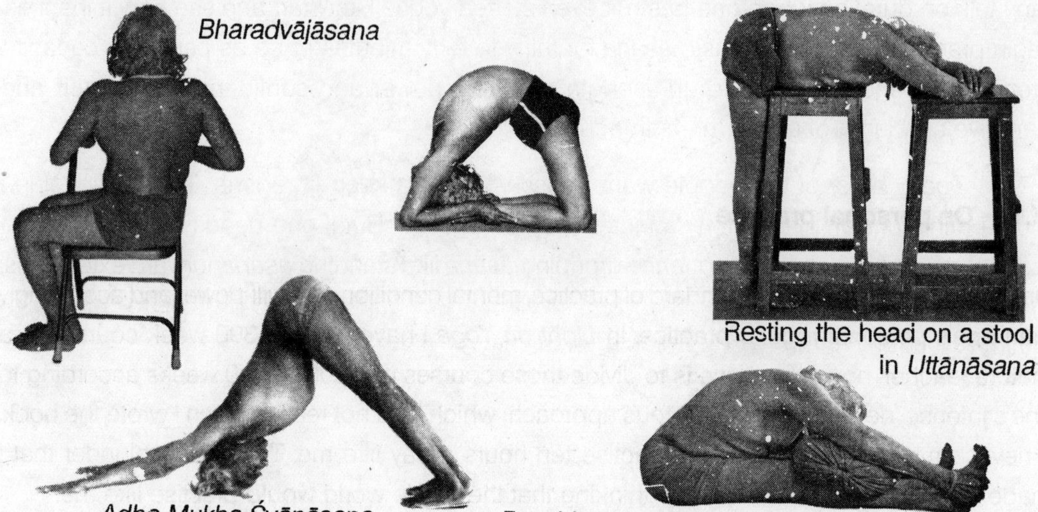

Bharadvājāsana

Resting the head on a stool in *Uttānāsana*

Adho Mukha Śvānāsana

Paschimottānāsana resting the head on bolsters

Plate n. 69 – Return to coolness and quietness after *Kapotāsana*

Some like to finish practice with *Śīrṣāsana* or to practise *Sarvāṅgāsana* before *Śīrṣāsana*. Hence, one has to find out what a healthy sequential order is and what is not through one's own experiences. *Śīrṣāsana* heats the body whereas *Sarvāṅgāsana* and *Halāsana* cool the body. So, my advice is to finish the practice with *Sarvāṅgāsana* cycle as it cools the brain and quietens the nerves. Let the sequence be such that yoga protects the *sādhaka*.

Actually I have sequenced in *Light on Yoga* the *āsana* practice showing where they are to be adapted. There is also a list of important *āsana* given at the end of each course so that one can practise according to one's physical and mental capacities. Practice of *āsana* is meant to sharpen the intelligence of the body, and when that intelligence is sharpened, then he may be able to make sequences for his daily practices. Until then, he cannot think of sequences, but follow the order as given in *Light on Yoga*, by extending the weeks practices longer than what I have mentioned.

As far as my study on several books on *āsana* goes, at present it is only *Light on Yoga* that gives the seeker a means for progressing from a good foundation with intelligence. Know that a good book is better than a bad teacher.

IX.2. - Duration of practice

The duration of practice can be thought of after getting some control over many *āsana*. How can I talk on duration when one has not even started yoga? First start and see how it inspires. Begin practice with certain basic *āsana* for thirty to forty minutes or so as per one's capacity, strength and endurance. Build up strength, enduring power and confidence in yourself, and then give a thought of giving more time for practice.

Today most of the people want to use yoga as a keep fit regime. For such people I think a minimum of thirty to forty minutes may be enough. But if one needs to know the real essence of yoga, one has to sequence grouping *āsana* like standing *āsana*, forward extensions, lateral twistings, backward extensions and inversions. The will to stay longer has to come from within, which may come when one stays in the āsana with comfort.

As an example, I give one sequence from *Tāḍāsana, Utthita Trikoṇāsāna, Utthita Pārśvakoṇāsana, Parivṛtta Trikoṇāsāna, Parivṛtta Pārśvakoṇāsana, Pārśvottānāsana, Uttānāsana, Adho Mukha Śvānāsana, Śīrṣāsana, Jānu Śīrṣāsana, Paśchimottānāsana, Uṣṭrāsana, Ūrdhva Dhanurāsana, Viparīta Daṇḍāsana* on a bench, *Bharadvājāsana, Marīchyāsana, Sarvāṅgāsana, Halāsana, Setu Bandha Sarvāṅgāsana, Viparīta Karaṇi* and *Śavāsana*. This way one can build up sequences as one progresses.

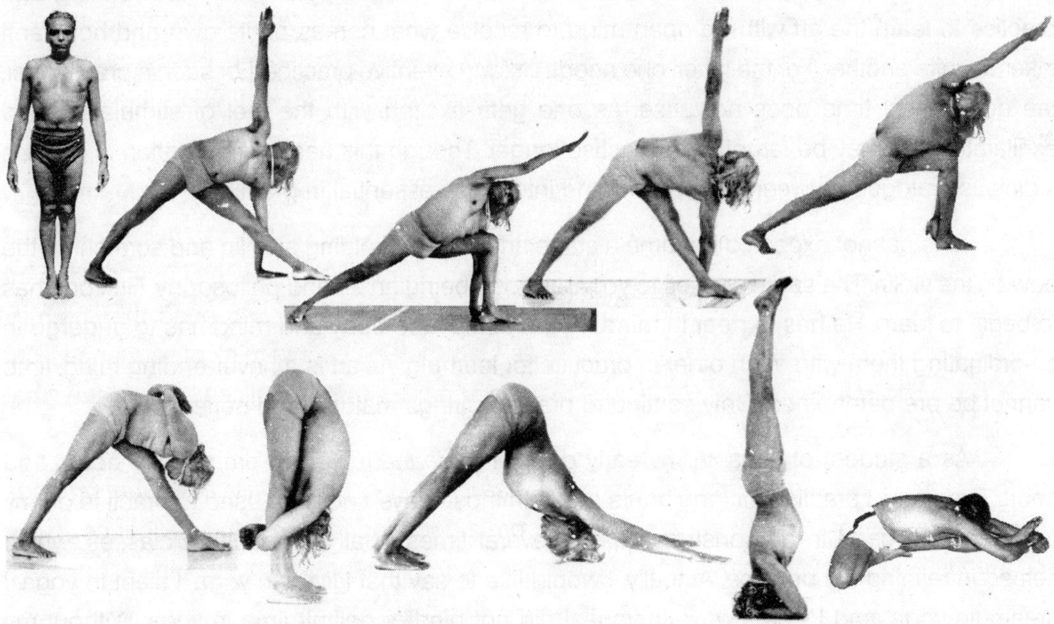

Plate 70a - Building of sequences - (cont. over)

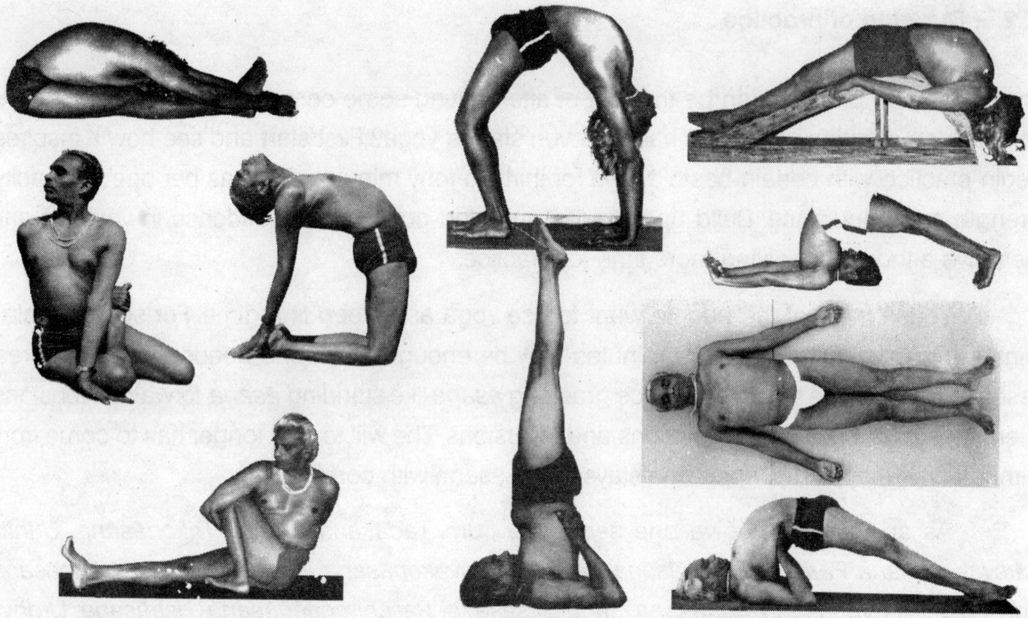

Plate 70b – Building of sequences

Duration of time for practice depends upon one's dedication and devotion to the art. First begin and let things take their own time. Practice for physical health is one thing and practice to learn the art with an open mind to receive what comes on its own and how far it takes is quite another. For the latter, one needs lifelong attentive practice. For such a practitioner, the question of time does not arise. As one gets excited with the feel of stimulation and exhilaration, he may be tempted to practise longer. Though this healthy temptation is good, a judicious dialogue between body, mind and intellect is essential in practice.

One cannot expect to become a stage artist just by holding a violin and scratching the bow on the violin. The same applies to yoga, as yoga being an art and philosophy. First one has to begin to learn. He has to bear in mind the hardships the body and mind has to undergo in co-ordinating them with each other in practice for learning. As art is a never-ending thing, time cannot be pre-determined. Only continued practice brings maturity and perfection.

As a student of yoga, in my early days of *sādhanā* I used to practise for hours and hours. Even now I practise for long hours a day. In those days, I not only used to practise on my own, but also used to demonstrate *āsana* several times in all my teaching classes, which helped in refining my practice. Actually, I would like to say that I lived in yoga, I slept in yoga, I dreamt in yoga, and I was always in yoga. I did not bind or delimit time in yoga. Without my yogic practice my life has no meaning, yoga is my life and my life is yoga.

IX.3. – On casual practice

Casual practice brings casual benefits and profound practice brings profound results. The beauty of yogic practice is that it does not leave any bad effects even if one practises inconsistently. Only one may feel the loss of sharpness in intelligence.

Even if one practises once or twice a week, its effects remain for two or three days. As one struggles hard to earn money, struggle in yoga is also needed to earn spiritual wealth. This spiritual wealth is the real essence of yoga. If one likes to experience that, then one has to do the practise daily keeping oneself in a religious state of mind.

If the mirror is not cleansed, it gathers dust and hence does not reflect the object clearly. It is the same with practice. If one does not maintain the body clean, it sullies the self and its reflection on one will be lost.

IX.4. – Is yoga shut to those who are disabled

First of all one has to find out whether this assumption is fiction or fact. How can one think that yoga is shut to those who cannot perform? Is not yoga meant for all? It is said clearly that yoga is for the young, old, ripe old, sickly and weak (*H.Y.P.*, I.64). Yoga is a practical experiencing subject. It has a bearing on both the physical practice and the mental practice.

In the history of the yoga-world, there were people who were physically disabled and yet were great saints and great yogis. It is not that a diseased or disabled body cannot do yoga, but it is the mind that finds ways of escape from action. One has to see how one can involve the disabled part of the body as well as the whole body. If the back is terribly painful, it can be reduced by correct yoga. Yoga makes one stand if he cannot stand; it makes one to sit if he cannot sit and move if he cannot move. I have taught bed-ridden persons nearing death, who lived more than they would have thought and died peacefully. Yoga is a life giver and not a life taker.

As such individuals suffering from asthma may say that they cannot breathe. But does it mean that they don't breathe at all? Then how do they survive? In fact, they breathe but laboriously. A paralysed person with deformity and disability can improve and becomes less dependent through yoga, which can help him in restoring the body. An asthmatic patient begins to breathe better after yoga. Yoga is a progressive self-improving subject. It teaches how to live with a positive mind by putting an end to negative thoughts.

One has to use the body as a tool to work on the mind and strengthen both body and mind. One has to learn to break the limitations that are dictated by the mind. One has to overlook the conditions of the mood and start yoga, which gradually builds confidence.

Ramakrishna Paramahansa and Ramana Maharshi were great individuals because they did not allow their mind to get caught in these negative thoughts like us in spite of their body being diseased. They accepted the disease and lived without complaining or escaping from it. Let us not forego good and worthy things like yoga in life with one pretext or the other. Let us take to yoga and bring the hidden energy to surface.

IX.5. – Does incorrect practice disturb the mental state

The feel of wrong practice is that one may become restless and irritable at first. Then this irritability leads towards disliking people and things and disgust in his surroundings. If such results are occurring, better to reflect on what went wrong in practice and then take advice from a mature teacher. It should not happen, as yoga calms the nerves and mind. If such things surface, one has to correct the mistakes in their *sādhanā* soon.

If one walks carelessly on the street, one is bound to meet with an accident. It is the same with yoga. If one climbs the ladder of yoga to one's capacity, constitution and strength, then yoga is a friend. Otherwise it is a foe. Hatred and disgust do not come by yoga. Non-attachment comes and in place of confusion, clarity dawns. So watch the practice and its reactions. If reactions are bad, seek advice from an experienced and matured teacher or use your discretion and find out ways with a dispassionate analysis.

IX.6. – Effort, adjustment and comfort

Views may differ to experiences. Practice has its comparative studies. One does not stay forever in the same state intellectually and emotionally. As the ways of doing differ from moment to moment as one progresses, they affect change in all the sheaths of the self. These effects may even change person to person, as his ways of thinking and quality of practice differ. Therefore, one has to use one's intellectual power and study and scrutinise the actions that take place in *sādhanā* to experience a non-conflicting state of comfort in positioning himself in all *āsana.* There should be no conflicting feeling between the right side and the left side in the corresponding parts of the body. Making the mind and intelligence run parallel to the action of the body and establish the self in the cells, tissues and the fibres of the body is comfort.

As *sādhanā* progresses experience varies. Take my own practice; changes are happening. Yet not once do I feel that I am struggling in the *āsana.* Even my cells ring their bells the moment some unhealthy movements take place. They alert my consciousness at once.

No doubt, the effort has its own value. Unwanted and unneeded efforts are not good. The cells are more honest than the mind. Therefore, when the cells ring for help, open the door of the mind to find out what sort of help they need. When they ask for help, act with a right mind and adjust at that moment, then the practitioner does not feel the action and adjustment at that time as an effort.

Patañjali's observations are very clear but problems arise in us from want of our understanding. It is true that Patañjali defines *āsana* in two words, *sthiratā* and *sukhatā,* and the cessation of duality between body, senses of perception, organs of action, mind intelligence and consciousness. It is important to observe when and where to establish the stability *(sthiratā),* and how to achieve comfort *(sukhatā).* Patañjali is not asking a beginner to experience this state. His statement of finality of the *āsana* is for the seasoned and matured practitioners.

He says, "When the mind and body reach and come close towards the infinite seer who is abiding within, he experiences perfection in *āsana* and at that time his efforts fade out due to that closeness with the seer".

Please re-read, digest and reflect on the words *yatna* to *prayatna* and *prayatna* to *śaithilya,* the cessation of effort (*Y.S.,* II.47).

When the practitioner reaches perfection in *āsana,* he does not feel the effort as effort. This is *sthiratā* and *sukhatā.* Here *sukhatā* means awareness of the Self, and *sthiratā* means the stable and alert body. In this state both body and Self unite in *āsana* in a natural way *(sahajatā).*

If *sthira sukham* is taken together, it means that as long as one is in an *āsana*, the flow of *sukhatā* has to run steadily without interruptions. When this uninterrupted flow of *sukhatā* is firmly established, there is no room for gross or subtle differences *(dvandvāḥ)*. This is what Patañjali means on *āsana*.

While doing the *āsana*, we are asked to correct our position and to translate the act to a state as required from the body. Instead of doing what the body needs, we strain the brain, tense it and think we have done the required job. Here the effort was on the brain and not at all on the needed areas. This creates a gap between the body and mind, which makes one to feel action as effort. If we co-ordinate body and mind in action, then the feel of effort fades out and practice appears effortless.

If the brain is kept as an observer while performing *āsana*, then the first step of effortlessness is felt. If stretch is needed in the leg, the leg has to act. If the chest has to open, the chest has to act. The brain has just to see whether its instructions are carried out by the concerned parts of the body and if not, then to make those parts act.

The effort to bring the dull aspect of the body at par with the intelligent facet is correct effort and correct adjustment. During these adjustments and efforts, let the brain be a witnesser, an observer and a guide. Let the body be the actor to reach maturity and perfection in *āsana*. This is effortlessness in the effort. This state of transformation is to be close to the infinite that is within *(anantasamāpattī)*.

The doer, the self, the instrument that is used in the body and the object *anantasamāpattī* is known. Here the subject, the instrument that is used and the object *(ananta-sthira* and *ananta-sukha)*, all unite as one. This is *anantasamāpattī*.

IX.7. – Effect of disproportionate practice of backbends

My advice to practitioners is to learn and study a balanced state of practice dividing uniformly the course of *āsana* each day. Plan to devote one day for standing *āsana*, one day for forward extensions, one day for twists, one day for backward extensions, one day for balancings, one day to take a few from each one from these and one day to concentrate on variations of inverted *āsana*. Do *Śīrṣāsana*, *Sarvāṅgāsana* and *Halāsana* daily for rejuvenating the system to maintain freshness.

Let me start with my own over zealous practice. As a stage performer I used to present more backbends to attract people towards my art and me. With my background and experience my advice would be not to devote time on back bends alone but to keep an overall touch of all *āsana*. Actually, my practices of overdoing or under doing served me to find out the hidden truth of each *āsana*. I experimented on myself a lot, before I worked on others. I myself was a guinea pig all the time and I am the same even now. If I do one hundred *Ūrdhva Dhanurāsana*, I can exactly tell how I performed each of them from the initial stage till the ending point. I was aware of the sources of energy as well as centre of gravity changing each time. I knew what to do and from where to do when I was coming towards the end of *Ūrdhva Dhanurāsana*. Whether I did the *āsana* quality-wise, quantity-wise or time-wise, I was observing, reflecting and noting changed in all movements and worked on building on them for further improvements. It was my sheer love for the subject that made me work like this. I never did *āsana* for muscle power. I was interested in the balance of energy and placement of intelligence in *āsana* to learn the right action.

I was touring from place to place, with my *gurujī* and some of his other pupils, to propagate yoga. Being the youngest in the group, my *gurujī* used to choose me for backbends, as the other members were aged, and they were not able to take the load of backbends. He repeatedly made me do backbends moving from *āsana* to *āsana* through jumpings, which today is considered by many as Power Yoga.

For example, from *Uttānāsana* to *Ūrdhva Dhanurāsana* to *Chaturanga Daṇḍāsana* to *Ūrdhva Dhanurāsana* and so forth. Being strong headed I did them. But as days and years went by, I realised that I was lacking endurance to stay in *āsana* for a long time. This made me re-think, re-adjust and re-learn to bring all parts of my body to get re-charged with life in quality, quantity and time-wise in all *āsana*. I began to concentrate on my forward bends, lateral twists and balancing *āsana* with priority. The backbends did not help me in holding the forward bends quality-wise and time-wise. So I had to analyse a lot on adjustments and re-adjustments in backbends and the importance of inversions in daily practices. This new thinking and re-adjustments helped me to regain balance and rhythm in all the *āsana* uniformly, quality-wise, quantity-wise as well as time-wise.

It is true that young practitioners being agile, energetic and flexible love to do more backbends. I appreciate their enthusiasm and advise them to pay equal respect to other *āsana* as well.

If only the back bending *āsana* are performed, then the spinal muscles get acclimatised to such movements and rebel against forward bends or balancing *āsana*. As I had stretched the spine in one direction through backbends, I had to train the spine to move laterally as well as posteriorly to develop with even growth and strength, so that it became accessible to all movements with ease and comfort. Actually when I started re-tooling the body for forward bends, the pain was such that it was as if someone is sledge hammering my back. The severe soreness and pain in my back took years to leave me. This unbearable pain made me practise with prudence and caution. Keep in mind the wholistic development of all parts of the body to function in unison and pay attention to be in touch with lateral, posterior, anterior and latitudinal movements of the body in daily practice. If one pays attention to do backbends one day, then do twists and finish with forward bends. One day do standing *āsana, Śīrṣāsana* and twists, ending with *Sarvāṅgāsana* and *Halāsana*. One day devote on balancing *āsana* with *Ūrdhva Dhanurāsana* or *Viparīta Chakrāsana* in each. One day begin with forward bends, do twists and end up with *Halāsana*. Each day increase staying in all *āsana* time-wise. Do two days *Śīrṣāsana* and *Sarvāṅgāsana* cycles. The other days, do only *Śīrṣāsana, Sarvāṅgāsana* and *Halāsana* without their cycles. Do *prāṇāyāma* for about thirty minutes concentrating on each type a day. This is just a general suggestion and an example, but one can think and adjust according to his level of *sādhanā*.

Only attentive practice is of prime importance in whatever *āsana* or *prāṇāyāma* one practices. In case the body or the mind fails to co-operate, do the *āsana* or *prāṇāyāma* that they accept and then go back to a normal routine. Concentrate intensively on certain *āsana* on a day and just casualy or lightly touch the other *āsana*. Devote The next day to intensively practise the previous day's lightly touched *āsana*. Whatever *āsana* are done with total attention, on a particular day, then do the other routine *āsana* as a secondary practice that day. This way one can change the cycles.

Experience the sense of delight in each *āsana*. Let the practice finally evolve from complexity to simplicity and from simplicity towards serenity.

IX.8. – On progressive and regressive practice

The body is a very mysterious instrument that we possess. It is very difficult to understand when it acts as a friend or a foe. Hence, our body and life are like a ladder with ascending and descending steps. It is the same in the yogic path also. This has happened to me on many occasions. In 1943, 1946, 1958 and 1979 I descended to such an extent that I almost lost control of my body and in my *sādhanā.* This affected my body and my mind a great deal. Though I was performing all the *āsana* in 1943, 46 and 58, I was not feeling the fragrance of excellence in the *sādhanā.* It was just an empty listless practice. I lost the mental and intellectual co-ordination with the movements of the body. Yet, I persisted on and on without any feel of sensitivity in my *sādhanā.* This state disappeared on its own after a gap of a year or so. The flavour of excellence reappeared to savour. But each time, it took more time to get back the fragrance of practice.

Recovery from regressions happened and remained constantly from 1955 to 1979. In 1979, two scooter accidents within a period of two weeks incapacitated me and put me out of gear for many years.

One thing was certain. After these accidents I touched the rock bottom in my *sādhanā,* the destiny and grace of yoga forced me to restart from scratch and I am happy that even though I am running eighty-nine, I do my *sādhanā* for many hours a day.

But with all these problems I was in peak practice from 1984 to 1998. Again I was afflicted, straining my heart. Yet I am happy, I do practice with zeal for hours each day even now.

In the beginning we see the progress happening fast. As one goes on practising, the effects do slow down. On account of this, one finds it tough to continue and maintain as the body gives way and the mind loses interest to pursue. Failures are bound to happen in *sādhanā* but one must accept them as steps towards success and persist in *sādhanā* as I did.

If the path was smooth, Patañjali would not have mentioned the obstacles and afflictions (*Y.S.,* I.30 & 31). The obstacles come to test the firmness of the *sādhaka.* So we have to march on facing the impediments with patience, faith, vigour and determination as Patañjali says (*Y.S.,* I.20). Then the rays of hope may flash again and ignite life force in our *sādhanā.*

We need not get disappointed with regression. I learnt a great deal in regressions and God was kind enough to grace me to pursue my *sādhanā.* I took regressions as providence to re-construct, rethink and rebuild the *sādhanā* afresh. As we are glad of success, we have to develop the attitude that regression is meant to ponder upon our *sādhanā.* Let us take the stagnations in our stride as a step to charge the battery of intelligence and energy to find out the reason for stagnations that crept in. We have to take them as God sent or as destiny's play. By such happenings we begin to know what to drop and what to keep. Regression and progression help us to learn, unlearn and relearn with new thoughts that spring out for new adjustments in presentation. If we progress uninterruptedly all the time, then the ego or pride gets inflated and this may lead us to our downfall.

In the third chapter of *Yoga Sūtra* Patañjali says that in spite of achievements and accomplishments the ultimate freedom may remain far away: *te samādhau upasargāḥ vyutthane siddhayaḥ* (*Y.S.*, III.38) – these attainments are impediments to *samādhi,* although they are powers in the active life. Therefore, one has to remain non-attached to successes and achievements. Otherwise involvement in these achievements tempt us to play on them which may rebound and we fall prey to them. This is dispassionate *sādhanā*. If one does not pay attention to success or failure, then illumination and emancipation are possible.

In *Kaivalya Pāda* Patañjali again cautions about the effects of success. He says the fissures may appear in the *sādhaka* which may create a divisible state between the *citta* and the seer: *tat chidreṣu pratyayāntarāṇi saṁskārebhyaḥ* (*Y. S.*, IV.27) – with this, the force of past impressions may disturb one's path towards emancipation.

Consider successes as signals that one is on the right path in the *sādhanā* and don't stop but continue with devotion to see what is in store for further experiences in the *sādhanā*.

IX.9. – On insensitivity and oversensitivity

When a man like Arjuna could not face the vision of the cosmic form of Sri Krishna *(Viśvarūpa darśana)* (*B.G.*, XI), at his request the Lord had to bless him with divine eyes *(divyacakṣu)* (*B.G.*, XI.8). Therefore I say, practise yoga well and earn the grace of God so that one can withstand to see or feel that divine force.

Yoga is like walking on a razor's edge. If we do properly it can uplift and if wrongly done, it can bring sorrow. We have to observe watchfully each step of our action so that no wrong takes place. Insensitivity can invite carelessness or heedlessness and make one lose intellectual sensitivity. We have been graced with discriminative intelligence so that both insensitivity and over-sensitivity are evenly weighed. Over-sensitivity heads towards inflated egoism, whereas under sensitivity may not ignite the *sādhaka* to continue practice. To be sensitive we need a controlled intelligence in order to check over-sensitivity with prudence.

IX.10. – On unhealthy sensitivity

Sensitivity is not a matter for comparative study. There is no such thing as healthy sensitivity and unhealthy sensitivity but disturbing sensitivity. When we don't react to the demand of sensitivity *(saṁvedanā)* it is non-sensitivity or a disturbing sensitivity and not an unhealthy sensitivity.

When consciousness *(citta)* feels the actions, it has to rethink to judge its aptness. This is sensitivity. A scientist is not just a brainy person. When he tries to explore or discover what is unknown to him, he has to be highly sensitive.

We are all aware and feel pain and complain. But how many of us try to find out the source of pain? To trace the source of pain, we need to use not only our logical intelligence but also its in-depth penetration. This way we have to develop sensitivity and work on the affected part to eradicate the pain by adjusting the muscles, the fibres, the tendons, the nerves and so forth. This is sensitive development.

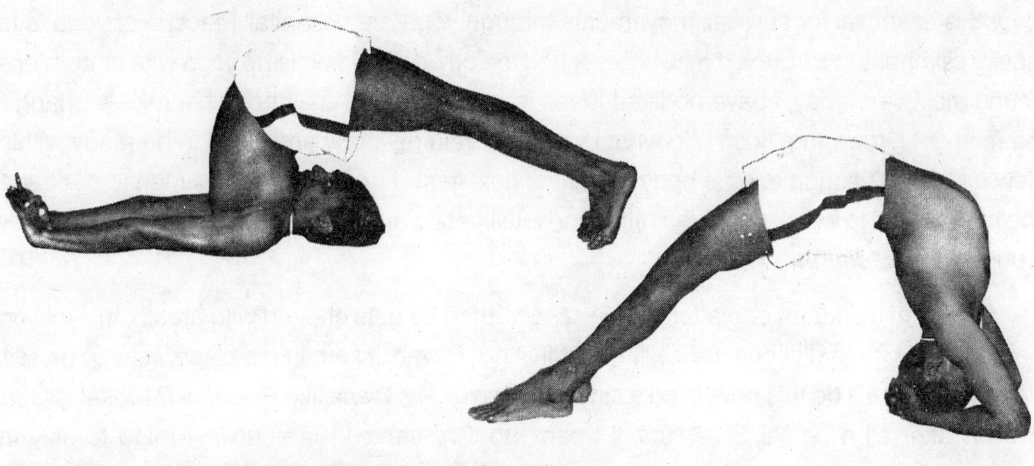

Plate n. 71 – *Halāsana* and *Viparīta Daṇḍāsana*

When we do *Halāsana*, the brain remains silent with a hypo-sensitive feeling. When we do *Viparīta Daṇḍāsana,* we are hyper-sensitive. The sensitivity in forward bends is average. By different *āsana* we learn different sensitivities and we must learn to alternate them to know not only the *āsana* well but their effects also.

In *Halāsana* some feel limited pain in the neck. It is not pain but the weight of the body that brings insensitivity and through this insensitivity brings heaviness, dullness and pain. There we have to adjust the head as well as neck and shoulders to sensitise the neck to stay longer. Then calmness and quietness increase.

Sensitivity is a faculty of consciousness. Feeling and observing whatever changes that occur and their imprints are the signs of sensitivity. The longer we stay in the *āsana*, the more we learn where stretch and touch is and where they are not. This learning and unlearning through observation and re-building is a sign of development in sensitivity.

Likes and dislikes are all signs of sensitivity. When we indulge in objects of enjoyments, we know that we are sensitive to them. It is also another sign of sensitivity when we realise the sorrowful ending of those very enjoyments.

IX.11. – Essentiality of regular practice

As food is essential for survival, movements through yoga are essential. Practice of yoga is to acquire calmness in a troubled mind. I never had the privilege of practising yoga with all comforts around me. Even today, I have no fixed ideas for practice. Each day body chemicals change. The moment I know that I can't do what I wanted, I train my body and mind to be ready within a few minutes. The moment the body and mind gets fresh, I proceed with my intense *sādhanā.* One has to learn to watch when the mind and intelligence are ready to cooperate with the body to pursue the *sādhanā.*

If, all of a sudden one attempts *Śīrṣāsana*, then he gets choked with breath; this feeling is enough for him to discontinue saying that it is not for me. If I am in his place, I say to myself, "Never mind. I can't do this now, I find a similar *āsana* to *Śīrṣāsana* like *Prasārita Padottānāsana,* which is after all a partial *Śīrṣāsana.* If I can't do *Śīrṣāsana*, I make up my mind to stay in *Prasārita Padottānāsana, Uttanāsana* and *Adho Mukha Śvanāsana.* By these *āsana* I get the feel of the effect of *Śīrṣāsana.* Then I try *Viparīta Karaṇi*, where the lower trunk is rested on a stool, and head on the floor to get the feel of *Śīrṣāsana.* This way, I work out to accommodate *Śīrṣāsana.*

Sometimes, legs may ache, and the mind might say, "Miss yoga"! But an intelligent mind has to find out why they are paining and work out how to remove that pain. One finds means to escape, but to persist and pursue needs a strong mind. Practice is like using a pin to remove a splinter in the hand. In the same way, one has to learn to use the intelligence to practise to remove the so-called pains and reform the practices so that these pricks do not occur at all. Use your intelligence to find the sense of soothness and calmness and then

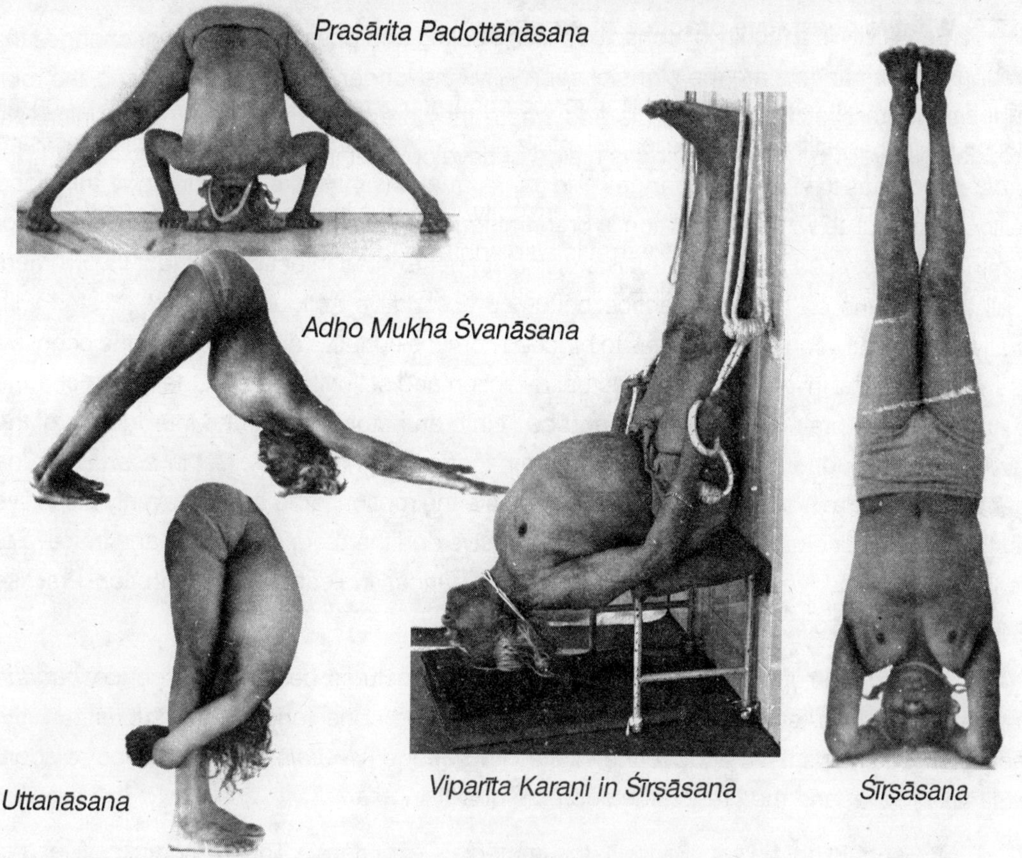

Plate n. 72 – Approach for the body, mind and intelligence to cooperate for *Śīrṣāsana*

extend and expand that soothe and calm feeling to all the other parts of the body in the *sādhanā*. Take advantage of such good changes and feelings with caution. This is how one has to practise maintaining regularity. Yoga philosophy is to rest the body through action and not to allow it to rust by inaction.

It is not good to drop routine practice but find alternative methods so that one maintains the *sādhanā* without a break.

If a medical treatment fails, doctors introduce an alternative treatment. In the same way, keep in mind how to substitute the main *āsana* by an alternative *āsana*, and when you can perform with ease, then you can go back to your practice. Practise uninterruptedly using your discretion, so that you punctuate your mind deep inside the body to experience its immeasurable depth in each *āsana*.

IX.12. - What is qualitative practice of an *āsana*

One has to practise *āsana* with total involvement. Each *āsana* has various facets such as balance, motion, repetitive action, reflection, intellectual penetration and elevation. While practising the *āsana* one has to study the changes and transformations that take place in body, mind and intelligence. Practise without reflection is predominance on motion and not action. It is easy for the mind to get excited in motion, but it is difficult to get excited in action. Without involvement on all the sheaths of the self, practice becomes a conative action. No doubt all start with conative action but soon each one has to proceed from the conative action towards the cognitive observation, mental involvement, intellectual reflection and self-witnessing. One has to change the attitude of the brain into a witness, and body into an actor keeping the intelligence of the heart present throughout. Normally it is the brain that acts on the body. But in *āsana*, it is the other way round. Each one must learn to co-ordinate the motions and actions evenly in the five sheaths of man. For example, if one part is aggressive and the other part is dull and inactive or one limb strong and the other weak, then such imbalances indicate lack of attention. Practise qualitatively with discrimination and reflection.

We are made up of five elements and their infrastructures, besides intelligence *(buddhi)*, consciousness *(citta)* and conscience *(antaḥkaraṇa)*. The conscience is the subtlest of all.[1] Practice of yoga helps us to acquire the exalted knowledge *(vivekaja jñāna)* to savour wisdom *(rasātmaka jñāna)*, and then reach the supreme quality in *āsana*.

One should not be satisfied with the immediate experience. Through practice filter and re-filter hundreds of times the same experience to reach the essence of knowledge (*rasātmaka jñāna*). Patañjali calls it *ṛtaṁbharā prajñā* or truth-bearing wisdom, which is considered as the peak of *rasātmaka jñāna*.

Does any one like to drink unfiltered coffee, which tastes like mud? But definitely one enjoys drinking a paper-filtered coffee which is full of aroma. Similarly, the subjective intelligence has to filter the experiences several times for the essence to come out as *rasātmaka jñāna* or divine experience. This is how one has to practise intelligently weighing the quality of experience every now and then. I consider this way of qualitative practice alone leads one towards *viveka khyāti* or the exalted state of knowledge filled with wisdom.

---

[1] The author refers here to the composition of *antaḥkaraṇa* as mentioned in *Triśikhibrāhmaṇopaniṣad*, 9. In Iśvarakṛṣṇa's *Sāṁkhyakārīkā*, *antaḥkaraṇa* is considered to be composed of *manas, buddhi* and *ahaṁkāra*, being synonymous with Patañjali's *citta*.

See what Patañjali says: *yogāṅgānuṣṭhānāt aśuddhikṣaye jñānadīptiḥ āvivekakhyāteḥ* (*Y.S.*, II.28) – by dedicated practice of the various aspects of yoga, the impurities of body, mind and intelligence are destroyed: the crown of wisdom radiates its glory.

IX.13. – How to understand one's own capacity in practice

Yoga is a demanding subject. Hence, to understand one's capacity for practice *asana* or *prāṇāyāma,* he has to judge his body's ability through his thinking mind. If the mind is reluctant to co-operate, yoga becomes a heavy and monotonous subject. Both body and mind must accept and be ready for practice. In case one is not able to decide on his own, he has to take the guidance from an experienced teacher what and how much to practise.

Sometimes body remains lethargic and at times mind remains inertic. As a psychologist treats depression and schizophrenia, and a physiotherapist treats the mal-developed or disabled body, in yogic *sādhanā* also one has to have will-power *(icchā śakti)* and trigger the mind and body for practice.

Āsana like *Adho Mukha Vṛkṣāsana, Pincha Mayūrāsana* or *Adho Mukha Śvānāsana,* if repeated twice or thrice recharge the body, mind and nerves with energy as they eradicate the dullness and non-cheerfulness and stimulate him with electrifying enthusiasm. Supported practice of *Dvi Pāda Viparīta Daṇḍāsana* and *Viparīta Karani* in *Śīrṣāsana* trigger the neurological body, which is the bridge between the physical and the mental bodies. When the nervous system is charged, one is freed from heaviness as well as monotony. When lightness sets in repeat these *āsana* in quick succession: *Ūrdhva Hastāsana – Uttanāsana* to *Adho Mukha Śvānāsana* and back to *Uttanāsana* and *Ūrdhva Hastāsana,* say ten times at a stretch. They do wonders.

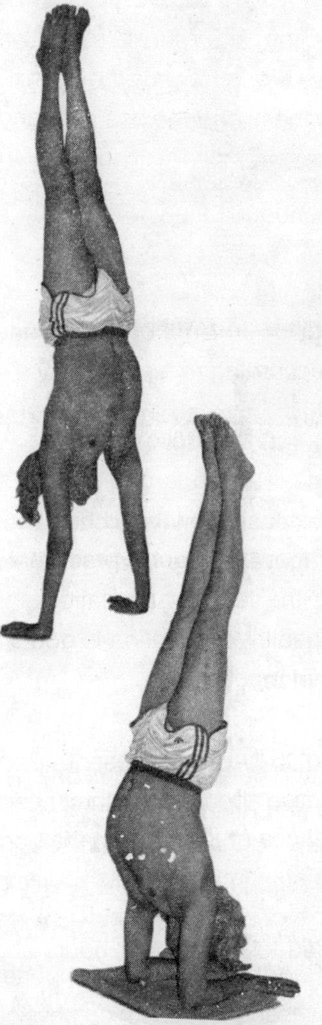

Plate n. 73a – *Adho Mukha Vṛkṣāsana* and *Pincha Mayūrāsana*

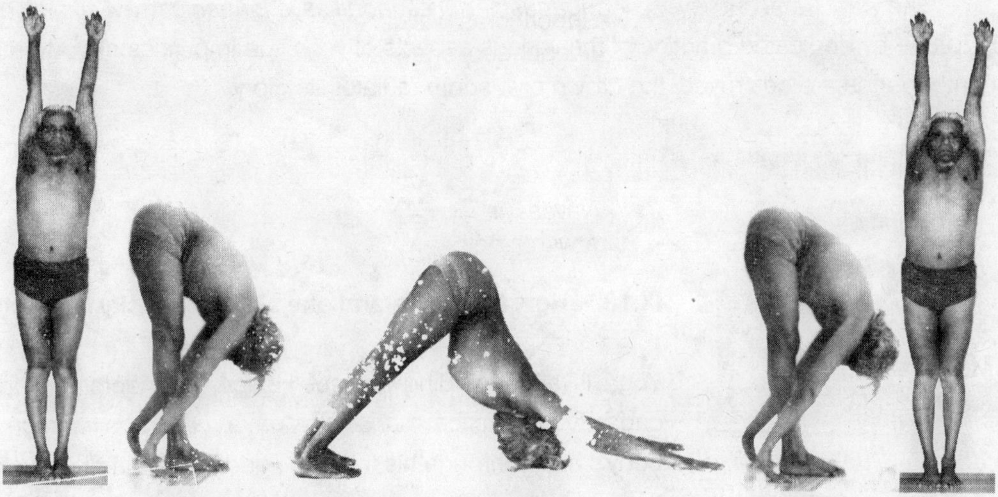

Plate n. 73b – *Āsana* in quick succession

How much to do, what to do, depends upon one's condition. In *Light on Yoga* I have given in appendix one, a weekly programme. One can follow it according to his capacity.

If there are any defects or deformities, then refer to appendix two and follow the sequence judging them to fit in according to your capabilities.

For general practice, a few standing *āsana,* forward extensions, inversions, a few backbends, lateral twists, resting and rejuvenating *āsana* and *prāṇāyāma* like *Ujjāyī* or *Viloma* would do. At least an hour is needed to do all these *āsana.*

a) – Does practice of *āsana* have to be limited age-wise

The tendency in old age is to speak of the glory of the past, but not to live in the present. *Āsana* practice makes aged persons to live in the present. They can practise according to their needs and capacity. Only judicious thinking is needed to study which *āsana* or *prāṇāyāma* the body can take and at the same time what fits in to that age.

Āsana like *Viparīta Daṇḍāsana, Setu Bandha Sarvaṅgāsana, Bharadvājāsana, Pavana Muktāsana, Vīrāsana, Supta Vīrāsana, Baddha Koṇāsana, Supta Baddha Koṇāsana,* supported *Nāvāsana, Sarvāṅgāsana* and *Halāsana* on stool, *Adho Mukha Vṛkṣāsana,* work both on physical and mental levels as well as on the nerves and brain. Only one has to do them understanding one's physical limitations. One has to judge his capacity or take guidance from experienced teachers.

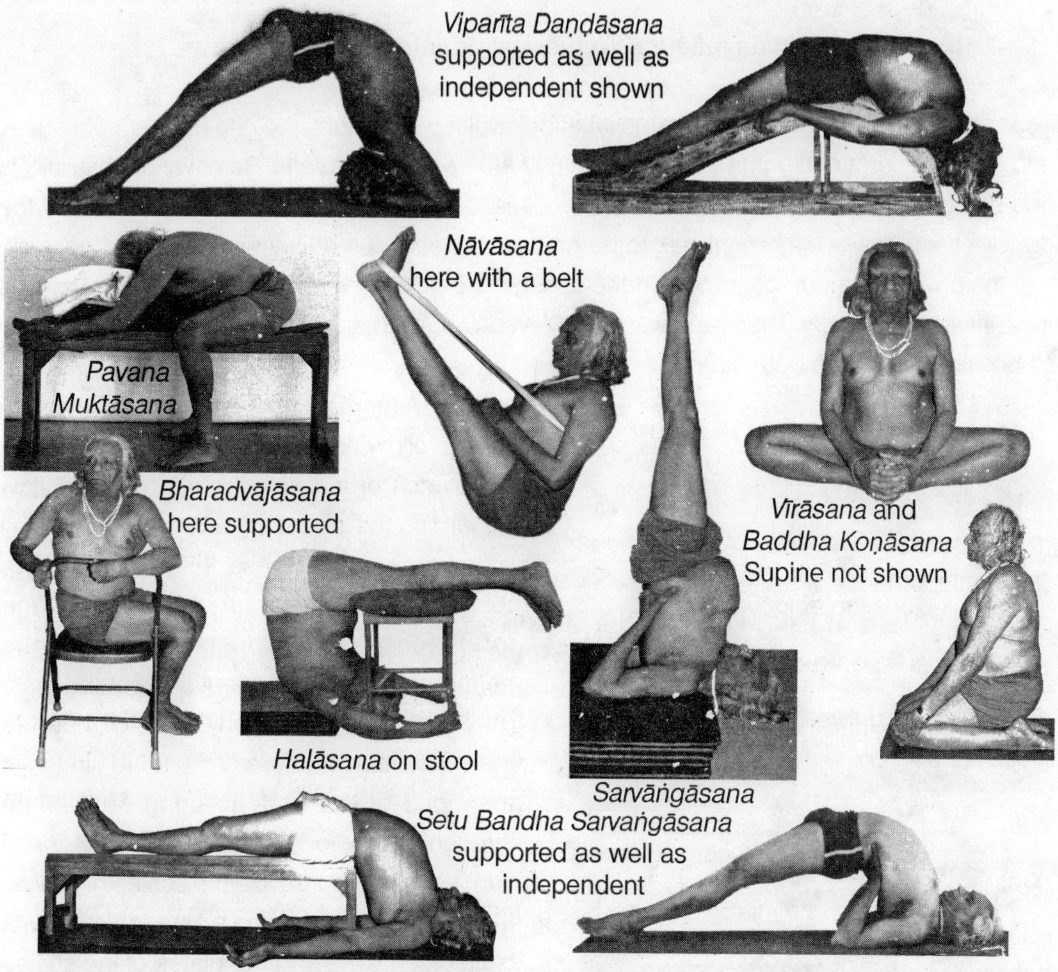

Plate n. 74 – Practice in old age, according to capacity and experience

A man suffering from cardiac problems may have limitations and may not be able to do backbends. With his limited approach, he has to see and work out how to derive maximum benefits with minimum efforts. For example, take *Sarvāṅgāsana.* In this *āsana* he may sink the chest, or he may not charge the back portion of the torso from his hands. Due to these wants, it may dull his brain, as the flow of blood and energy does not reach the glands to produce secretions. In such situations, aged people should take the teacher's guidance and learn how to pressurise the arms on the back to derive the benefit of the *āsana.* Please see the *āsana* through a magnifying glass from *Light on Yoga,* to understand the accuracy of the *āsana* to practise. This way one can learn and improve to practice the *āsana.* Knowing one's limitations he can do the *āsana* courageously and judiciously with the help of a chair or with ropes against the wall.

b) – Are the *āsana* meant as a therapy or something more

Āsana are not meant only for the removal of deformities. No doubt, they do correct deformities and eliminate wrong alignments. Several things are involved in *āsana*. Removal of deformity is one part of it. Take scoliosis. Here the spine loses its alignment, disturbing the carriage of the body. In such cases alignment has to be brought by judicious adjustment. It is also possible that there would be non-alignment in the senses of perception, mind and intelligence as well as in the flow of energy. Therefore even such persons have to adjust to balance the body as far as possible evenly on both sides.

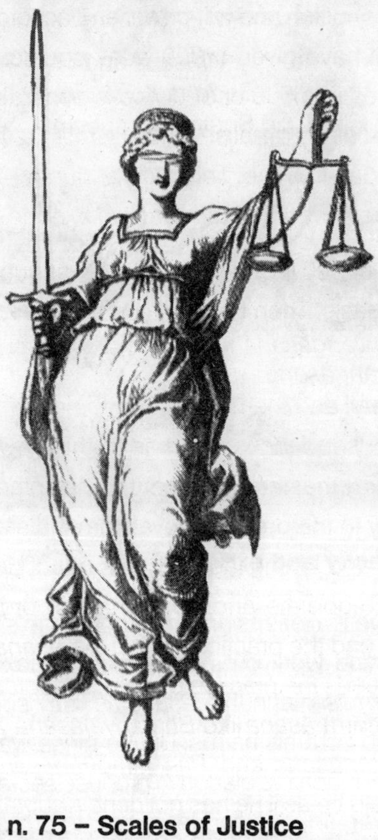

Plate n. 75 – Scales of Justice

Alignment of mind and intelligence has to follow as one aligns the body. Even in the stretch of a finger, the mind should flow equally on the inner and outer edge of the nail with attentive awareness. All disparities have to be studied and attended to by the intelligence and consciousness while performing an *āsana*. Attention from the brain guides to stretch the body from the head to the feet, and awareness of the mind stretches the sides of the body to bring equilibrium throughout the body. I say that *āsana sādhanā* should be measured like the scales of justice. Many of us have seen the statue of justice with blindfolded eyes and the plates of the scales balancing evenly, showing that justice cannot go wrong. This way each one has to be a judge for himself in practice so that he does not go wrong.

One has to use his consciousness and intelligence to weigh each *āsana* by observing and bringing equanimity of intelligence *(samānatva buddhi)* and spread of consciousness *(samānatva citta)* throughout the length and breadth of the body, without creating artificial limitations. One should not be whimsical, but weigh evenly fearlessness and caution in practice. This way of practice is the prudent approach in yoga to one's capacity.

IX.14. – Feel of mind in practice

The mind changes from one place to another place of the body while practising *āsana*. One has to train the mind to become aware and get involved with the feel of action and adjustments that take place while doing the *āsana*.

Practise the *āsana* repeatedly to watch where the unattended dark holes exist in the body and find out how to reach these remote areas and think how to work to illuminate those dark spots. If one feels the mind in certain *āsana*, it means that he notices that part of the body well in those *āsana*. He has to learn to recharge his battery of the intellectual torch to pierce those non-perceivable and un-noticeable and un-conceivable areas of the body and while performing *āsana* has to make himself to reach those intangible areas.

As the doctor performs endoscopy with instruments to find out the defective area in the inner body, the practitioner has to use his intelligence to perform that endoscopy. If he is not feeling anything within, it means that his intellect is insensitive. As one uses a torch if the room is dark, he has to use the torch of intelligence to beam on the mind to attend, perceive and conceive to reach those insensitive parts.

If the house drainage system is blocked, we try within our means to clear it and if it doesn't clear, we call a plumber who can clear the drainage system. In the same way, wrong imprints may be accumulating in the body, which block the flow of intelligence. Let us use our energy with intellectual force and flush those parts so that they are washed out and pave the way for the mind to feel those neglected areas in the body that remain non-perceptible. Otherwise you have to contact a senior teacher for this guidance.

At the beginning of practice, the body is just like a mass. The chances of perceiving the effects of action in *āsana* take time. First one has to start breaking the mass into molecules and molecules into atoms before experiencing their effects.

Choose parts of the body like legs, knees, arms or elbows in an *āsana* and pay attention to feel where the stretch and attention is. Perceive those parts well and then move the mind and intelligence close to the perceivable parts. This way, ignite your sensitivity slowly part to part so that they are able to reach the inner and the innermost subtle body.

Even for those who do not activate their muscles in the way they should be activated, through yogic means a sense of well-being arises in those muscles. Then they do derive the benefit of lightness in body and freshness in mind. One should not be contented with this exhilaration. It is just like striking a matchstick to feel the arena of yoga. Later one has to light the lamp from the matchstick to brighten his mind and energy on correct alignment of body with its mind, mind with its intelligence and intelligence with the Self.

IX.15. – From *vinyāsa krama* to *avinyāsa krama*

Yoga practices have both motion and action. Moving from one position to sequentially reach the final position and to return back to the starting point is motion or *vinyāsa krama*. Here the outer mind is active. If one holds the *āsana* for a longer period of time, the outer mind automatically moves inside the body to touch the inner mind, the consciousness and the self. It also makes the intelligence and consciousness to penetrate the unknown or unrecognisable parts of the interior body. Here, one has to act with patience, perseverance, forbearance, courage, confidence, faith and endurance to interpenetrate the mind and intelligence in positioning the body judiciously in each *āsana* to experience sobriety and serenity as one gets accustomed to stay with comfort and ease.

Vinyāsa krama is a series of motions for an action by arranging and distributing the body energy to act in an *āsana* according to one's perceived ideas; whereas *avinyāsa krama* of *āsana* is like an artisan who arranges and sets precious stones without showing the signs of metals he has used to set these stones.

As there are ascending and descending scales and score in music, there are forward movements to reach the final *āsana*. Moving from *Tāḍāsana* and reverse movements from the final *āsana* to *Tāḍāsana* is *vinyāsa krama*. For example, take *Paschimottānāsana*. Here, one moves from *Tāḍāsana* to *Uttānāsana, Chaturaṅga Daṇḍāsana, Ūrdhvamukha Śvānāsana, Adhomukha Śvānāsana* and jump to *Lolāsana* to *Paschimottānāsana*. These are the ascending movements. After the final position the practitioner has to go back to *Tāḍāsana*. Here the sequence is *Lolāsana, Chaturaṅga Daṇḍāsana, Ūrdhvamukha Śvānāsana, Adhomukha Śvānāsana* and jump to *Uttānāsana* and then to stand up to *Tāḍāsana*. These are the descending movements. In *avinyāsa karma* one goes straight to the final position with proper measured alignment of the muscles, joints and bones in par with the extension and expansion of the mind, intelligence and consciousness to run parallel to the centre point of the body, which is the centre of the core. All of us have to try and fix the body in each āsana so that the right side, the left side, the corners of the body, the back and front are close to the core with equi-distance to it.

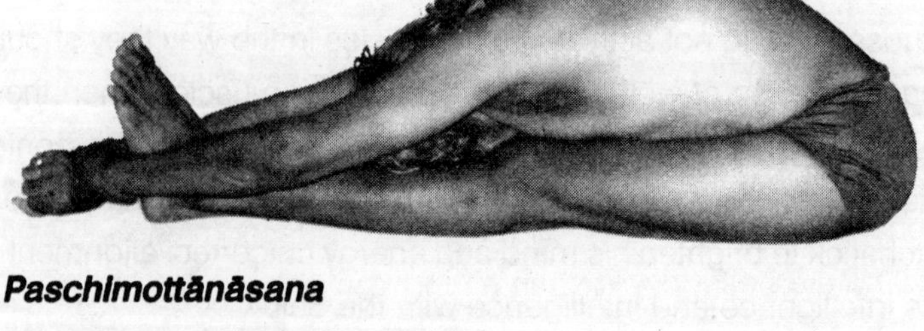

Plate n. 76a – *Paschimottānāsana*

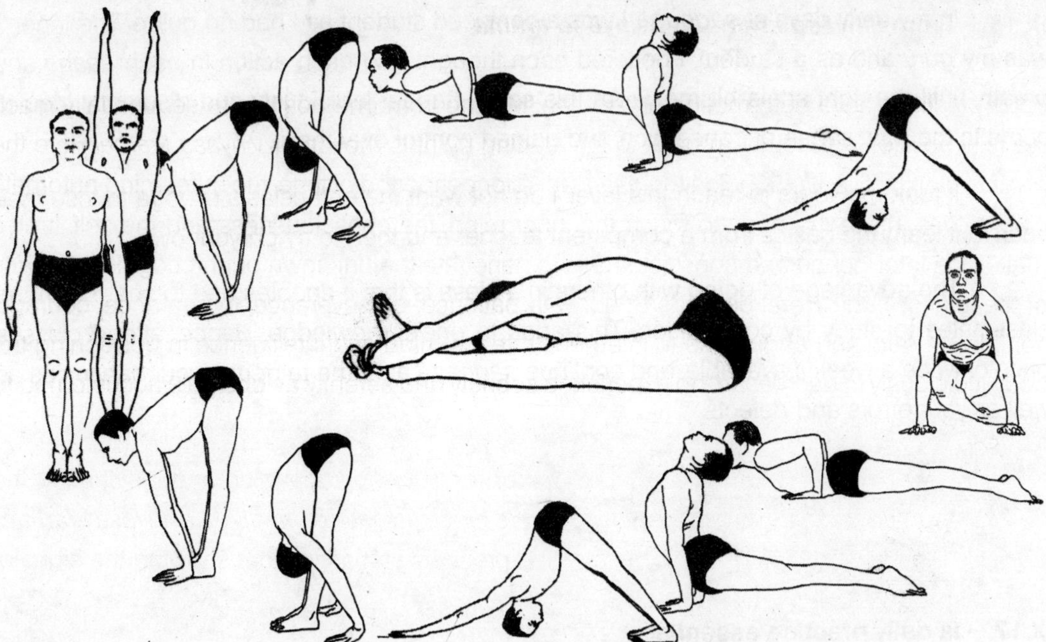

Plate n. 76b – Ascending and descending order in *vinyāsa krama*

IX.16. – Can one practise alone

No doubt, it is possible but really hard and difficult to practise alone. To achieve control over the *āsana* and for *prāṇāyāma* it demands a special quality of intellectual attention and awareness. In order to grasp them soon, it is better to go to classes where teachers explain and bring attention on what to learn and how to attend to each *āsana.*

As parents, we like to send our children to good and reputed schools so that they earn knowledge in the shortest time. Without going to school, children may learn and acquire knowledge, but it may take a long time to reach the goal, as he alone has to work with pros and cons to arrive at a correct solution. As I had no peers to share or a guru to guide me, it took me years to learn, whereas my students pick up fast, as the right guidance's are available. Practise alone is not only time consuming but often depressing and melancholic. Hence it is better to learn from an experienced teacher. As we find hard to find a good teacher, I say *Light on Yoga* or *Light on Prāṇāyāma* are better books than many good teachers.

In my early days of *sādhanā*, I was a confused student as I had no guide. The inner 'I' was my *guru* and as a student, I bettered each thought and each action in each *āsana* and breath, until the right scale hit me. From this scale, I again judiciously and discreetly tried to come to the right sense of conception and gained control over them.

It took me years to reach this level. I do not want the enthusiasts of yoga to lose their heart, but learn the basics from a competent teacher and then to try on your own.

The advantage of doing with others in a class is that it enables one to share with the classmates to study by comparison. This adds to one's knowledge. Hence, attend classes once or twice a week if available, and continue *sādhanā* at home to gauge your capacities as well as your errors and defects.

IX.17. – Is daily practice essential

Yoga is a life-long educative and instinctive subject as it guides one to live in contentment and satisfaction in spite of discontentment and dissatisfaction in our lives, due to economic and social situations. Its practice is an everyday affair, like taking food, and its aim is to refine one's life and to remain in peace within oneself as well as with family, society and community.

Unfortunately, today people practise yoga to become teachers whereas it takes years just to scratch and search out the essence of the subject. If all aspire to be teachers, then where would be pupils?

In daily practice, perceive as much as possible from the frame of the body, and then proceed to penetrate the intelligence towards the consciousness to reach the latent unknown content – the Soul.

I teach what I have digested and I use the rest of my time for *sādhanā* to learn for tracing that which is not yet surfaced. Very often new thoughts, new ideas and new actions appear on their own, which strikes me in my *sādhanā* to get myself refined each day.

So, with full involvement I maintain my regular practice, the illuminating light of knowledge may dawn on me as I become fit and ripe *(pātran)*.

IX.18. – Is yoga fun

Yoga is neither an amusement nor is it fun. It is not a serious or monotonous subject, but it is an intense subject. That makes one to travel inwards and journey towards the sight of the soul. So in it there is fun and there is sensitivity. The problem with us is that we are blind in our intellectual eyes. Yoga practice not only exhilarates us but makes us to perform with joy for the sake of opening those intellectual eyes to see well. We should not mistake this feel of exhilaration that comes out of practise as fun, but continue practice to transform that to turn into spiritual enlightenment.

We may be curious to start practise on the anatomical sheath without penetration of the mind. Attention at the physical level makes one mechanical, but the aim of yoga is to use it at the mental and intellectual levels to unfold avenues to intelligise, so that it helps to penetrate further to understand its depth for understanding the real aim of life. Seriousness does not mean grabbing, forcing, pulling and pushing while practising yoga. We should not feel the burden of seriousness. We should use our developed qualitative intelligence in practice to experience that unalloyed inner joy, which is far beyond the "fun".

IX.19. – Does change of sequence disturb physical and mental sheaths

Change of sequence in *āsana* does not disturb the physical or mental bodies but brings new thoughts and new ideas. In order to change the sequential order of *āsana*, one needs a logical mind which comes only when one has a hold on the subject. But most of us restrict *āsana* to on only the physical level. One has to proceed to churn the energy and intelligence to penetrate the depth of yoga as well as the depth of the body. The subject has to saturate into the mind for interest to set in. Yoga has to act like a mirror on the body, mind and soul to make one understand the perfection in body, stability of the mind on emotions and clarity in intelligence. Permutations and combinations may run into infinite numbers, hence yoga has to be learnt by trials and errors for right sequencing to reach a state of maturity in *sādhanā*.

It starts from the known physical frame of the self and takes one to know the subtle aspects like mind, intelligence and consciousness so that the practitioner experiences the subtlest and finest part of himself – the Soul. It is but natural for one to start first from the physical level in order to move towards the psychological, emotional and intellectual levels.

Even the elements, namely earth, water, fire, air and ether present their sequential order as per the progress in *sādhanā*. The element of earth is felt first and ether the last. As *sādhanā* progresses *prakṛti* gradually unfolds from distinguishable to non-distinguishable and from differentiable to non-differentiable. It is the same in the yogic *sādhanā* also. It is a journey from outside to inside or from distinguishable and differentiable *prakṛti* to non-distinguishable and non-differentiable *puruṣa*.

The distinguishable particles of nature are the five elements (*pṛthvi, āp, tej, vāyu* and *ākāśa*), five organs of action (legs, arms, speech, genital and excretory organs), five senses of perception (ears, eyes, tongue, nose and skin) and mind.

The non-distinguishable principles of nature are the subtle manifestations of the elements, (sound, touch, form, taste and odour), and the individual 'I', a power (*śakti*), which shines in all of us as *ahaṁkāra*. This 'I', though eternal is mutable. These non-distinguishable principles are mentally conceptual. They can be apprehended but not interpreted.

Both these interpretable (*viśesa*) and non-interpretable (*aviśesa*) principles of nature are closely connected to the universal consciousness (*mahat*) as mark (*liṅga*). All of these revolve around the qualities (*guṇa*) of nature, namely; *tamas, rajas and sattva*.

When the *sādhaka* reaches the state of *sthira sukham* in his presentation of the *āsana*, then he is no more a 'seeker' attempting with searching something or someone but reaches the state of a 'seer' by developing insight through the process of remaining silent in himself, keeping the principles of *prakṛti* active, steady and non-oscillating in the *āsana*.

This is what I understand when Patañjali defines *āsana* with *tataḥ dvandvāḥ anabhighātaḥ* (Y.S., II.48), wherein he says that the dualities and disparities cease between the nature and the soul (*pakṛti* and *puruṣa*). This implies that one has reached the most exciting climax point with perfect presentation in the performance of the *āsana*. Patañjali coins this state of climax with the phrase *ananta samāpattibhyām* (*Y.S.*, II.47).

In one word, the journey of yoga is from the known towards the unknown.

Correct sequencing is an education to the body, mind and intelligence, by which the steps of that journey are traced to reach the final destination.

IX.20. – How to know whether one is ready for *prāṇāyāma* and *dhyāna*

Yoga Sūtra says that one can practice *prāṇāyāma* only after gaining perfection in *āsana*; *tasmin sati śvāsa praśvāsayoḥ gativicchedaḥ prāṇāyāmaḥ* (*Y. S.*, II.49).

An artist carefully and accurately models. A musician produces an accurate melody from his instrument; a vocalist produces the exact sound. Similarly practitioners of *āsana* should perform the *āsana* accurately. The extension and expansion should be measured very precisely from the head to the feet and from the right side to the left side in each *āsana*, from the centre of the body and they should not vary.

In order to know whether practice of *āsana* is perfect or not, please refer to my book *Light on Yoga*, where you find *āsana* are neither overstretched nor under stretched. Learn to reach such a quality in each *āsana* practice. Listen to the vibrational sound of energy in the body according to its correct stretch in each *āsana*. Learn to evenly weigh the activity and passivity of the extension and expansion in the body. Keep the brain alert and yet passive and let the brain look at the functioning of the body, mind and intelligence in each *āsana*. Spread the awareness throughout the body, both inside and outside, by making the mind and intelligence to move inwards. This is the even spread of intelligence *(samabuddhi)* and balance in all parts of the body (*samakāyā*).

Regarding *prāṇāyāma*, first learn to sit correctly. The spine should be straight and firm. The respiratory organs should be free from stress. The spine must be ready, the nervous system must have the power to endure and the lungs the capacity to bear the load of sustained deep inhalation and exhalation. No doubt, *prāṇāyāma* is a fascinating subject, but it demands these qualities.

The lungs are like balloons. If we blow a balloon beyond its capacity, it bursts. If we know its capacity, then we fill it carefully. We have two balloons in the form of two lungs which have to be trained carefully by *āsana*.

Patañjali suggests that all the eight aspects of yoga have to be followed by the practitioner to tread on the path of yoga. As far as *prāṇāyāma* is concerned, he indicates a definite step. The *sūtra* guides us to proceed towards *prāṇāyāma* after gaining perfection in *āsana*.

Vyāsa too, while commenting, says; *śati āsana jaye....* When one has conquered the *āsana...*, then only he has to practise *prāṇāyāma*. Even the *Haṭhayoga Pradīpikā* has mentioned:

> *Athāsane dṛḍhe yogi vaśī hitamitāśanaḥ* I
> *Gurūpadiṣṭamārgeṇa prāṇāyāman sambhyaset* II (*H.Y.P.*, II.1)

Having perfected himself in the *āsana,* the yogi with his senses under control and by an agreeable moderate diet, should practise *prāṇāyāma* according to the instructions of his *guru.*

So *prāṇāyāma* is clearly a step after *āsana.* There is an indirect indication in *Sādhana Pāda,* where Patañjali sows the seed of *dhāraṇā* as an effect of *prāṇāyāma: dhāraṇāsu ca yogyatā manasaḥ* (*Y.S.,* II.53) – with *prāṇāyāma* the mind becomes a fit instrument for concentration. This way one finds a clear-cut step for *prāṇāyāma* and *dhāraṇā.* This clearly means that when one has perfected the *āsana,* he is eligible for *prāṇāyāma* and *prāṇāyāma* leads him towards *dhāraṇā.* Today's teaching is all topsy-turvy.

Pratyāhāra is an aspect or a platform to stabilise what has been practised and accomplished through *yama, niyama, āsana* and *prāṇāyāma.*

When the brain does not cooperate with the body or the body does not listen to the dictates of the intelligence of the brain, it means that duality exists in the individual. Duality ceases when the *āsana* is perfect. Then there is no more depletion of energy. The spine is retained straight and firm without effort. One remains in a state of zero tension. When this state is achieved, one is fit to commence *prāṇāyāma.*

In *prāṇāyāma* one has to keep the thoracic diaphragm and intercostal muscles free from stress. One has to perform chin-lock *(Jālandhara bandha)* to keep the brain passive. The brain should remain as an unbiased observer and lungs as a pious observant. Watch all these things. If they co-ordinate, then one is ready for *prāṇāyāma.* Body has its own *vṛtti.* So it is better to bring first *samavṛtti* or evenness in body through *āsana. Āsana* teach how to let go of stress in the brain, chest and diaphragm and prepare one for *prāṇāyāma.*

The mind wanders here and there and hence one likes to meditate. Concerning meditation *(dhyāna),* when one sits for an examination, he knows in his head and heart whether he passes or not, but his teacher may not. Yet the student consults his teacher whether he passes or not. He must know that it is he who has to answer the questions and not the teacher, so why take teacher's opinion. If a teacher like me says that you are unfit, then you think that I am a useless teacher, and if I say yes, you are happy and think me to be a good teacher. For fitness for *dhyāna* a certificate is not needed. It happens only when one learns to remain quiet and still. Before leaping to *dhyāna,* one has to purge the intelligence of its veils, and when the intelligence is stable and clear, then one is fit for *dhyāna.*

Sugar is sweet. But can anyone explain its sweetness? One can experience its sweetness but cannot explain. This is *dhyāna.*

IX.21. - Difficulties in sitting *prāṇāyāma*

In most of us the right and left sides of the body do not run parallel to each other in the sitting position. The sitting posture is difficult for those who have lordosis, hunchback, spinal defect or short neck. In hunchback, the sternum caves in and breathing becomes shallow. Backbends like *Uṣṭrāsana, Ūrdhva Dhanurāsana, Viparīta Daṇḍāsana* and *Setu Bandha Sarvāṅgāsana* are good for a hunchback and caved-in sternum. Those with such defects have to concentrate on the dorsal spine and chest to rectify these. Hence, correct them first before thinking of *prāṇāyāma*.

In *prāṇāyāma,* normally one side of the shoulder blade lifts up in turn compressing that side of the lung. In inhalation the frontal ribs do not open as many move the back ribs up. While practising *prāṇāyāma,* the back ribs should move down and the front ribs should move up. Hence, start with *āsana* and correct the frame of the torso and then proceed towards *prāṇāyāma*. Meanwhile one can begin *Ujjāyī* and *Viloma* lying on a bolster. Learn to rest the lower palate and keep the tongue passive during *prāṇāyāma* practise. Do not inflate or thicken the tongue. Let the lungs be attended in *prāṇāyāma*.

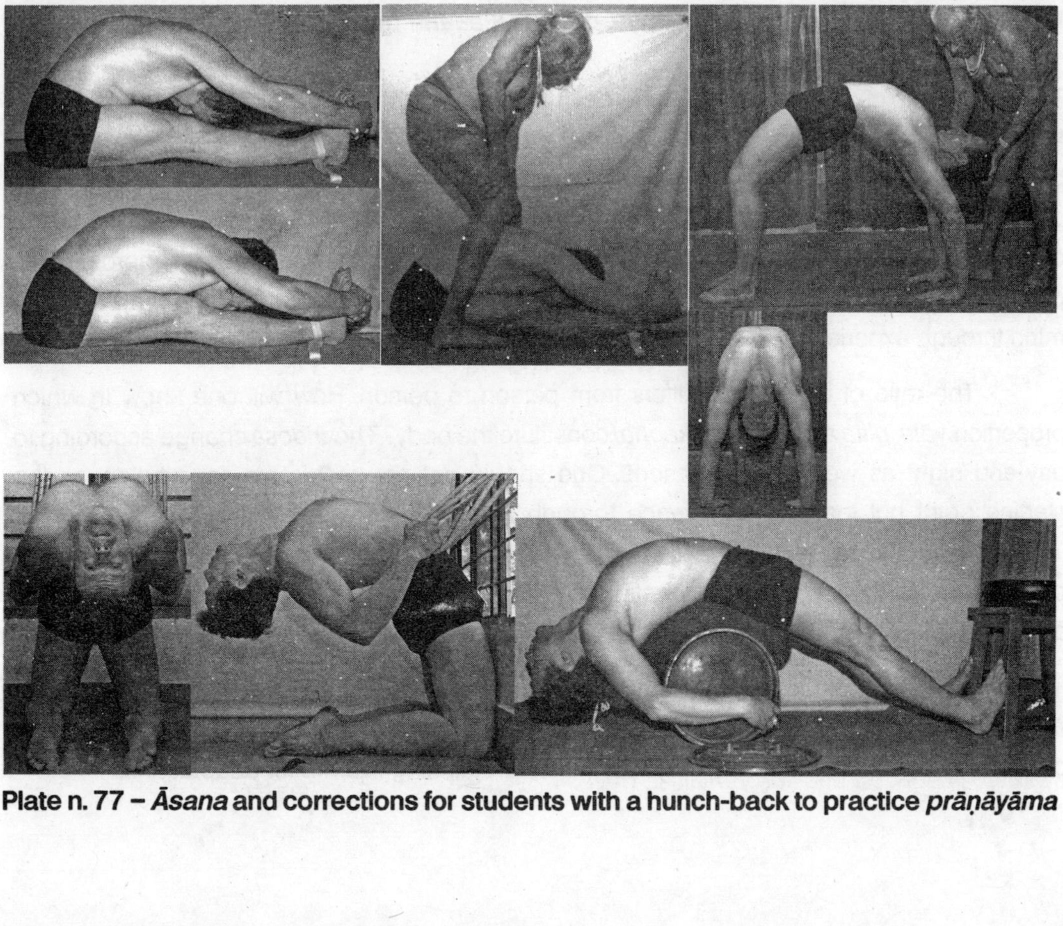

Plate n. 77 – *Āsana* and corrections for students with a hunch-back to practice *prāṇāyāma*

IX.22. – Can one practise *prāṇāyāma* without a teacher

When a student of yoga has no regular teacher but attends sporadic classes, my advice is that as soon as he is capable of performing *Śīrṣāsana, Sarvāṅgāsana, Halāsana, Setu Bandha Sarvāṅgāsana*, with their possible cycles, he/she can begin *prāṇāyāma* as explained in *Light on Prāṇāyāma*. Keep in mind the cautions that are given in the book. Grasp the points well. Then begin with ease *Viloma Prāṇāyāma* and *Ujjāyi prāṇāyāma* in *Śavāsana*, and gradually follow the steps as explained in the text. I have explained from the base how to start *prāṇāyāma*. Read and re-read several times the detailed explanations and technique before practising. As the stages and sequences are dealt with clearly in it, one can commence *prāṇāyāma* without fear, or without a teacher.

IX.23. – Based on the *āyurvedic doṣa,* does the *āsana* practice differ?

There is a distinct difference in the approach to *āsana* practice on the basis of constitutional types with regard to *vāta, pitta* and *kapha doṣa*. Slight variations, modifications with required balance and duration of stay in *āsana* are necessary to be worked out. But if one thinks of constitution according to *āyurvedic doṣa* theory and plans the yoga *sādhanā,* then one has to condition his mind before beginning yoga *sādhanā*. One cannot judge and approach the practice on *tridoṣic* constitution, but one has to work on himself to understand the body and mind through experience.

The ratio of the *tridoṣa* differs from person to person. How will one know in which proportion *vāta, pitta* and *śleṣma (kapha)* constitute the body? The *tridoṣa* change according to day and night as well as the seasons. One should not pre-decide his constitution, as the starting point but learn to experience through *āsana*. For example, I am teaching *Utthita Trikoṇāsana* for fifty students in a class, have not my students seen me adjusting differently to different people according to their constitution? I say with assurance that I certainly use prudence and judge without conditioning the minds of the students.

Many mistake me as an immature teacher as I adapt various techniques in each *āsana* for the benefit of the students. Instead of finding mistakes in me, if they learn to study the constitution of theirs and others, they too will start rethinking like me for adaptations.

A man of *vāta doṣa* loses control on the muscles, his body throbs and feels shaky. Person of *pitta* constitution perspires soon. A person of *kapha doṣa* feels dull heavy and slow. *Doṣa* are known conditions. *Āsana* practice first takes one to correct these known conditions and leads him further to find out the hidden unknown space that is within. This is the soul or the *puruṣa* – the Light of Lights.